PHONETIC SCIENCE
FOR CLINICAL PRACTICE

PHONETIC SCIENCE FOR CLINICAL PRACTICE

Kathy J. Jakielski, PhD, CCC-SLP
Christina E. Gildersleeve-Neumann, PhD, CCC-SLP

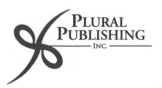
PLURAL
PUBLISHING
INC.

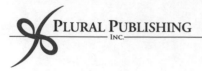

5521 Ruffin Road
San Diego, CA 92123

e-mail: info@pluralpublishing.com
Website: http://www.pluralpublishing.com

Typeset in 10/13 Stone Informal by Flanagan's Publishing Services, Inc.
Printed in the United States of America by McNaughton & Gunn

Library of Congress Cataloging-in-Publication Data

Names: Jakielski, Kathy J., author. | Gildersleeve-Neumann, Christina E.,
    author.
Title: Phonetic science for clinical practice / Kathy J. Jakielski, Christina
    E. Gildersleeve-Neumann.
Description: San Diego, CA : Plural, [2018] | Includes bibliographical
    references and index.
Identifiers: LCCN 2017037176| ISBN 9781597567312 (alk. paper) | ISBN
    1597567310 (alk. paper)
Subjects: | MESH: Speech Therapy | Phonetics | Child | Speech
    Disorders--therapy | Language Therapy
Classification: LCC RC424.7 | NLM WL 340.3 | DDC 616.85/5--dc23
LC record available at https://lccn.loc.gov/2017037176

CONTENTS

Let's face it: Phonetics is a difficult and potentially tedious course, for both the instructor and the students. Although it may seem like a shallow and trivial topic—something one could learn from the key at the bottom of a dictionary page—there are multiple complexities that challenge many students who are accustomed to doing well easily in all of their classes. Concepts from anatomy and physiology are needed to describe the articulators and their speech production functions. Concepts from physics are needed to explain the acoustics of speech sounds and prosody and how these are manifested in sound waves and spectrograms. Concepts from linguistics, including sociolinguistics, are needed to account for variable pronunciations of phonemes in different phonetic contexts and by different groups of speakers, as well as phonemic differences across languages. And, at the same time, students must develop a so-called "good ear" for detecting subtle nuances among speech sounds. Somehow, the professor of phonetics must maintain the interest and motivation of groups of undergraduates while leading them through the inter-relationships amongst all of these disparate aspects of our field.

Why should we bother? Because an understanding of all of these aspects of speech and of their interrelationships is key to the assessment and treatment of speech sound disorders, which account for the majority of speech-language services provided to preschoolers as well as services to many older children and to adults. To provide successful, high-quality, evidence-based services, speech-language pathologists must be more than competent in understanding and using phonetic concepts and skills. This mission is made all the more difficulty by the growing diversity in our country. No longer is it sufficient for the SLP to recognize and understand the phonemes and allophones of English. Our caseloads are becoming increasingly linguistically diverse, so we also must be able to tease apart the influences not only of disparate dialects but languages as well, including the additional impacts of being bilingual.

Having just reviewed my Phonetics student course evaluations for the past semester—one of a large number of sets of Phonetics course evaluations I have reviewed over the past three decades—I am keenly aware that many students find all of this overwhelming, as it is typically presented in current phonetics texts. In this book and workbook, Kathy Jakielski and Christina Gildersleeve-Neumann have taken a different approach to presenting this information that will make the material both easier to digest and more engaging to our students. They present articulatory phonetics first—the anatomical and physiological foundations for consonants, vowels, and diacritics—as the basis for a chapter dedicated to each of these. Chapters on prosody and then acoustics come next. Only once students have a solid foundation in these more basic concepts about speech do the authors focus on concepts from phonology—phonemes, allophones, etc. Finally, they close with a lively review of the many respects in which languages differ from each other phonetically. Thus, students will be able to process and master the various components of the field of phonetics one by one. As the reader progresses through the book, the material from the earlier chapters is reviewed and related to the new concepts. As a result, there are many opportunities to re-visit ideas from more basic aspects of phonetics and to integrate them into more complex concepts for a deeper understanding of the whole. This organization should be far less intimidating and far more reinforcing for students.

Another innovation in this book is that each chapter includes frequent "Did you get it?" reviews, which encourage the student to answer a small number of short answer or multiple-choice questions that reinforce the material just covered. These, in addition to the excellent, varied exercises in the accompanying workbook and also the mnemonic flashcards that are included, give the students many engaging opportunities to interact with the material and thus to master it at a far deeper level than they would by merely reading the text.

The organization of the material is definitely not the only innovative aspect of this book-workbook set. Most motivating for the students are the "Applied Science" sections that begin and end each chapter. Some are fascinating phonetic puzzles that will increase the students' curiosity about the topic of the chapter from the get-go. Others are clinical mini-case studies that raise interesting questions, the answers to which depend upon the material in that chapter. These are not trivial; they involve key clinical issues, such as identifying covert contrasts (Chapter 4), detecting production-based versus perception-based speech errors (Chapter 6), and differentiating the impacts of bilingualism from speech disorder (Chapters 7, 8, and 9). Despite the basic level of understanding that the undergraduate readers will have, the authors have managed to include accessible real-life clinical conundrums with "Aha!"

solutions, based upon the recently-learned material, revealed at the end of the chapter.

The clinical case studies are only one of the means by which Jakielski and Gildersleeve-Neumann introduce intriguing information about languages other than English into the text. Throughout the book, especially in Chapter 9, they provide fascinating phonetic details, not just about Spanish, German, and Chinese but also about Guarani, Navajo, Quichua, Xhosa, Tlingit, and Taa, to mention just a few. Students completing a course taught with this textbook should have a much wider appreciation of phonetics as a human trait, well beyond the speech sounds of English.

Don't be misled by the comfortable conversational style in which this book is written. These two authors "know their stuff"; both have many years of hands-on experience in clinical phonetics as well as in teaching this subject. The information in the book, for all of the aspects of phonetics that are covered, is solid as well as accessible.

[dɪg ɪn ænd ɛn'd͡ʒɔɪ]!

Shelley L. Velleman, PhD, CCC-SLP
Chair & Professor
Communication Sciences and Disorders
University of Vermont

The idea for this textbook originated in 1998, when one of us turned to the other and said, "One day, we are writing our own phonetics textbook." That statement was born out of our frustration of not finding an introductory phonetics textbook that maintained the powerful science material that underlies phonetics, while weaving the application of it into the speech and hearing sciences. As clinical and research speech-language pathologists ourselves, we experience daily how understanding the science that underlies the artful tool of phonetic transcription increases our success in the classroom, clinic, and lab. So, when Valerie Johns and Kalie Koscielak from Plural Publishing approached us about co-authoring an introductory phonetics textbook, it appeared that it was time to give substance to an idea that began almost 20 years ago.

Each of us has been teaching phonetics to students majoring in speech-language pathology and audiology for over 20 years, and practicing as clinical and research speech-language pathologists for even longer. *Phonetic Science for Clinical Practice* mirrors the courses we have crafted over those two decades, containing the information that speech-language pathologists and audiologists need to build a foundation in phonetic science, as well as to become accurate phonetic transcribers. Knowing how to transcribe is a practical skill. But knowing how to think like a phonetician is arming oneself with practical knowledge.

You would not be holding this book in your hands if not for the support we have received throughout our long careers. Our list of people to acknowledge is extensive. We first thank our academic mentors, including Leo Engler, Julie Ries, Barbara Davis, Peter MacNeilage, and Björn Lindblom. Their passion for teaching phonetic science was contagious. We thank the hundreds of students we have taught; their desire to dive into the inquiry of phonetics continually keeps us on our toes to remain current. This book also is the result of the support we have received during the actual writing process. Our many anonymous reviewers read early and late drafts, giving their valuable time to provide welcome feedback along the way. We gave every comment consideration, and we hope that our reviewers see their efforts to improve this book reflected on the pages that follow. Our non-anonymous reviewers also played a significant role in the development of this book, including Shelley Velleman and Andy McMillin. Many of our current and past students served as reviewers and contributors, including Jillian Adkins, Kristina Cruz, Cara Dick, Tania Giorgis, Nathan Hartleben, McKenzie Hendricks, Jessica Leff, Heather Mason, Bethany Miller, Jennifer Otwell, Evelyn Pulkowski, Micaela Quintana, and Jordan Siegel. Added to the mix of talented reviewers, the creative mind of Summer Zeimetz brought our ideas to life with all her figures and drawings. Given that this entire project spanned several years, it required the unwavering support of our families. To Jonathan, Simona, and Elijah, and David and Byron, we say thank you for believing in us, cheering us on, and making countless sacrifices.

Kathy J. Jakielski, PhD, CCC-SLP
Rock Island, Illinois
February 2017

Christina E. Gildersleeve-Neumann,
 PhD, CCC-SLP
Portland, Oregon
February 2017

REVIEWERS

Plural Publishing, Inc. and the authors would like to thank the following reviewers for taking the time to provide their valuable feedback during the development process:

Joy McKenzie, MS, CCC-SLP
Assistant Professor
Department of Communication Sciences and
    Disorders
St. Cloud State University
St. Cloud, Minnesota

Andy McMillin, MA, CCC-SLP
Clinical Associate Professor
Department of Speech and Hearing Sciences
Portland State University
Portland, Oregon

Heather L. Ramsdell-Hudock, PhD, CCC-SLP
Assistant Professor
Department of Communication Sciences and
    Disorders
Idaho State University
Pocatello, Idaho

Heather L. Rusiewicz, PhD, CCC-SLP
Assistant Professor
Department of Speech-Language Pathology
Duquesne University
Pittsburgh, Pennsylvania

Shelley L. Velleman, PhD, CCC-SLP
Chair & Professor
Communication Science and Disorders
University of Vermont
Burlington, Vermont

What follows are our suggestions for maximizing your learning while using this textbook. Your learning will be enhanced if you engage in the material as you read each chapter, so we hope that you take advantage of the methods we have included to help increase your active engagement.

Learning Objectives

Each chapter begins with a list of learning objectives. Before you begin reading the chapter, go over the objectives so you know the topics that will be covered. After you have finished reading the chapter, we recommend that you return to the list of learning objectives as a means of testing yourself on the major concepts.

Applied Science

Each chapter also begins with a question designed to motivate your thinking about the topics that will be discussed in that chapter—prior to learning about the topics. We employ this strategy to draw you into the topics, asking you to pause to consider possible answers to the question before you jump into the reading. We also include applied science questions to connect your learning to clinical scenarios. We encourage you to think about the clinical question while you read the chapter.

Applied Science: Revisited

We return to the Applied Science clinical question at the end of each chapter. All of the questions ultimately can be answered by applying the phonetic science concepts covered in that chapter, so we walk you through each step of solving the problem. By answering the questions, you will have learned how to apply the concepts in the chapter to solve a real-life clinical problem.

Did You Get It?

Throughout each chapter, you will find many "Did You Get It?" mini-quizzes for checking your comprehension of the material just presented. If you cannot answer a question, then you know that you missed an important concept and should re-read that section until you can answer the question. Once you have answered each question in a Did You Get It? quiz, you will find the answers at the end of each chapter. If you answered any questions incorrectly, then re-read the material until you comprehend it.

Bolded Text

There are bolded words throughout the textbook to indicate that a new term was just introduced. Definitions of these words can be found in the Glossary at the end of the book.

Audio Files

Whenever you see a sound, syllable, word, or phrase highlighted in burgundy text, you can find an accompanying audio file on the textbook's companion website. Listening to the file, you can hear exactly how it is pronounced.

Interest Piqued?

At the end of each chapter, you will find a section called Interest Piqued? There you will find a list of suggested print and online materials that illustrate or expand the materials covered in the chapter. Check out the suggested materials to help further your understanding of the topics.

Companion Website

Take some time to go to the companion website for the textbook. You will find an assortment of materials designed to support your learning. Materials include links to the Interest Piqued? resources, flashcards of the Glossary terms, flashcards of the mnemonic resources, and audio files of highlighted text.

Companion Workbook

Nothing aids learning like practice! We published *Phonetic Science for Clinical Practice: A Transcription and Application Workbook* to provide you with abundant opportunities to apply the knowledge and practice the skills you will learn by reading this textbook. You will find that the workbook parallels the structure of the textbook chapters and topics, making it easy for you to follow along. From our decades of experience teaching beginning phonetics students, application of concepts and more transcription practice are what students request.

This book is dedicated to two of our most appreciated academic mentors,
Barbara L. Davis and Peter F. MacNeilage.

1

INTRODUCTION TO PHONETIC SCIENCE

Learning Objectives

By reading this chapter, you will learn:

1. the scientific fields of phonetics and phonology
2. the concepts of phonemes, phones, and allophones
3. the difference between orthographic and phonetic symbols
4. about the International Phonetic Alphabet and its applications
5. the continuum of different styles of speech, including speech registers
6. skills underlying phonetic transcription
7. the phonotactic structure of words
8. the concept and types of word stress

Applied Science

A mother calls a local speech-language pathologist to request an evaluation of her four-year-old son, whose speech "is immature for his age and sometimes difficult to understand." The mother explains that even though she cannot always understand his speech, "he talks in sentences and understands what is said to him." When asked to describe her son's speech, the mother reports that "he can't pronounce all of his 't' and 's' words." The speech-language pathologist arranges to test the little boy's speech.

- Give examples of words you think the child cannot correctly pronounce.
- Make a list of words the speech-language pathologist could use to test the child's speech.
- How will the speech-language pathologist unambiguously write down the child's pronunciations?

The Study of Speech: Phonetics and Phonology

Phonetics is the study of speech sounds. Speech sounds are the consonant and vowel sounds that make up the words in a spoken language. Scientists who study this fascinating field are called **phoneticians**. Phoneticians are interested in the physical properties of speech sounds. Some phoneticians are interested in the production aspects of speech sounds, determining exactly how humans produce sounds, while others are interested in how humans recognize sounds as speech. Others still are interested in understanding how our brains process speech, and others in how speakers combine sounds to make words in their language. There are different branches of phonetics, and within each domain of inquiry, phoneticians focus a specific lens on production, recognition, perception, or use. We will introduce you to five of the branches of phonetics: articulatory, acoustic, auditory, linguistic, and clinical.

Articulatory phonetics is focused on the actual movements needed to produce speech sounds. When we talk about how and where in the vocal tract the "s" sound, for example, is produced, we are practicing articulatory phonetics. **Acoustic phonetics** is the study of the actual auditory signal generated when speech sounds are produced. For example, when we examine a speech waveform to compare the loudness of the "s" sound with other sounds, we are practicing acoustic phonetics. **Auditory phonetics** is the study of how humans hear, perceive, and categorize speech sounds. When we study the age at which infants can tell the difference between the "s" and "f" sounds, we are practicing auditory phonetics. **Linguistic phonetics** is focused on understanding the articulatory, acoustic, and auditory characteristics of speech sounds in different languages. When we study how these physical characteristics influence how the "s" sound is used in words, we are practicing linguistic phonetics. Finally, **clinical phonetics** is the study and practical application of phonetics to solving real-life problems affecting the diagnosis and treatment of individuals who exhibit speech sound errors. When we attempt to determine the most effective intervention for "s" sound errors, we are practicing clinical phonetics. Clinical and research speech-language pathologists and audiologists, as well as speech and hearing scientists, utilize phonetics to better understand the nature of speech sound disorders and differences.

There is another area of study that is particularly important to clinical and research speech-language pathologists—an area that is entwined with linguistic phonetics. This area of study is called **phonology**. Phonology is a distinct branch of linguistics, separate from, but related to, phonetics. Scientists who study phonology are called **phonologists**. Phonologists are interested in how speech sounds are mentally represented in the human brain. Whereas phoneticians study the spoken sound, phonologists study the thought of a sound. Phonologists study the sounds that hold meaning in a language, as well as the rules for how those sounds can be combined into words. The rules are the phonological grammar of a language. When we determine, for example, that the consonant cluster "sf" cannot occur at the beginning of a word in a language, such as English, we are studying the phonology of that language. An overlap between phonetics and phonology occurs when there are articulatory and acoustic factors that motivate a specific phonological rule, resulting in a phonetic explanation for an observed phonological systematicity. Throughout this textbook, we will discuss the inquiry into these varied domains while weaving in examples of how to apply the information to clinical situations.

? 1–1. Did You Get It?

1. Name the branch of phonetics—articulatory, acoustic, auditory, or linguistic—that each example describes.

    a. Determining if a puff of air is typically emitted during production of a "p" sound when in initial position of English words. _____

    b. Determining if a puff of air that was produced during production of a "p" sound could be heard by a panel of listeners. _____

    c. Determining if a puff of air was emitted during production of the "p" sound by examining a speech spectrogram (a visible representation of sound). _____

    d. Determining if a puff of air was emitted during production of the "p" sound by placing your hand near the speaker's mouth to feel the airflow.

        _____

2. A phonetician studies the _____ of a language.

3. A phonologist studies the _____ of a language.

The Sounds of Speech: Phonemes, Phones, and Allophones

Speech sounds that establish meaning when used in words are called **phonemes**. Phonemes are not interchangeable in words, because when a phoneme is changed, so is the meaning of the word. For example, the word *pat* holds specific meanings. *Pat* can refer to an action we perform with our hand to congratulate someone, the name of a friend, or a dab of butter. If we replaced "p" with "b" to make *bat*, a new word, with its own meanings, is formed.

Being able to create meaningful words is what establishes "p" and "b" as phonemes in English. In Chapter 7, we will detail how phoneticians and phonologists determine which sounds are phonemes in languages.

In addition to phonemes, there are speech sounds called **phones** that do not change the meaning of words. Phones are the physical product of producing speech. When we want to say the word *go*, for example, the mental representation of *go* is a specific sequence of a consonant phoneme + a vowel phoneme. When we actually produce that consonant + vowel sequence, the phonemes move from being abstract thoughts to concrete sounds (i.e., phones) having measurable physical properties. For example, we can measure the loudness of the two phones or the tongue strength required to say them. Because of the dynamic nature of speech production, we never say the same sound the exact same way twice, and phoneticians love to study these intricate details of speech production within and across speakers and languages. In addition to careful listening and using acoustic methods, we also have tools for seeing sound production as it is being produced. Some of these tools include cinefluoroscopy (imaging using motion x-rays), ultrasound (imaging using sound waves), and electropalatography (an artificial mouth plate fitted with contacts that detect when the tongue touches the roof of the mouth).

Within a language, some of the differences in pronouncing sounds are systematic and predictable, and other differences are less predictable. For example, we can say the "t" sound in the word *pat* with a little burst of air at the end. Or, we can say the "t" sound without the burst of air. Even though the pronunciation of the word *pat* would sound differently in the two productions, the meaning of the word *pat* remains the same. Nonetheless, those two variations of "t" are different phones: one with a burst of air and one without. They are two phones that represent the single phoneme "t." We call these production variations **allophones**. Therefore, the "t" with a strong burst of air and the "t" without a burst of air are considered allophones of the phoneme "t." The term *allophone*, like phone, refers to the actual spoken production of a phoneme. Therefore, every phoneme mentally represents a set of phones. In Chapters 4, 7, and 8, we will provide detailed information about the production and usage of phonemes, phones, and allophones.

> **? 1–2. Did You Get It?**
>
> Match the following terms.
>
> **1.** phonemes _____   a. the sounds articulated when a child says *no*
>
> **2.** phones _____   b. the different ways the sound "s" can be articulated
>
> **3.** allophones _____   c. the mental sound units that make up the word *chair*

The Written Representation of Speech: Orthographic and Phonetic Symbols

Orthographic Symbols: The Latin Alphabet

Because in English there is not a one-to-one correspondence between alphabet **graphemes** (i.e., letters) and the sounds they represent, it is important to distinguish between how phonemes are written using **orthographic** alphabet graphemes and how those phonemes are produced as phones. For example, consider the written word *bow*. The written word *b-o-w* could mean the pretty decoration that you tie around a gift box, or it could mean the action of bending at the waist at the end of your fine performance. In the first example, the decoration that you tie around a gift box, the word *bow* is pronounced as a "b" sound plus a long "o" sound. In the second example, the word *bow* is pronounced as a "b" sound plus the sound you yell when you bang your knee on the corner of a table, "ow" (as in *ouch*). Simply reading the word *bow*, written by itself, you have no way of knowing to which *bow* the word refers; thus, you have no way of knowing which pronunciation to use. These two words are spelled the same way, yet they mean different things and they have different pronunciations. The alphabet letters used to spell them do not offer any help in knowing which pronunciation to utter. Orthographic spellings often do not help us with pronunciation. Words that are spelled the same way but have different meanings are called **homographs**, and some homographs are pronounced differently (as in the above examples of *bow*), while others are pronounced the same (as in *bat*, which could refer to the animal, the club used to hit a ball, or the action of striking something).

There also are examples of two words that are spelled differently, yet pronounced the same way. These words are called **homophones**. Such is the case with the word that means the action of bending at the waist at the end of a fine performance, *bow*, and the word *bough* that means a tree branch. Both words are pronounced as a "b" sound plus an "ow" sound. But now another confusion using orthographic alphabet letters to represent sounds emerges. Can you identify it? Yes, there is no single way of using alphabet letters to represent the "ow" sound. We could use the alphabet letters "ow" (*owl*), "ough" (*bough*), "ou" (*foul*), or in some dialects, "a" (*gal*). Confusions such as these are common.

Phonetic Symbols: The International Phonetic Alphabet

Phoneticians help us to understand that while spelling is focused on the orthographic graphemes used to write a word in a language, phonetics is focused on capturing how a word was pronounced, or articulated, by a speaker. To **articulate** speech is to produce it. When we read a dictionary, we can study the special pronunciation spellings that were developed to tell us how a word typically is pronounced. For example, in the Encarta Dictionary for North American English (Microsoft Corporation, 2009), pronunciation of the word *example* is listed as "ig 'zæmpl." There also is a Pronunciation Key that serves as a guide for how to pronounce each of the letters. When examining the key, we find a variety of letters representing the pronunciation for each of the 50+ different speech sounds; therefore, not even the Pronunciation Key represents a one-to-one correspondence of one letter for one sound. And even if you were so inclined, you would not want to spend your time memorizing those letters and associated sounds, because each dictionary has its own abstruse pronunciation key!

There is hope, however, for students who are interested in unambiguously capturing phonemes, phones, and allophones using written symbols. That hope comes in the way of the International Phonetic Alphabet (IPA). The IPA is a set of symbols used to represent the speech sounds across the world's languages. Each symbol represents one, and only one, consonant or vowel. The IPA was developed in 1886 by a group of scholars interested in speech sound articulation who had formed an organization called the International Phonetic Association. The International Phonetic Association also is abbreviated as IPA. For clarity, every time we refer to the International Phonetic Association we will write out the name of the organization throughout this textbook, and every time we refer to the International Phonetic Alphabet, we will use the abbreviation IPA. The IPA periodically is updated, with the most recent version published in 2015. Even though the IPA represents sounds in all the world's languages, it is biased toward English and other Indo-European languages and largely uses symbols from the Latin alphabet; therefore, you will recognize many of the phonetic symbols. Most of the phonetic symbols we will use in this textbook will be from the IPA; however, we also will introduce a few other symbols that we believe better represent phonetics for clinical use in speech-language pathology and audiology.

One major benefit of learning the IPA is to be able to capture, using written symbols, how words in a language are pronounced. When determining how words are pronounced, we may be interested in knowing how a word is typically pronounced by speakers of the language and/or we may be interested in knowing how an individual actually articulates a word. The former is important to establish common pronunciations of words in a language, so that even speakers with different dialects within one language can be understood. The latter is important so that when an individual **misarticulates** (i.e., mispronounces) a word, there is an unambiguous way of writing down just how the person said a word.

We utilize the same basic symbol set, the IPA, to write phonemes, phones, and allophones. We designate phonemes, phones, and allophones, as such, by enclosing the letter symbols in-between either **virgules**, / /, or **brackets**, [ ]. When we write using IPA symbols that represent a word, we place the symbols within virgules, which represents a phonemic transcription. For example, we could transcribe the mentally stored word *no* as /no/. When we write using IPA symbols that represent an actual production of a word, we place the symbols within brackets, which represents a phonetic transcription. For example, if we transcribed a child's correct articulation of the word *no*, we would transcribe it as [no]. In summary, a phoneme is enclosed in-between virgules and a phone is enclosed in-between brackets.

? **1–3. Did You Get It?**

1. List an example of one consonant sound that is spelled with different graphemes in two different words.

   _____

2. List an example of one vowel sound that is spelled with different graphemes in two different words. _____

3. List a pair of homographs. _____

4. List a pair of homophones. _____

5. Would you transcribe the following words using virgules or brackets?

   a. *book*, as said by a child   _____

   b. *book*, as the object itself   _____

   c. the word *kitten*   _____

   d. the spoken word *kitten*   _____

The Registers of Speech

To paraphrase the renowned linguist Roman Jakobson, "we speak to be heard to be understood." Driven by a desire to communicate, speakers will talk just clearly and loudly enough to be heard, so they have a chance of being understood. The styles in which speakers talk vary along a continuum of **speech registers**. Registers vary from frozen (using unchanging archaic language, as in reciting the Pledge of Allegiance) to formal (one-way communication, as in giving a speech) to consultative (communicating with an authority figure, as in a student–professor conversation) to casual (speaking to peers) to intimate (speaking to close friends and family members). We change registers by changing the way we articulate sounds. During any conversation, we may move back and forth across this continuum, using listener feedback and our own intentions to guide exactly how formally or informally we articulate our words. The same speaker produces the same speech sound differently—even in the same word—as speaking registers change.

The fact that the articulation of every phoneme varies so greatly within and across speakers presents many challenges to speech researchers, and they have given this phenomenon a name: the invariance problem. The invariance problem also captures the nature of speech sound variance as phonetic contexts change. For example, we might think that the long "i" vowel sound (pronounced as the word *eye*) is one invariant sound, but if we pay attention to how this vowel sounds when we speak aloud the words *I* and *bite*, we will hear that the two vowels sound slightly different. The difference is because the phonetic contexts are different: the vowels and/or consonants between the two words vary. For example, *I* has only a single vowel sound, so we say it has a single vowel (V) **word shape**, while *bite* contains three sounds, resulting in a consonant-vowel-consonant (CVC) word shape. We articulate the long "i" vowel sound—and every other speech sound—slightly differently based on the consonants and vowels coming before and after it. The result is a multitude of possible productions for every phoneme, and for every speaker.

Pronouncing words using very precise articulation, as you would when speaking in frozen and formal, and sometimes consultative, registers, is called **citation-form speech**. Citation form is over-articulated speech. It is speech on which a word's dictionary pronunciation form is based. We use citation-form speech when we need everyone to hear our words clearly and unambiguously. Citation form typically refers to single word productions; however, it also can be used on a single sound or syllable to ensure understanding, as in, "The vocal folds <u>ab</u>-duct during breathing and <u>ad</u>-duct to produce sound," or to emphasize a particular point, as in, "<u>No</u>, <u>you</u> <u>may</u> <u>not</u> <u>go</u>." Citation-form speech is typically articulated slightly slower and is produced with greater effort and attention on the structures used to produce speech: the articulators, such as the tongue and lips. If we use citation-form speech for too long, our listeners might become fatigued hearing all our overarticulations. Dictionary forms of words are prescriptive by nature, telling a reader exactly how to pronounce any given word. As you will discover in later chapters, there are many reasons why an individual may articulate a word differently than its dictionary citation form specifies. It is important to understand that as clinical scientists we are more interested in descriptive phonetics than prescriptive rules. That is, we are more interested in *how* people speak than how they *should* speak, even while we compare their productions to the speech of other members of their linguistic community.

The most common form of speech production is casual. Casual speech is highly intelligible in most speaking contexts. Speech sounds are articulated clearly; however, we do not overarticulate sounds, decreasing the effort we expend producing speech. It is easy to listen to casual speech. Speech produced in a significantly relaxed style, such as when speaking intimately to very close friends and family, is characterized by omitting some sounds, syllables, and words (e.g., *Are you coming?* becomes *Comin'?*), mixing two sounds into one (e.g., *Don't you want to go?* becomes *Donchu wanna go?*), and substituting one sound for another (e.g., *I see you* becomes *I see ya*).

The linguist Björn Lindblom referred to over- and underarticulated styles of speech as hyper- and hypo-speech, respectively. Lindblom hypothesized that variations in articulation are a speaker's adaptations not only to changes in speaking situations, but also to the consonants and vowels that come before and after any particular sound, creating phonetic contexts that continually change from one syllable to the next (e.g., Lindblom, 1983, 1990). Lindblom explains this occurrence as **economy of articulation**, a factor in speech production that linguist Peter Ladefoged called the principle of ease of articulation (Ladefoged, 2005). Researchers have conducted numerous studies over recent decades to identify factors related to the degree of articulatory effort put forth by speakers. In one of the first such studies, Philip Lieberman in 1963 discovered that speakers used less articulatory precision when saying words that could be considered predictable in a sentence, and that those words were less intelligible to naïve listeners hearing only the predictable words spoken. Contrastively, speakers used more articulatory precision when saying the unpredictable words, and those words were more intelligible to the naïve listeners. For example, in Lieberman's study, the word "nine" was considered to be predictable in the sentence "A stitch in time saves nine," whereas the word "nine" was considered to be unpredictable in the sentence, "The number you will hear is nine." Another interesting study was conducted by Carol Fowler and Jonathan Housum in 1987. In their study, articulatory features of words produced the first time (called "new words") and a second time (called "old words") by speakers giving a monologue were compared. New words produced the first time were articulated approximately 40 to 70 milliseconds more slowly on average than during their second production, and the new words were more intelligible to listeners who heard the words in isolation. These findings elucidate what we seemingly do unconsciously.

Remember, though, Jakobson's assertion that speakers not only want to be heard, they also want to be understood. Lindblom explained that speakers attempt to strike a balance between their own desire to make articulation as easy as possible and their listener's need for intelligible speech. Ladefoged referred to this additional factor as the principle of sufficient perceptual separation. Ladefoged observed that languages preserve auditory distinctions across speech sounds, allowing listeners to be able to distinguish one phoneme from another with minimal difficulty. "Rose may be a rose may be a rose may be a rose" (Stein, 1990), but when it comes to speech production, "P is not a p sound is not a p sound is not a p sound." Talking to be heard and then to be understood is achieved by a speaker successfully balancing the diverse forces presented by his or her own inclination toward articulatory ease and demands from various listeners, speaking environments, and phonetic contexts.

? 1-4. Did You Get It?

1. Practice saying each of the following sentences using a formal register, a casual register, and an intimate register.
   a. Hi, how are you doing today?
   b. Please, let me help you with that!

Seeing Letters, but Hearing Sounds

The IPA is a powerful tool that is used to capture actual speech production; however, to phonetically transcribe speech correctly, you must first learn to hear the speech sounds that actually were produced, and largely ignore the orthographic spellings of words. Beginners of phonetic transcription often let written orthographic spelling guide their transcriptions, which frequently results in incorrect phonetic transcriptions. Think back to the problems we discussed earlier about the many difficulties of pronunciation and spelling using the orthographic alphabet. You want to begin to improve your listening skills right away, so that you will be able to identify correctly the number of sounds—not letters—in words.

Let's revisit some of the words we looked at previously, beginning with *bow* (the decoration) and *bough* (a tree branch). Say each word aloud using citation-form speech. How many sounds did you hear in each word? The correct answer is that there are two sounds pronounced in each word, either "b" + long "o" or "b" + "ow." If you incorrectly answered that you heard three sounds, you probably said that you heard the consonant sound "w" at the end of each word. If that is the case, then you may have grossly overarticulated your pronunciation of the vowel sound. Both the long "o" and "ow" vowel sounds require that you round your lips to make them, and that lip rounding can sound as though you are making a "w" sound, when you are saying the vowel only, thus, only one sound.

We now will consider a different type of problem when determining the number of speech sounds articulated in a word: saying speech sounds that are not represented in the spelling of a word. For example, say the word *one* aloud. How many speech sounds do you hear? The correct answer is that there are three speech sounds in the articulation of *one*: "w" + vowel "uh" + "n." Even though the word *one* is spelled orthographically as vowel + consonant + vowel, it is pronounced as consonant + vowel + consonant.

It is helpful to practice counting the number of sounds in words. We will start with easy words. Remember to listen to how the words sound, not to how they are spelled.

A	B	C
in	fin	skin
egg	leg	dreg
am	bam	spam
us	bus	plus
op	top	crop

How many sounds did you hear in each of the words in each column? Hopefully you heard two sounds in the words in Column A, three sounds in the words in Column B, and four sounds in the words in Column C. All the words in Column A begin with a vowel sound and end with a consonant sound. All the words in Column B begin with a consonant sound, have a vowel sound in the middle, and end with a consonant sound. Last, all the words in Column C begin with two consonant sounds, have a vowel sound in the middle, and end with a consonant sound.

Next, try segmenting intermediate-level words into individual sounds.

A	B	C
edge	any	tread
la	blah	smock
who	you'd	glued
duh	none	ahead
off	cough	golf

How many sounds did you hear in each of the words in each column? Again, hopefully you heard two sounds in the words in Column A, three sounds in the words in Column B, and four sounds in the words in Column C. In Column A, *edge* and *off* begin with a vowel sound and end with a consonant sound, and *la*, *who*, and *duh* begin with a consonant sound and end with a vowel sound. In Column B, *any* is the only word that begins with a vowel sound, followed by a consonant and then a vowel sound. Also in Column B, *blah* begins with two consonant sounds and ends with a vowel sound, while *you'd*, *none*, and *cough* begin with a consonant sound, have a vowel sound in the middle, and end with a consonant sound. Last, the first three words in Column C begin with two consonant sounds, have a vowel sound in the middle, and end with a consonant sound; *ahead* alternates from vowel sound to consonant sound to vowel sound to consonant sound, and *golf*, which begins with a consonant sound, has a vowel sound in the middle, and ends with two consonant sounds, "l" + "f."

Last, try a few challenging words. Remember, try to not let the spelling trick you.

use

cue

taxi

special

column

shriek

friend

ghost

height

colleague

Below are the correct number of sounds in each word. Note that the sound made by the letter is listed, and specific vowel sounds are not listed because there are multiples ways to write vowel sounds using the orthographic spelling.

use (noun)	= 3	"y" + vowel + "s"
use (verb)	= 3	"y" + vowel + "z"
pew	= 3	"p" + "y" + vowel

? 1–5. Did You Get It?

1. How many consonant and vowel sounds do you hear in each of the following words?

   a. dog _____ doggie _____ doghouse _____

   b. win _____ window _____ windowsill _____

   c. in _____ inside _____ inside-out _____

   d. hon _____ honey _____ honeybee _____

   e. bass _____ basket _____ basketball _____

taxi	= 5	"t" + vowel + "k" + "s" + vowel
special	= 6	"s" + "p" + vowel + "sh" + vowel + "l"
column	= 5	"k" + vowel + "l" + vowel + "m"
shriek	= 4	"sh" + "r" + vowel + "k"
friend	= 5	"f" + "r" + vowel + "n" + "d"
ghost	= 4	"g" + vowel + "s" + "t"
height	= 3	"h" + vowel + "t"
colleague	= 5	"k" + vowel + "l" + vowel + "g"

The Phonotactic Structure of Speech

Another skill that underlies the ability to master phonetic transcription is being able to specify the sound structure of syllables and words, that is, the shapes of syllables and words. Specifying the sound structure or permissible combination of sounds is called **phonotactics**. Every word has a **phonotactic structure** that is based on its actual production, not its spelling. The phonotactic structure of a word has an underlying value in a language and is constrained by the phonological rules of the language—concepts that we will discuss in detail in Chapters 7 and 8. Let's practice using the easy words of *in*, *fin*, and *skin*. We established that *in* has two sounds, *fin* has three, and *skin* has four. Because *in* begins with a vowel sound and ends with a consonant sound, its phonotactic structure is vowel (V) + consonant (C), abbreviated as VC. The phonotactic structure of *fin* is CVC and *skin* is CCVC. Now, we will try the challenging word *one*. Because we determined previously that *one* begins with a consonant sound, followed by a vowel, and followed by another consonant sound, its phonotactic structure is CVC. Phonotactic structure is defined for each language. For example, in English we have a phonological rule that permits words to begin with "s" + "p" (as in *spot*), "s" + "t" (as in *steak*), and "s" + "k" (as in *skip*), but not with "s" + "b," "s" + "d," or "s" + "g." Contrastively, in Spanish no words can begin with "s" + another consonant.

? 1–6. Did You Get It?

1. What is the phonotactic structure of each of the following words?

   a. dog _____ doggie _____ doghouse _____

   b. win _____ window _____ windowsill _____

   c. in _____ inside _____ inside-out _____

   d. hon _____ honey _____ honeybee _____

   e. bass _____ basket _____ basketball _____

Consonants and Vowels by Position

When we talk about the consonant sounds that make up a particular word, we need to specify where in the word those sounds occur. Consonant sounds that occur at the beginning, middle, and end of words are said to be in initial, medial, and final positions, respectively. For example, in the word *hot*, "h" is word initial and "t" is word final; there is no consonant in word-medial position. However, in the word *hotel*, we find that "h" is word initial, "t" is word medial, and "l" is word final.

When determining the position of consonants, it is important to understand how we classify consonants that are abutting (i.e., not separated by a vowel), such as "sk" in the word *skip* or "nd" in *hand*. Sequential consonants in a word are called **consonant clusters**. Consonant clusters are considered to be represented in our brain's speech system as a single "unit;" therefore, all of the consonants in a cluster occupy the same position in a word. For example, in the word *skip*, "sk" is a word-initial cluster. There are no medial consonants in the word *skip*. Similarly, in the word *hand*, "nd" is a word-final cluster and there are no medial consonants. When consonant clusters occur at the beginning and/or end of a word, it is useful to consider them as an inseparable unit of speech. When consonant clusters occur in the middle of words, things become more complicated, as we will discuss later in the chapter.

Attempting to better understand speech representations and productions, phoneticians and other researchers also can study consonants by their syllable position in words. Returning to the example of the word *hotel*, if we wanted to specify its consonants by syllable position instead of by word position, we would begin by determining the number of syllables in the word *hotel*, which is two: CV + CVC or "ho" + "tel." We then would specify that "h" is in initial position in the first syllable, and that "t" is in initial position and "l" is in final position in the second syllable. Therefore, when we specify phonotactic structure by syllable position, consonants can occur in initial and final positions only. Consonant sounds that occur in syllable-initial position are called syllable initiating; the "h" and "t" consonant sounds in the word *hotel* are syllable initiating. Consonant sounds that occur in syllable-final position are called syllable arresting, such as the "l" sound in the second syllable of *hotel*.

It is not always easy to determine to which syllable a sound belongs. One such difficulty occurs when a consonant is produced across a syllable boundary. Why does this happen? It is helpful to understand that speech is a series of articulations that are sequential, but that also overlap. We do not produce speech by saying only a single speech sound at a time, like pearls strung on a necklace. Instead, while we are saying one speech sound, we simultaneously are finishing saying the sound before it and getting ready to say the sound after it. Our speech gestures overlap. This phenomenon is called **coarticulation**. Because of the overlapping movements during coarticulation, some sounds are produced across two syllables. Take, for example, the two-syllable word *silly*. The "l" sound in *silly* seems to span both the first and second syllables; it seemingly is syllable arresting (in syllable one) and syllable initiating (in syllable two). However, given that there are four speech sounds produced in the CVCV word *silly*, and "l" is produced only once, it cannot occupy two positions. Consonant sounds such as the "l" in *silly* are called **ambisyllabic** because they sound like they belong to two syllables. Ambisyllabic consonants can occur only in words that have more than one syllable and when the vowel following the consonant in question is unstressed, as in the word *silly*. The word *silly* satisfies both conditions, because it has two syllables and the first vowel, not the second vowel, carries the stress. Ambisyllabic consonants can increase the difficulty of transcribing phonetically, especially for beginner transcribers.

Segmenting words into syllables is called **syllabification**. Specifying how many syllables a word has is a relatively easy task, even for young children; however, determining where those syllables begin and end is a difficult task, even for some adults. Let us begin by again considering the word *silly*. Because "l" is ambisyllabic, the options for dividing *silly* into two syllables could include "sil" + "y" and "si" + "ly," and you might even be tempted to use "sil" + "ly" (however, do not give in to this temptation, because you already determined that *silly* has a CVCV phonotactic structure). How do you know which syllabification to use? As a starting place, you might consult the dictionary. Prior to providing the definition(s) of words, dictionaries list the syllabification of each entry two ways. The first way is with syllables separated by dots, as in *ho · tel*. This type of syllabification reflects the established practice of editors and printers who need a conventional way of breaking words that fall at the end of a line of type, as at the end of a line of words in a newspaper column with a set number of spaces. The second way that dictionaries list the syllabification of words is based on language rules that are specific to the language; however, confusingly, dictionaries sometimes list more than one way to break a word into syllables. It is important to understand that dictionaries divide written words into their linguistic forms, dividing words into prefixes, root words, suffixes, and the like. In linguistics, this study of word structure and how words are formed is called **morphology**. Dictionaries do not divide words into syllables *as they are spoken*. Therefore, consulting the dictionary to discover a word's syllable components may not be useful if your goal is to divide words into syllables in spoken language.

Syllabification of spoken language is largely accomplished by following a few phonetic principles. One key concept for dividing words into syllables in speech is called the **maximal onset principle**. An **onset** is the sound that occupies the syllable-initiating position. As previously discussed, the word *hotel* contains two syllables, "ho" + "tel"; "h" and "t" are the syllable onsets. The maximal onset principle applies to words containing one or more medial consonants. Employing this principle, a word-medial consonant would be assigned to the syllable that follows it, so that the word-medial consonant occupies the syllable-initiating, or onset, position. We will use the word *cookie* to illustrate this principle. The word *cookie* has two syllables, and it contains the word-medial consonant sound "k." We divide *cookie* into the syllables "coo" + "kie," so that "k" occupies the syllable-initiating position in syllable two, thus maximizing the syllable onsets (which also has a resulting effect of decreasing syllable-arresting consonants). Let us practice dividing another word, *spinach*, into its spoken syllables. *Spinach* has one word-medial consonant and two syllables. Following the maximal onset principle, we would divide *spinach* into the syllables "spi" + "nach."

Let us now practice dividing two words, each containing word-medial consonant clusters. The word *mistake* has a CVCCVC phonotactic shape. Following the maximal onset principle, to which syllable, syllable one or two, do we assign the medial "st" consonants? Yes, we would divide the spoken word *mistake* into the syllables CV + CCVC, "mi" + "stake." Consider now the word *stanza*, which has a CCVCCV phonotactic shape. To maximize syllable onsets, we would divide *stanza* into the syllables CCV + CCV, "sta" + "nza." But wait, is that really correct? Say the two syllables aloud. Hopefully you can hear how that division does not represent how we say the word *stanza*. We say the word *stanza* in the syllables "stan" + "za." So why can we not apply the principle to this example? Because there is an exception to the principle: you can only place consonants in onset position that follow the phonology of the language. English does not permit the cluster "nz" to occur in syllable-initiating position (that is, no words in English begin with "nz"); therefore, we need to break the word into syllables that follow the phonological rules of English.

One other guideline should prove helpful for dividing spoken words into syllables. It is important for you to know that one vowel sound equals one syllable. Therefore, every vowel represents one syllable and every syllable contains one, and only one, vowel. This is where our previous practice of identifying the phonotactics of a word becomes useful. Whenever you see a vowel in a word, you know to count that sound as representing one syllable.

In phonetics, the convention for writing the syllabification of words is to use a period in-between syllables. For example, the word *hotel* would be written as CV.CVC. The word *cookie* would be written as CV.CV. Last, the word *spinach* would be written as CCV.CVC. With practice, you will develop this skill over time. Following these guidelines, the correct syllabification of the spoken word *silly* is CV.CV, or "si" + "ly."

Our final consideration is how to determine word position for clusters. If you classify consonant sounds by their position in words because you are interested in the actual production of those sounds, then abutting consonants in the middle of words would be considered word-medial clusters. For example, the word *window* would be considered to have a word-medial "nd" cluster, and the word *basket* would be considered to have a word-medial "sk" cluster. However, if you want to classify consonant sounds by their position in *syllables*, then no opportunity ever exists for a medial cluster to occur. In syllables, clusters can occur in initial and final positions only. To exemplify, *window* has two syllables: "win" + "dow." In the first syllable, "n" would be syllable arresting, and in the second syllable, "d" would be syllable initiating. In the example of *basket*, the "sk" cluster would be initiating syllable two: "ba" + "sket." How you decide to classify consonants positionally is based largely on the purpose of your analysis. For example, if you are focused on understanding how someone articulates the continuous movements of speech, then you would be less concerned about the syllable structures in the word, and more concerned about how the speaker moved from one speech sound to another. Thus, you would be likely to classify the cluster "sk" as a word-medial cluster:

basket. Alternatively, if you are interested in creating an inventory of the different syllable shapes that someone produces, then, following the maximal onset principle for spoken language, you likely would classify the "sk" cluster as syllable initiating in the second CCVC syllable: "sket."

Unlike consonants, vowels are described positionally by syllable only. Vowels are not described as being in initial, medial, and final positions in words. Instead, vowels are described positionally by syllable number. In the example of the word *hotel*, the first vowel, long "o," is designated as belonging

---

? 1–7. Did You Get It?

1. Describe each of the consonant sounds in the following words by their positions in *words*. Two examples follow.

   it = VC   contains a word-final "t"

   into = VCCV   contains a word-medial "nt" cluster

   a. dog   _____

   b. doggie   _____

   c. in   _____

   d. inside   _____

   e. bass   _____

   f. basket   _____

2. Next, describe the same consonant sounds by their positions in *syllables*. Two examples follow.

   it = VC   contains a syllable-arresting "t"

   into = VC.CV   contains a syllable-arresting "n"

                   contains a syllable-initiating "t"

   a. dog   _____

   b. doggie   _____

   c. in   _____

   d. inside   _____

   e. bass   _____

   f. basket   _____

in syllable one and the second vowel, short "e," is designated as belonging in syllable two. Remember that every syllable must contain a vowel. Therefore, words with a single vowel sound always have a single syllable.

Contrastive, Linguistic, and Grammatical Stress

Stress is the amount of emphasis we place on a sound, syllable, or word. In American English, stress is the result of us increasing our speaking effort. Compared with unstressed productions, we exhibit stress by slowing down and overarticulating stressed sounds, producing stressed sounds using a louder voice, and/or producing stressed sounds using a higher or lower vocal pitch. Slowing down and hyperarticulating our speech requires excellent control of our articulatory muscles, making our voice louder requires excellent control of our **respiratory** (breathing) system, and changing our vocal pitch requires excellent control of our **phonatory** (voicing) system.

We will consider three types of stress: **contrastive**, **lexical**, and **grammatical**. Contrastive stress is when we emphasize a sound, syllable, or word because we want our listener to pay attention to that sound, syllable, or word. For example, if I were at a cookout with you and I wanted you to pass me the hot sauce and not the hot dogs, I might emphasize (as shown by capitalization) the word *sauce* by saying, *Please pass me the hot SAUCE.* By stressing the word *sauce* in the sentence, I am more likely to get what I want—the hot sauce. Or maybe I am mildly upset because you, specifically, showed up late to my party, and I let you know that I am upset by saying, *I am not unhappy that Emma came late to my party, but I AM unhappy that YOU came late.* By using contrastive stress, I am conveying what I think is important in what I am saying by how I'm saying it. The speaker has the flexibility to use contrastive stress as he or she likes, depending on the message the person wants to send. A person also may purposely overexaggerate, or stress, a single sound so two words are not confused by a listener. For example, an anatomy instructor may overstress the "b" sound in the word *aBduct* and the "d" sound in the word *aDDuct* when describing the opening and clos-

ing of the vocal folds, so students will be able to disambiguate the two words. A speech-language pathologist may overstress a sound a child has a difficult time articulating as a means of drawing attention to that sound, as in the example of: *Listen carefully to how I say SSSSSStar.*

There is no flexibility in how we use the other types of stress—lexical and grammatical. Lexical and grammatical stress are the patterns of emphasis inherent in each **multisyllabic** word. All examples of grammatical stress fall under the broader category of lexical stress; however, not all lexical stress is grammatical in nature. **Lexical stress** is the underlying, unchanging stress pattern of a word. In two-syllable words, such as in the word *laughter*, "laugh" + "ter," one of the two syllables carries more stress than the other. Say the word *laughter* aloud by first stressing the first syllable, "laugh," and then by stressing the second syllable, "ter." Which way sounds correct? Yes, *LAUGHter* has stress on the first syllable. The stress on the syllable with the most emphasis is called **primary stress**. In words that are three or more syllables long, it can be said that each syllable carries a different degree of stress. The heaviest emphasis is called primary stress, the second-heaviest is called secondary stress, and the third is called tertiary stress. It can be difficult to discern between secondary and tertiary stressed syllables, and there is some disagreement as to how we produce these lesser degrees of stress. For now, let's focus only on primary stress. In Chapter 5, we will go into more detail about how we produce stress, how stress functions, and how we use it to communicate.

Not everyone differentiates between the terms "lexical" and "grammatical" stress; however, we think it's important for you to understand that each word has an underlying stress pattern (i.e., lexical stress) and that in some words changing the stress pattern results in words with different syntactical functions (i.e., grammatical stress). Every multisyllabic word has an underlying stress pattern. Consider again the word *laughter*. We established that *laughter* is a two-syllable word with the first syllable carrying the primary stress, a pattern called STRONG-weak. Therefore, the correct pronunciation of *laughter* includes producing a STRONG-weak stress pattern. However, if you produced *laughter* with a weak-STRONG stress pattern, as in *laughTER*, the word's meaning would not change. It would sound odd, but it would still mean a vocal expression of pleasure. This is what we mean by the term "lexical stress."

Grammatical stress indicates a word's syntactic category. For example, let's think about the two-syllable word *content*. The word *content* is a homograph—a word spelled one way that has two meanings—a concept that we discussed previously. *Content* can be produced with a STRONG-weak pattern: CONtent. A production of CONtent signals a noun, as in the sentence, *The CONtent in the box was unknown*. But wait, *content* also can be produced with a weak-STRONG pattern: conTENT. This latter production indicates an adjective, as in, *The conTENT baby slept all night long*. Grammatical stress is emphasis that, if changed, results in a change in word meaning and in the syntactical category of the word. We hope that you can see that stress is important—to the speaker, to the listener, and to the meaning of the message intended to be sent.

There is one last consideration of stress in words, and that is its effect on vowels. Vowels in stressed syllables typically are fully articulated, whereas vowels in unstressed syllables often are what are referred to as weak forms of the vowel. Consider the two-syllable word *apply*. *Apply* has a weak-STRONG stress pattern, with the second syllable carrying the primary stress. The first vowel, "a," is produced as the short "u" vowel, "uh." The second vowel, "y," however, is fully articulated as the long "i" vowel sound. Using this notation system, we might spell its production as "uh-pli." But what happens when you lengthen the word *apply* into the word *application*? Say both words aloud: *apply – application*. Which syllable carries the primary stress in the four-syllable word *application*? Yes, the third syllable: appliCAtion. How is the vowel "a" produced in the first syllable of *application*? Is it still produced as "uh" like in the word *apply*? No, it has changed. The first-syllable vowel in *application* is produced as the short "a" vowel, as in *hat*. What about the vowel "i" in the second syllable—is it still articulated as the long "i" vowel sound? No, in the word *application*, the long "i" sound is casually articulated as "uh." The articulatory changes are the result, in part, of syllable stress. We will talk extensively about the effect of stress on vowel production in Chapters 3 and 8.

Understanding the different types of stress is important information for speech-language pathologists and audiologists. There are various populations of individuals with speech, language, and hearing disorders that have difficulty producing, hearing, and using stress correctly. For example, individuals with speech disorders due to motor-based problems often have trouble producing stress correctly. Individuals with certain types of language disorders exhibit difficulty interpreting and using stress correctly. Individuals with hearing impairments who cannot hear stress patterns can have difficulty producing and interpreting stress. In addition, many individuals learning a second language have difficulty learning to produce and interpret stress in their second language.

We have found that many of our phonetics students have trouble identifying the syllable that carries the primary stress. If this is a difficult task for you, below are some guidelines that may make the task easier as you get started.

1. In one-syllable words, there is one vowel, and that vowel is stressed.

2. In two-syllable nouns, adjectives, and adverbs, primary stress is *typically* produced on the first syllable.
   - Examples of nouns include *student* (STUdent), *mother* (MOther), and *table* (TAble).
   - Examples of adjectives include *quiet* (QUIet), *funny* (FUnny), and *useful* (USEful).
   - Examples of adverbs include *never* (NEver), *slowly* (SLOWly), and *often* (OFten).

3. In most two-syllable verbs and prepositions, primary stress *typically* is on the second syllable.
   - Examples of verbs include *embrace* (emBRACE), *decide* (deCIDE), and *relax* (reLAX).
   - Examples of prepositions include *between* (beTWEEN), *aside* (aSIDE), and *among* (aMONG).

4. In most compound nouns (i.e., two words combined to make a new word), primary stress *typically* is on the first syllable.
   - Examples include *moonlight* (MOONlight), *bathtub* (BATHtub), *grandfather* (GRANDfather), and *basketball* (BAsketball).

? 1–8. Did You Get It?

1. Say the following sentences by stressing the capitalized syllables and words. What type of stress is represented in these examples: contrastive or grammatical?

   No, I wanted the PENCIL.

   _____

   That sounded like an INsult to me, too.

   _____

   HE thinks he's really funny.

   _____

   You MUST meet my new roommate.

   _____

   Do you have to preSENT in class today?

   _____

2. Write the lexical stress pattern, in terms of strong and weak syllables, for each of the following words. One example follows.

giraffe	weak-STRONG
pizza	_____
scissors	_____
counter	_____
balloon	_____
candle	_____
baby	_____
pretty	_____
machine	_____
brochure	_____

3. Say the following words aloud. How many syllables are in each word? Which syllable carries the primary stress in each word? One example follows.

table	2 syllables	STRONG-weak
January	_____	_____
mother	_____	_____
garage	_____	_____
pencil	_____	_____
telephone	_____	_____
mist	_____	_____
dancing	_____	_____
nothing	_____	_____
community	_____	_____

4. Say the following homographs first as nouns. Then say each of them as a verb. What is the pattern of stress that marks these words grammatically as either nouns or verbs?

   contest
   produce
   envelope
   address
   increase
   refuse
   impact
   insult
   object
   incline

   The nouns have a stress pattern of _____

   The verbs have a stress pattern of _____

Putting It All Together

When you first read that phonetics is the study of speech sounds, it may have seemed straightforward and uncomplicated. Hopefully you are discovering that phonetics is quite complex and encompasses many different areas of spoken language. In practicing as a clinical or research speech or hearing scientist, possessing knowledge of phonetics will provide you with a solid foundation for understanding typical and disordered speech. You likely will meet many professionals who equate phonetics with phonetic transcription, because often in the speech and hearing sciences, phonetics is taught only as a tool for phonetic transcription. That is a shame, for phonetics is a science in and of itself, and one that can inform many aspects of our clinical practice and research, from differential diagnosis to goal setting to theory development and testing. As you continue to read, you will discover the science behind the tools we call the IPA, as well as practical ways to employ it.

References

Example. (2009). In Microsoft Encarta (Version 2.1) [Software]. Redmond, WA: Microsoft Corporation.

Fowler, C. A., & Housum, J. (1987). Talkers signaling of "new" and "old" words in speech and listeners' perception and use of the distinctions. *Journal of Memory and Speech, 26,* 489–504.

Ladefoged, P., & Johnson, K. (2014). *A course in phonetics* (7th ed.). Boston, MA: Wadsworth.

Lieberman, P. (1963). Some effects of semantic and grammatical context on the production and perception of speech. *Language and Speech, 6,* 172–187.

Lindblom, B. (1983). Economy of speech gestures. In P. F. MacNeilage (Ed.), *Speech production* (pp. 217–245). New York, NY: Springer-Verlag.

Lindblom, B. E. F. (1990). Explaining phonetic variation: A sketch of the H & H theory. In W. J. Hardcastle & A. Marchal (Eds.), *Speech production and speech modelling* (pp. 403–439). Dordrecht: Springer Netherlands.

Stein, G. (1990). *Selected writings of Gertrude Stein.* New York, NY: Random House.

Interest Piqued?

Recommended materials to further your understanding of topics covered in this chapter.

Print Resources

A particularly useful dictionary for phonetics students is *Longman Pronunciation Dictionary* (3rd ed.) by John Wells, published in 2008 by Pearson ESL.

Online Resources

http://www.antimoon.com/how/pronunc-sounds ipa.htm
Site for IPA symbols.

https://blogonlinguistics.wordpress.com/2013/10/12/phoneme-sound-allophone-phone
Concepts of phones, phonemes, allophones.

http://enjoyphonetics.weebly.com/uploads/5/3/5/9/5359376/definitionsseminar1.pdf
Concepts of phones, phonemes, allophones.

http://www.genconnection.com/English/ap/LanguageRegisters.htm
Examples of different speech registers.

http://www.internationalphoneticsassociation.org
The official website of the International Phonetic Association, which has a wealth of information for students (and others).

http://people.umass.edu/scable/LING201-SP13/Slides-Handouts/Syllables-Phonotactics.pdf
Site explaining word syllabification.

http://www.saypyu.com
An interesting writing system based on phonetics is called SaypYu: Spell as You Pronounce Universal Project.

https://westonruter.github.io/ipa-chart/keyboard/
Site for IPA symbols.

https://www.youtube.com/watch?v=L16i2enJA_w
Listen to speech registers.

https://www.youtube.com/watch?v=FgfSTwagHyc
Phonotactic structure of words.

https://www.youtube.com/watch?v=1Up5hSm7LYI
Phonotactic structure of words.

Applied Science: Revisited

Summary

Now that you've read this introductory chapter, do you want to make any changes to the list of words you think the child cannot say? Do you want to make any changes to the list of words you think the speech-language pathologist could use to test the child's speech? If so, go ahead and make those changes.

Let's see what the speech-language pathologist found when she tested the child.

One Step at a Time

1. When the speech-language pathologist tested the boy's speech, she used play and objects of words that tested all the speech sounds in English in the beginning and ending of words, so that she could obtain a full understanding of his speech. But she paid particular attention to "t" and "s" words that the mother reported as being difficult for him to say.

2. The speech-language pathologist found that the child made the following speech errors.

    top/stop (read as, "He said 'top' for the word 'stop.'")

    tep/step

    no/snow

    pill/spill

    fum/thumb

    fink/think

    fin/thin

    duh/the

    dat/that

    dem/them

    All other speech sounds were articulated correctly.

3. The mother reported that her son had difficulty pronouncing "'t' and 's' words." Looking at the child's speech errors, how would you describe the sounds the child did not produce correctly?

Answer

Your descriptions are correct if you said that the child misarticulated the speech sounds "th" and s-clusters at the beginning of words. The child did not have difficulty with "t" words. Instead, he had difficulty pronouncing words that started with the "th" sound. Similarly, the child did not have difficulty pronouncing words that started with the "s" sound, but instead, his difficulty was isolated to words that started with s + another consonant (i.e., s-clusters).

Science Applied

Applying phonetics to this problem was the solution to understanding how to capture the child's speech errors. Being able to use one symbol, and only one symbol, in the IPA permits the unambiguous capturing of speech production.

? Did You Get It?

ANSWER KEY

1–1.

1. Name the branch of phonetics—articulatory, acoustic, auditory, or linguistic—that each example describes.

    a. Determining if a puff of air is typically emitted during production of a "p" sound when in initial position of English words.   <u>linguistic</u>

    b. Determining if a puff of air that was produced during production of a "p" sound could be heard by a panel of listeners.   <u>auditory</u>

    c. Determining if a puff of air was emitted during production of the "p" sound by examining a speech spectrogram (a visible representation of sound).   <u>acoustic</u>

    d. Determining if a puff of air was emitted during production of the "p" sound by placing your hand near the speaker's mouth to feel the airflow.   <u>articulatory</u>

2. A phonetician studies the <u>phonetics</u> of a language.

3. A phonologist studies the <u>phonology</u> of a language.

1–2.

Match the following terms.

1. phonemes   <u>c</u>   a. the sounds articulated when a child says *no*

2. phones   <u>a</u>   b. the different ways the sound "s" can be articulated

3. allophones   <u>b</u>   c. the mental sound units that make up the word *chair*

1–3.

1. List an example of one consonant sound that is spelled with different graphemes in two different words.

    <u>Answers will vary; examples include "s" sound in *mass* and *face*, "k" sound in *kite* and *cat*, etc.</u>

2. List an example of one vowel sound that is spelled with different graphemes in two different words.

    <u>Answers will vary; examples include the long "e" sound in *feet-beat*, the long "a" sound in *hey-hay*, etc.</u>

3. List a pair of homographs.
    <u>Answers will vary; examples include *dove, wind, close*, etc.</u>

4. List a pair of homophones.
    <u>Answers will vary; examples include *blue-blew, bear-bare, sell-cell*, etc.</u>

5. Would you transcribe the following words using virgules or brackets?
    a. *book*, as said by a child   <u>brackets</u>
    b. *book*, as in the object itself   <u>virgules</u>
    c. the word *kitten*   <u>virgules</u>
    d. the spoken word *kitten*   <u>brackets</u>

1–4.

1. Practice saying each of the following sentences using a formal register, a casual register, and an intimate register.

    a. Hi, how are you doing today?

    b. Please, let me help you with that!

<u>This is a verbal practice task, so there is no written response needed.</u>

1–5.

1. How many consonant and vowel sounds do you hear in each of the following words?

    a. dog <u>3</u>   doggie <u>4</u>   doghouse <u>6</u>

    b. win <u>3</u>   window <u>5</u>   windowsill <u>8</u>

    c. in <u>2</u>   inside <u>5</u>   inside-out <u>7</u>

    d. hon <u>3</u>   honey <u>4</u>   honeybee <u>6</u>

    e. bass <u>3</u>   basket <u>6</u>   basketball <u>9</u>

1–6.

1. What is the phonotactic structure of each of the following words?

    a. dog <u>CVC</u>   doggie <u>CVCV</u>   doghouse <u>CVCCVC</u>

    b. win <u>CVC</u>   window <u>CVCCV</u>   windowsill <u>CVCCVCVC</u>

    c. in <u>VC</u>   inside <u>VCCVC</u>   inside-out <u>VCCVCVC</u>

    d. hon <u>CVC</u>   honey <u>CVCV</u>   honeybee <u>CVCVCV</u>

    e. bass <u>CVC</u>   basket <u>CVCCVC</u>   basketball <u>CVCCVCCVC</u>

1–7.

1. Describe the consonant sounds in the following words by their positions in *words*. Two examples follow.

it = VC   <u>contains a word-final "t"</u>

into = VCCV   <u>a word-medial "nt" cluster</u>

    a. dog   <u>a word-initial "d"</u>
                 <u>a word-final "g"</u>

    b. doggie <u>a word-initial "d"</u>
                 <u>a word-medial "g"</u>

    c. in   <u>a word-final "n"</u>

    d. inside <u>a word-medial "ns" cluster</u>
                 <u>a word-final "d"</u>

    e. bass   <u>a word-initial "b"</u>
                 <u>a word-final "s"</u>

    f. basket <u>a word-initial "b"</u>
                 <u>a word-medial "sk" cluster</u>
                 <u>a word-final "t"</u>

2. Next, describe the same consonant sounds by their positions in *syllables*. Two examples follow.

it = VC   <u>a syllable-arresting "t"</u>

into = VC.CV   <u>a syllable-arresting "n"</u>
                 <u>a syllable-initiating "t"</u>

    a. dog   <u>a syllable-initiating "d"</u>
                 <u>a syllable-arresting "g"</u>

    b. doggie <u>a syllable-initiating "d"</u>
                 <u>a syllable-initiating "g"</u>

c. in   <u>a syllable-arresting "n"</u>

d. inside   <u>a syllable-arresting "n"</u>
                <u>a syllable-initiating "s"</u>
                <u>a syllable-arresting "d"</u>

e. bass   <u>a syllable-initiating "b"</u>
                <u>a syllable-arresting "s"</u>

f. basket   <u>a syllable-initiating "b"</u>
                <u>a syllable-initiating "sk" cluster</u>
                <u>a syllable-arresting "t"</u>

1–8.

1. Say the following sentences by stressing the capitalized syllables and words. What type of stress is represented in these examples: contrastive or grammatical?

    No, I wanted the PENCIL.   <u>contrastive</u>

    That sounded like an INsult to me, too.
    <u>grammatical</u>

    HE thinks he's really funny.   <u>contrastive</u>

    You MUST see my new puppy.   <u>contrastive</u>

    Do you have to preSENT in class today?
    <u>grammatical</u>

2. Write the lexical stress pattern, in terms of strong and weak syllables, for each of the following words. One example follows.

giraffe	weak-STRONG
pizza	<u>STRONG-weak</u>
scissors	<u>STRONG-weak</u>
counter	<u>STRONG-weak</u>
balloon	<u>weak-STRONG</u>
candle	<u>STRONG-weak</u>
baby	<u>STRONG-weak</u>
pretty	<u>STRONG-weak</u>
machine	<u>weak-STRONG</u>
brochure	<u>weak-STRONG</u>

3. Say the following words aloud. How many syllables are in each word? Which syllable carries the primary stress in each word? One example follows.

table	2 syllables	STRONG-weak

January	<u>4</u>	<u>STRONG-weak-weak-weak</u>
mother	<u>2</u>	<u>STRONG-weak</u>
garage	<u>2</u>	<u>weak-STRONG</u>
pencil	<u>2</u>	<u>STRONG-weak</u>
telephone	<u>3</u>	<u>STRONG-weak-weak</u>
mistal	<u>2</u>	<u>weak-STRONG</u>
dancing	<u>2</u>	<u>STRONG-weak</u>
nothing	<u>2</u>	<u>STRONG-weak</u>
community	4	<u>weak-STRONG-weak-weak</u>

4. Say the following words (i.e., homographs) first as a noun. Then say each of them as a verb. What is the pattern of stress that marks these words grammatically as either nouns or verbs?

    contest

    produce

    envelope

    address

    increase

    refuse

    impact

    insult

    object

    incline

    <u>The nouns have a stress pattern of STRONG-weak.</u>

    <u>The verbs have a stress pattern of weak-STRONG.</u>

2

ARTICULATORY PHONETICS OF CONSONANTS

Learning Objectives

By reading this chapter, you will learn:

1. ways we classify consonant sounds
2. anatomical processes we use to produce consonant sounds
3. the concept and production of voicing
4. anatomical structures we use to produce consonant sounds
5. the concept and examples of cognates
6. place classes and associated consonants in American English
7. manner classes and associated consonants in American English
8. phonetic symbols for the consonants in American English

Applied Science

Thinking in terms of consonant sounds, what is interesting about the pairs of words in each of the four sets that follow?

Set 1	Set 2	Set 3	Set 4
kit – cat	gym – hymn	carrot – cereal	axis – axes
kwanza – quick	box – socks	thigh – thy	gas – Arkansas
young – Jung	bus – fuss	chase – chaos	cough – bough
shell – charade	moose – juice	chair – chic	rage – beige
sycamore – psyche	rough – huff	mutt – muse	smooth – booth
hope – who	until – sill	suit – suite	braise – base
fast – phase	bet – debt	few – food	Texas – taxes
note – knot	lift – laughed	gum – gem	epoch – poach
not – gnat	beak – back	scene – scare	based – phased

Consonants in American English

There are 24 consonant phonemes in American English. These 24 consonants can be classified across three different articulatory domains: voicing, place of articulation, and manner of articulation. **Voicing** refers to whether a consonant is produced while the vocal folds are vibrating or being held apart. **Place of articulation** refers to where in the vocal tract a consonant is produced. **Manner of articulation** refers to how a consonant is produced. Each phoneme has its own unique combination of categorizations that specify the ways in which each speech sound is made. No two consonant phonemes share the exact same set of categorizations.

? 2–1. Did You Get It?

1. Voicing results because the vocal folds are _____.

2. Place of articulation refers to _____ a sound is produced.

3. Manner of articulation refers to _____ a sound is produced.

Anatomical Processes of the Speech System

In this chapter, we will detail five anatomical processes and a variety of physical structures that humans use to produce speech. They include the **respiratory**, **phonatory**, **resonatory**, **oro-nasal**, and **articulatory processes**. All five of these interactive processes combine to make up the **speech system**. An overview of the speech system is illustrated in Figure 2–1.

There also are two very important additional processes that affect speech production, the auditory (hearing) system and the neurological (brain) system. Both processes are critical to speech production; however, due to the scope of this textbook, we will not be covering the intricacies of audition or neurology. These topics typically are covered in their own courses in the speech and hearing sciences.

The power supply for speech is air, and in American English we use air from our lungs, called **pulmonic** air, to power speech. Pulmonic airflow is part of the respiratory system. Pulmonic air is pushed out of our lungs by the **diaphragm** and **abdominal muscles**, up through the **trachea** (the windpipe) and into the **larynx** (the voice box), where the **vocal folds** (the vocal cords) are housed. The vocal folds

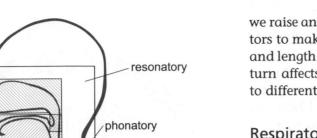

FIGURE 2–1. Sagittal view of the five anatomical processes used to produce speech.

are paired and they are made of muscle fibers that have a lot of elasticity. When the vocal folds are held apart, airflow passes silently between their medial edges. When the vocal folds are closed and airflow blows them apart, setting them into vibration, sound waves are created. Sound waves originating from the vocal folds are part of the phonatory system. From the laryngeal region, sound waves and/or silent airflow travel upward into the **vocal tract**. The vocal tract is a region containing the **pharynx** (the throat), **oral cavity** (the mouth), and **nasal cavity** (the nose). As sound travels through the vocal tract, it resonates in these different cavities, shaping the sound as part of the resonatory system. The oro-nasal process determines if the upward-moving airstream will travel through the oral and/or nasal cavities. Air in the oral cavity is shaped into speech sounds by a variety of structures that are part of the articulatory process. Speech sounds traveling primarily through the oral cavity are called **oral** sounds and speech sounds traveling primarily through the nasal cavity are called **nasal** sounds. As

we raise and lower the velum and move the articulators to make different sounds, we change the shape and length of the cavities of the vocal tract, which in turn affects the resonation of sound, permitting us to differentiate one sound from another sound.

Respiratory Process

The respiratory system includes the anatomical structures and their functions for breathing. Breathing is vitally important—it keeps us alive. But did you realize that it is also vitally important for producing speech? Without the respiratory system, English would have no consonant or vowel sounds. Not only does the respiratory system keep us alive, it also keeps our language alive.

Breathing is an exchange of air that takes place in the **alveoli** (tiny air sacs) in the lungs. Breathing air into the body is called **inhalation** (or **inspiration**) and breathing air out of the body is called **exhalation** (or **expiration**). You may find it interesting to count the number of inhalation-exhalation cycles you complete in the next 60 seconds; we encourage you to take a minute to do so. Look at a clock with a second hand or a stopwatch while your breathe quietly for one minute. How many full cycles did you complete? While breathing in a relaxed and quiet manner, we typically complete 10 to 18 cycles in one minute. During quiet breathing, inhalation is an active process that begins when the dome-shaped **diaphragm** contracts. The diaphragm is the primary muscle of respiration and is situated in the **abdominal area** (the stomach) below the lungs. Contraction of the diaphragm flattens out this muscle, increasing space in the **thorax** (the chest) and causing the rib cage to expand. Because a covering over the lungs "adheres" to a covering over the ribs, the lungs also expand with the rib cage. This expansion of the lungs creates a decrease in the air pressure in the lungs, compared with the atmospheric air pressure. Air moves from areas of high pressure to low pressure, so air flows into the lungs. During quiet breathing, one inhalation takes about 1½ to 2 seconds to complete.

Exhaling during quiet breathing takes about the same amount of time as inhaling. The breath cycle is completed when the diaphragm relaxes, causing it to raise and fill the cavity. The rib cage and lungs lower back to rest position, and air flows outward.

That outward flow of air is an exhalation. During quiet breathing, exhalation is a passive process of muscle relaxation. However, during physical exertion, such as when we are exercising, and during speech, we actively engage the muscles of respiration to help us control how much and how fast air flows outward. We encourage you to pause a moment now to ponder: why do you think we turn exhalation into an active process during speech, instead of letting the respiratory system passively complete the breath cycle?

To help you answer the above question, try this quick experiment. Slowly say the word *me* while gently exhaling. Now say *me* while gently inhaling. Which was the easier production? Yes, it was much easier to say *me* on exhaled air. All speech sounds in English are produced on exhaled air. Next, time yourself with a stopwatch while you casually say the following sentence aloud: *It's interesting studying all the different aspects of phonetics and I'm looking forward to learning more.* How long did it take you to say that sentence? We already established that a typical exhalation would have taken approximately 2 seconds to complete. It probably took you at least twice as long to say that sentence, so if you had spoken on passive exhalation, you would have run out of air about halfway through the sentence. But you didn't run out of air—because you actively controlled the rate of your exhalation. When we talk, we engage our respiratory muscles to be able to control the rate of expiratory airflow to be able to speak longer on each breath. The respiratory system supplies the power needed to produce speech—and that power is air. However, the rest of the speech system is needed to turn that expiratory airstream into sounds we call speech.

Phonatory Process

The larynx consists of six different cartilages and connects the inferior portion of the pharynx with the trachea. The vocal folds are housed in the larynx. When we are preparing to speak, we bring our vocal folds close together. It is called **adduction** when the vocal folds are approximating one another, as diagrammed in Figure 2–2. In contrast, it is called **abduction** when the vocal folds are wide apart, with the space between the folds called the **glottis**, as diagrammed in Figure 2–3. There are 17 muscles in the

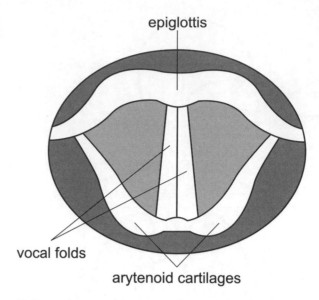

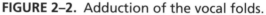

FIGURE 2–2. Adduction of the vocal folds.

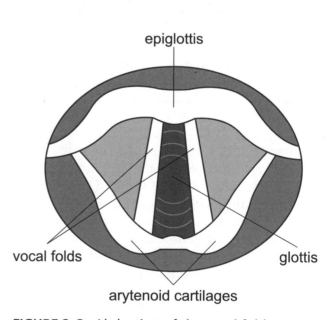

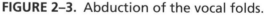

FIGURE 2–3. Abduction of the vocal folds.

laryngeal area: 11 are involved in opening the vocal folds for breathing and 6 are involved in producing **phonation** (sound).

When we adduct our vocal folds, we cause pulmonic air to build up beneath the folds. The diaphragm drives the pulmonic airstream, blowing the vocal folds apart and increasing the velocity of the airstream as it blows through the narrow space between the vocal folds. The air pressure in the trachea decreases as the velocity increases, and the decreased air pressure serves to pull the folds together, closing them—an aerodynamic effect known as the **Bernoulli principle**. This open-close vibratory cycle is repeated over a hundred times a second as the vocal folds are blown apart and then brought back together because of the elasticity of the muscles and the Bernoulli principle. Vibrating vocal folds produce air pressure waves that we perceive as sound. When the vocal folds vibrate during the articulation of speech sounds, the phenomenon is called voicing. Sounds produced when the vocal folds are vibrating are called **voiced**, and when the vocal folds are abducted and not vibrating, the sounds are called **voiceless**. Approximately 60% of American English consonants, such as "v," are voiced, as are all the vowels. The other 40% of the consonants, such as "f," are voiceless, that is, produced when the vocal folds are not vibrating.

Practice producing voiced and voiceless sounds now. To begin, prolong saying an "h" sound for several seconds. Be certain not to say "h" plus a vowel sound, as in "haaaaaa," but instead, say "hhhhhhh" without a vowel sound. When you say a prolonged "h" sound, you are holding your vocal folds in a slightly adducted position, which lets the air from your lungs pass through the small space created by the open vocal folds. Next, lightly place the four fingertips of one hand vertically on your larynx and say "hhhhhhhh" again. Did you feel anything on the surface of your larynx? Contrast that feeling to the one you have when you prolong saying the "ee" vowel sound (as in *bee*) while your fingertips lightly touch your larynx. With your fingers still on your larynx, alternate saying "hhhhhhhh" and "eeeeeeee," as in "hhhhh/eeeee/hhhhh/eeeee." What did you feel in the throat region this time? You should have felt a slight vibration of the laryngeal cartilages during the productions of "eeeeeeee," the vibrations created because the vocal folds were adducted while air passed over their lateral edges. Those vibrations are what we call voicing. Another way to help you discern voicing is to gently push on the flap of cartilage (called the **tragus**) situated in front of your ear canal, which will serve to block sound from entering your ear canal. While plugging your ears this way, say "hhhhhhhh" and "eeeeeeee." You should be able to hear the difference in voicing quite easily.

Resonatory Process

The human vocal tract is approximately 17 cm long in adult biological males and approximately 15 cm long in adult biological females. Think of the vocal tract as an air-filled tube that can be subdivided into a series of smaller chambers of dynamically changing lengths during speech production; for example, when we pucker our lips, we make the oral tube longer. When the vocal folds vibrate, the resulting bursts of air set the molecules in the air-filled pharyngeal, oral, and nasal tubes into acoustic vibration. Each tube serves as a resonating chamber to amplify and dampen particular vibrations, permitting listeners to differentiate one sound from another. When a speech sound is voiceless, that is, produced without the vocal folds vibrating, acoustic vibrations are created when air flowing from the lungs moves through the constricted space where the sound is created during the articulatory process, which we will discuss below. We will discuss the resonatory process in much more detail in Chapter 3, because we find it easiest to explain in the context of vowel production.

Oro-Nasal Process

The airflow travels from the laryngeal region up into the pharynx, where it can move into the oral and/or nasal cavities. The direction of the airflow is dependent on a membranous structure called the **velum**, or the soft palate. The velum is directly behind the hard palate, on the roof of your mouth. Unlike the hard palate, the velum consists of soft tissue only, including muscle fibers covered by mucous membrane. At the posterior portion of the velum is a piece of tissue called the uvula, which hangs down the back of the throat. Using a flashlight, look in a mirror to identify your velum and uvula. When the muscles of the velum are in a relaxed state, the velum is lowered, permitting air flowing up from the lungs to enter the nasal cavity. If you are breathing quietly through your nose as you silently read this sentence, then your velum is in a relaxed state now. The velum in this lowered position is illustrated in Figure 2–4. When the velum is in a raised position, it touches the back and side walls of the pharynx, blocking air from entering the nasal cavity, as illustrated in Figure 2–5. When the muscles of the velum are contracted, we cannot breathe through our nose,

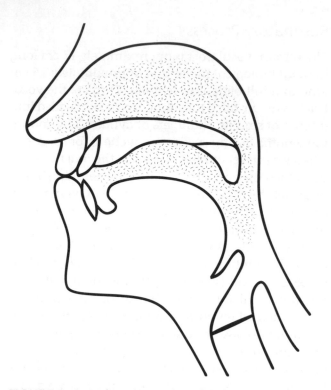

FIGURE 2–4. Velum in a relaxed state with air flowing into nasal cavity.

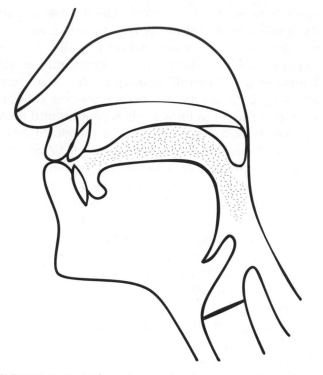

FIGURE 2–5. Velum in a raised state with airflow blocked from entering nasal cavity.

instead, we must breathe through our mouth. We articulate most speech sounds with the velum in a raised position, which causes the sound to come through our mouth. We lower the velum to produce a small set of three speech sounds in American English, which permits the sound pressure waves to flow into the nasal cavity.

If we speak entire words and sentences with our velum relaxed, then too much air will flow into our nasal cavity. Too much nasal airflow results in what we call **hypernasal** speech. Alternatively, if not enough air flows into our nasal cavity, such as when we raise our velum or when we have a cold and our oral and pharyngeal tissues are swollen, blocking airflow and sound waves from entering the nasal cavity, we characterize the speech as **hyponasal**. These two terms often are used incorrectly; as a student of phonetics, you want to understand both terms. To have too much nasal sound quality results in hypernasal, or nasal, speech. To have too little nasal sound quality results in hyponasal, or denasal, speech. Take a moment to practice producing exaggerated hypernasal and hyponasal speech.

First, say the sentence, *Buy Bobby a puppy*, with your velum lowered; your speech should sound hypernasal. Practice saying the sentence several times, each time with increased nasality. Now say the sentence, *Mama made some lemon jam*, while holding your velum in a raised position; your speech should sound as though you have a bad head cold. With practice, you will be able to feel the slight muscle movements involved in raising and lowering your velum on command.

Articulatory Process

The articulatory system refers to the structures used to produce speech sounds. Humans use a variety of anatomical structures in the vocal tract to produce speech sounds, some of them actively, others passively. The structures include our lips, upper teeth, various parts of the tongue, upper **alveolar ridge** (the bony ridge behind the upper incisors), hard palate, velum, uvula, pharynx, **epiglottis** (the cartilage that protects our airway), and vocal folds. You will want to become familiar with these speech structures, as illustrated in Figure 2–6. Note that we have illustrated the vocal folds in the figure as vibrating, therefore creating phonation.

Looking at the anatomical speech structures, take a moment to try to think of at least one speech sound that is made using each structure. If you cannot think of a sound that you make using a particular anatomical part, it may be because English does not have speech sounds that use that structure. As we will see in Chapter 9, different languages have different speech sounds, and we produce those sounds by using different structures in the vocal tract.

One of the most used structures for speech is the tongue. The tongue is a muscular organ involved in the production of most speech sounds. Eight different muscles make up the tongue. Four of these muscles originate and insert into the tongue itself (called the intrinsic muscles), and four tongue muscles insert into the tongue but originate at bone (called the extrinsic muscles). Two-thirds of the tongue is visible in the oral cavity when you open your mouth wide, but one-third of the tongue is not visible because it courses back and down into the pharynx. We produce different speech sounds using different areas of the entire tongue, so for phonetics purposes, we name these different areas. As shown in Figure 2–7, anteriorly to posteriorly the areas include the tongue tip (also called the apex), blade, front, back, and root. We also can refer to the tongue body, which consists of the front and back of the tongue.

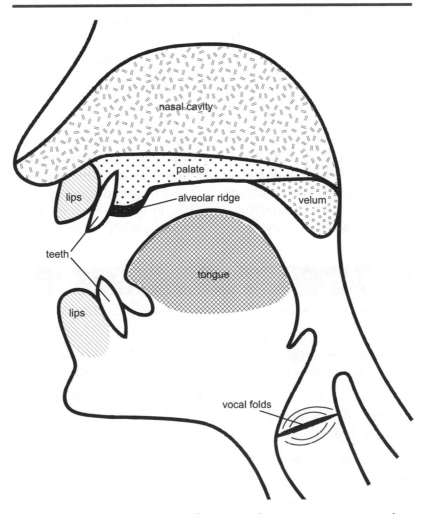

FIGURE 2–6. Sagittal view of the vocal tract structures used to produce speech.

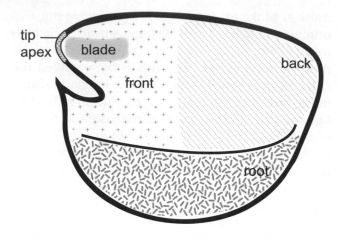

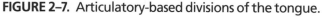

FIGURE 2–7. Articulatory-based divisions of the tongue.

Sonorant and Obstruent Sounds

We articulate some consonant and vowel sounds using a primarily open vocal tract. We call these sounds **sonorants**. Pressure waves travel through the vocal tract largely unobstructed, creating a nonturbulent, continuous airflow. Examples of sonorants include consonant sounds such as "m," "w," and "l," and all the vowel sounds. When airflow is impeded completely but temporarily, creating a moment of silence, or impeded partially, creating turbulence, we produce consonant sounds called **obstruents**. Obstruents are created when we obstruct airflow during the articulation of some consonants, such as "p," "z," and "ch."

Cognates

Two consonant sounds are called **cognates** when they are articulated in the same place and in the same manner, but one is voiceless and the other is voiced. The consonant sound "p" is made with the vocal folds held apart, therefore not vibrating, so "p" is a voiceless sound. Say a string of "p" sounds, "p p p p p"—but not "papapapapa"— while your fingertips are lightly touching your larynx; you should feel no laryngeal vibration. Next, can you think of a sound that is articulated similarly to "p," but with voicing? Try to articulate a "p" sound while your voice is turned on. The sound you make should be "b." These two sounds, "p" and "b," are articulated in the same place and manner; however, "p" is a voiceless consonant and "b" is a voiced consonant. Because "p" and "b" differ only on voicing, they are a pair of consonant cognates.

Let's try to identify one more pair of cognates. Begin by saying the voiced sound "g." Can you figure out its cognate—a similarly produced sound that is voiceless? Yes, it is the sound "k." The sounds "k" and "g" are cognates. It is important to know that not all sounds have a cognate. For example, the voiceless sound "h" does not have a voiced cognate. When we list a pair of cognates, it is conventional to list the voiceless sound first, followed by its voiced counterpart. So, for example, when we list the cognate pair "k" and "g," we list it as "k, g," and when we list the cognate pair "p" and "b," we list it as "p, b."

?   **2–2. Did You Get It?**

1. Airflow that originates in the lungs is called _____ air.

2. All speech sounds in American English are produced on an inhaled/exhaled airstream.

3. We _____ the vocal folds so they vibrate and produce sound.

4. We _____ the vocal folds to keep them from vibrating.

5. When the velum is in a raised position, where can air flow?

6. When the velum is in a lowered position, where can air flow?

7. In what position is the velum when we are breathing quietly through our nose?

8. Name a word that begins with a sound produced using each of the following anatomical structures.

   both lips   _____

   tongue tip or blade   _____

   upper teeth   _____

   hard palate   _____

? 2–3. Did You Get It?

Circle the correct word and name the cognate of the following sounds to complete each sentence.

1. The voiceless/voiced cognate of the "t" sound is _____.

2. The voiceless/voiced cognate of the "v" sound is _____.

Consonant Place Classes in American English

Place of articulation is used to classify consonants based on where in the vocal tract they are articulated and which anatomical structures are used to articulate them. Speakers of English articulate consonants using a variety of different vocal tract structures. The structures include the upper and lower lips, upper teeth, various regions of the tongue, upper alveolar ridge, post-alveolar ridge, hard palate, velum, and vocal folds.

In American English, there are nine place-of-articulation classifications for consonants. The nine place categories include **bilabial** (both lips), **labiodental** (upper teeth on lower lip), **interdental** (tongue tip or blade through upper and lower teeth), **alveolar** (tongue tip or blade on or near upper bony ridge that is just behind the upper teeth), **post-alveolar** (tongue blade immediately behind the alveolar ridge, near the front of the hard palate), **alveopalatal** (tongue tip or blade movement starts at the alveolar ridge, ends with tongue front at the hard palate), **palatal** (front of tongue near the hard palate), **velar** (back of tongue on soft palate), and **glottal** (space between abducted vocal folds). A summary of the pairings of structures and places of articulation can be found in Table 2–1. As we have already discussed, some of the consonants that are articulated at each place are classified as voiceless sounds, while others are classified as voiced.

Bilabial

Consonants produced using the upper and lower lips are called bilabials. There are four bilabial phonemes in American English, including one cognate pair. One bilabial phoneme is "p," as in the word *pay*. The sound "p" is produced by momentarily closing

TABLE 2–1. Descriptions of Place Classes for Consonants in American English

Place of Articulation	Description
Bilabial	Upper and lower lips involved
Labiodental	Upper incisors resting on the lower lip
Interdental	Tongue tip or blade lightly touching the upper teeth and protruding slightly through the upper and lower incisors
Alveolar	Tongue tip or blade on or near the upper gum (alveolar) ridge
Post-alveolar	Tongue blade just behind the alveolar ridge, near the front of the hard palate
Alveopalatal	Beginning with the tongue tip or blade at the alveolar ridge, ending with tongue front near the hard palate. This is the only place category that describes articulator movement.
Palatal	Front of the tongue near the hard palate
Velar	Back of the tongue near the soft palate
Glottal	Vocal folds involved

the lips and then quickly opening them. While the lips are closed, air pressure builds up behind the lips in the mouth because the velum is raised, blocking air from entering the nasal cavity. When the lips are quickly opened, the built-up air bursts outward through the lips. It is that burst of air that creates the "p" sound. There is no simultaneous vocal fold vibration occurring, so "p" is classified as a voiceless bilabial sound. The phonetic symbol for the phoneme "p" is /p/. Articulation of [p] is illustrated in Figure 2–8. Its cognate is the phoneme "b," as in the word *bay*, symbolized as /b/. [b] is articulated in the same way as [p], except that [b] is produced with the vocal folds vibrating, as shown in Figure 2–9.

Another sound produced using both lips is the sound "m," as in *may*. The sound "m" is produced in the same way that [b] is produced, with both lips momentarily closed while the vocal folds are vibrating; however, the velum is lowered during the articulation of "m," causing the air to flow through the nasal cavity and out of the nostrils instead of through the lips. Articulation of "m" is shown in Figure 2–10. The symbol for this voiced bilabial phoneme is /m/.

The fourth consonant produced using both lips is the sound "w," as in the word *way*. This sound is articulated by protruding the lips slightly and then opening them using a circular gliding motion while the vocal folds are vibrating, as seen in Figure 2–11. If you produce a string of "w" sounds, you look like you're imitating fish lips. The symbol for this voiced bilabial phoneme is /w/.

We would like you to be aware, though, that the articulation of [w] is a little more complicated than

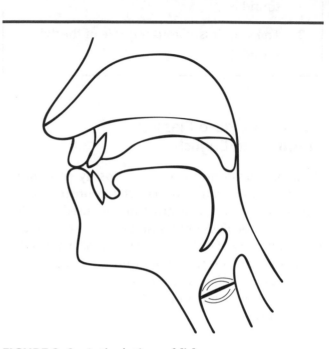

FIGURE 2–9. Articulation of [b].

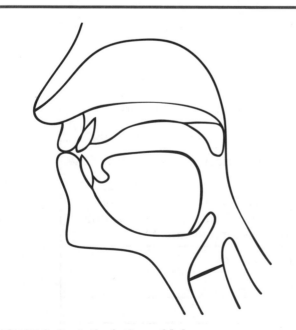

FIGURE 2–8. Articulation of [p].

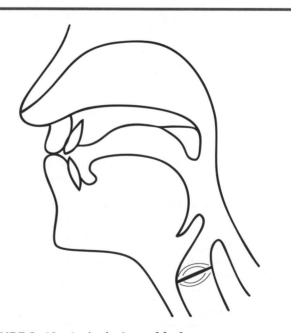

FIGURE 2–10. Articulation of [m].

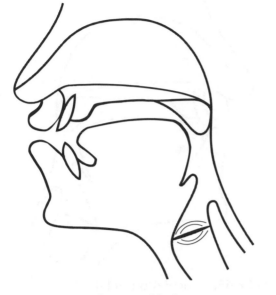

FIGURE 2–11. Articulation of [w].

only moving the lips. Producing [w] also involves raising the back of the tongue. Technically, /w/ is classified as a labiovelar consonant, because its production involves both places of articulation. It is important that you realize that the back of the tongue is involved in the correct articulation of [w], because the raised tongue posture affects how [w] sounds. However, typically developing children, as well as children with speech sound disorders and individuals learning English as a second language, rarely have difficulty acquiring correct production of [w]. But even if individuals do misarticulate [w], they can be taught to produce [w] correctly by teaching only the movement of the lips. Therefore, for practical applications in speech-language pathology, we will classify /w/ as a labial consonant throughout this book.

? 2–4. Did You Get It?

1. Name a word that has /p/ in medial position.

2. Name a word that has /b/ in final position.

3. Name a word that has /m/ in both initial and medial positions.

4. Name a word that has /w/ in initial position.

Labiodental

There are two consonants in American English produced with the upper incisors resting lightly on the lower lip while blowing air through the space created by this articulation. To produce these two sounds, a speaker raises the lower lip to the upper incisors. Can you guess which sounds we're describing? One sound is "f," as in the word *fan*, and the other is "v," as in *van*. One of these sounds is voiceless and the other is voiced; therefore, the two sounds are cognates, as illustrated in Figures 2–12 and 2–13. Try prolonging "ffffffff" and then prolonging "vvvvvvvv." Next, try saying "ffffffff/vvvvvvvv/ffffffff." Can you tell which consonant sound is voiceless and which is voiced? If you remember to lightly place your fingertips on your larynx while articulating both sounds, you will feel laryngeal vibrations only during production of the sound "v" because "f" is voiceless and "v" is its voiced cognate. The phonetic symbols match their orthographic spellings: /f/ and /v/.

? 2–5. Did You Get It?

1. Name a word that has /f/ in medial position.

2. Name a word that has /v/ in final position.

Interdental

There are two consonants in American English produced with the tip of the tongue protruding slightly between the upper and lower incisors. The two sounds are spelled the same orthographically as "th"; however, one "th" sound is voiceless and the other is voiced, as shown in Figures 2–14 and 2–15. The voiceless "th" is in the words *think*, *thumb*, and *thirty*, and its phonetic symbol is /θ/ (Greek letter theta). The voiced "th" cognate is in the words *they*, *that*, *the*, and *those*, and its phonetic symbol is /ð/ (Latin letter ethe). Practice saying both versions of the interdentals by varying voicing while articulating [θθθθθθθθθðððððððððθθθθθθθθθ]. To hear the difference in voicing between these two sounds, say the words *thigh* and *thy*. The "th" in *thigh* is the voiceless interdental consonant, and the "th" in *thy* is the voiced interdental consonant. The voiceless cognate, /θ/, occurs in **content words**, such as nouns, verbs,

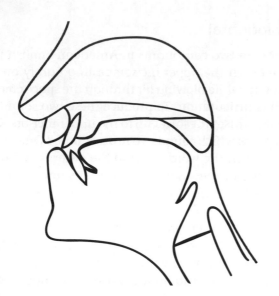

FIGURE 2–12. Articulation of [f].

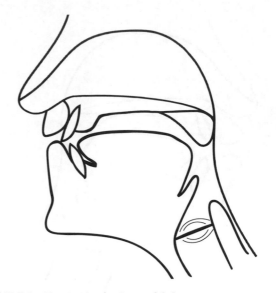

FIGURE 2–13. Articulation of [v].

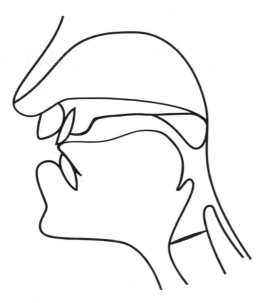

FIGURE 2–14. Articulation of [θ].

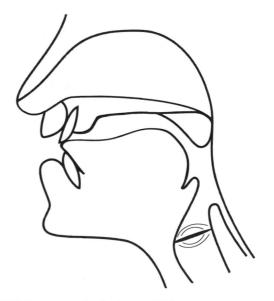

FIGURE 2–15. Articulation of [ð].

adjectives, and adverbs; whereas /ð/ occurs in **function words**, such as determiners, prepositions, and pronouns.

Students learning phonetics often have difficulty differentiating between /θ/ and /ð/ in words. One way to help you hear which version of "th" is in a word is to say the word two times, once with [θ] and once with [ð]. It tends to be easy to pick out the correct version as soon as you hear both words spoken aloud, but this strategy won't work unless you teach yourself to use it. This strategy can help you differentiate voicing between any pair of cognates, so make a habit of employing it. To help you remember these non-Latin alphabet phonetic symbols, see Figure 2–16 for a mnemonic of *th*umbnail for /θ/ and Figure 2–17 of fea*th*er for /ð/.

? 2–6. Did You Get It?

1. Name a word that has /θ/ in final position.

2. Name a word that has /ð/ in medial position.

Alveolar

There are more consonant sounds articulated on or near the upper alveolar ridge than any other ana-tomical structure. In American English there are six alveolar phonemes, including two pairs of cognates. The first cognate pair includes the "t" and "d" sounds, as in *too* and *do*, respectively. To produce these two consonants, you raise your tongue tip or blade to the alveolar ridge and then quickly lower it while pushing out air, as shown in Figures 2–18 and 2–19. The "t" sound is voiceless, so when you say the "t" sound, be certain to say only the consonant—do not add a vowel to it. The phonetic symbol is /t/. The voiced "d" sound is written with the phonetic symbol /d/.

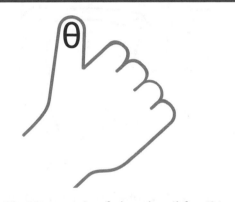

FIGURE 2–16. Mnemonic of *th*umbnail for /θ/.

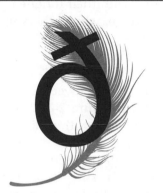

FIGURE 2–17. Mnemonic of fea*th*er for /ð/.

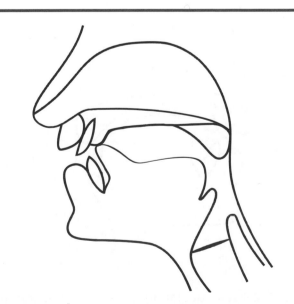

FIGURE 2–18. Articulation of [t].

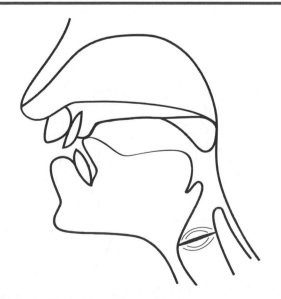

FIGURE 2–19. Articulation of [d].

Another sound produced by raising your tongue tip or blade to the alveolar ridge is "n," as in *new*, shown in Figure 2–20. Place your fingertips lightly on your larynx while you prolong "nnnnnnnn." Hopefully you can feel the vibration of the vocal folds. The sound "n" is a voiced alveolar phoneme and its phonetic symbol is /n/.

The second cognate pair produced at the alveolar ridge is "s" and "z," as in the words *sue* and *zoo*, respectively. The sound "s" is voiceless and "z" is voiced. These two sounds match their orthographic representations: /s/ and /z/. Unlike the articulation of [t], [d], and [n], [s] and [z] are produced by moving the front of the tongue close to, but not touching, the alveolar ridge. Interestingly, some people articulate these two sounds with their tongue tip raised to the upper alveolar ridge, while others use more of the tongue blade. There also are individuals who lower their tongue tip to articulate [s] and [z]. These three methods are shown in Figures 2–21, 2–22, and 2–23 for articulation of [s]. An alveolar tongue placement for [z] is shown in Figure 2–24. Speech-language pathologists who work with individuals who have difficulty producing "s" and "z" sounds teach these sounds by trying all three methods. One method likely will garner more success for an individual, but speech-language pathologists won't know which approach will work best until they experiment by trying all three. Try now to determine which method you use by slowly articulating [s] and [z], paying close attention to which part of the tongue you use and whether it moves up or down in your mouth. You also can try producing [s] and [z] using all three articulator positions; one should feel more natural to you.

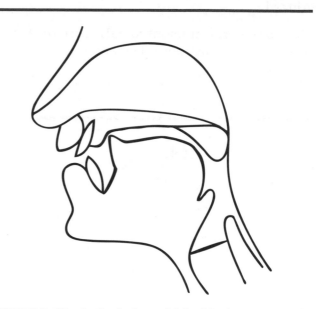

FIGURE 2–21. Articulation of [s] with the tongue tip approximating the upper alveolar ridge.

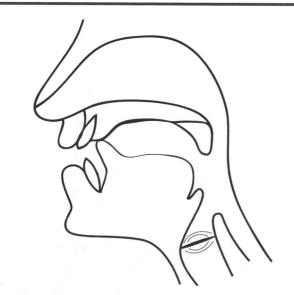

FIGURE 2–20. Articulation of [n].

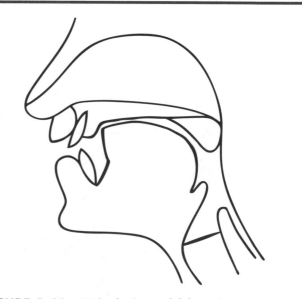

FIGURE 2–22. Articulation of [s] with the tongue blade approximating the upper alveolar ridge.

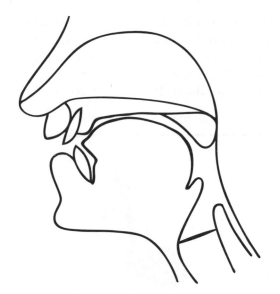

FIGURE 2–23. Articulation of [s] with the tongue tip lowered.

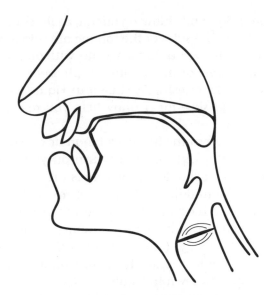

FIGURE 2–24. Articulation of [z] with the tongue tip approximating the upper alveolar ridge.

The consonant sound "l," as in the (British) word *loo*, also is an alveolar production. Say a prolonged "lllllllll" and feel the vocal fold vibration with your fingertips on your larynx. That's because "l" is a voiced alveolar phoneme; it is represented as /l/. The phone [l] is a unique consonant production because it is the only sound in American English that has air flowing over the sides of the tongue during its production. A two-dimensional diagram of the alveolar production of [l] is shown in Figure 2–25.

?	**2–7. Did You Get It?**

1. Name a word that has /t/ in final position.

2. Name a word that has /d/ in final position.

3. Name a word that has /n/ in medial position.

4. Name a word that has /s/ in final position.

5. Name a word that has /z/ in initial position.

6. Name a word that has /l/ in medial position.

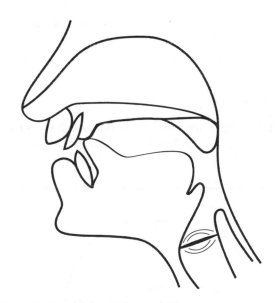

FIGURE 2–25. Articulation of [l].

Post-Alveolar

There is one pair of post-alveolar cognates. The voiceless sound in the pair is symbolized orthographically as "sh," as in *shoe*. This is the sound we make while holding one index finger in front of our lips to quiet children. The "sh" is articulated by holding the blade of the tongue close to the back of the alveolar ridge while blowing out air, as illustrated in Figure 2–26. The sides of the tongue are raised from the area post-alveolar to the palate, with air flowing over the middle of the tongue. Its phonetic symbol is /ʃ/ (Latin letter esh). As shown in Figure 2–27, a mnemonic of *sh*oe for /ʃ/ may help you remember this symbol.

To try to determine the voiced cognate of esh, prolong saying [ʃʃʃʃʃʃʃʃ] and then turn on your voice. The sound you should be making is the consonant sound in the middle of the word *mea̱sure*. See Figure 2–28 for a diagram of this sound's articulation. This voiced post-alveolar phoneme, symbolized phonetically as /ʒ/ (Latin letter ezh), occurs only rarely in American English. Its mnemonic is measuring cup, as shown in Figure 2–29.

?	2–8. Did You Get It?

1. Name a word that has /ʃ/ in final position.

2. Name a word that has /ʒ/ in medial position.

Alveopalatal

There are two alveopalatal cognates. We produce both alveopalatals by starting with the tongue tip

or blade at the alveolar ridge and ending with the tongue front at the hard palate. We spell the voiceless alveopalatal consonant orthographically as "ch," as in the words *cheese* and *choose*. Its phonetic symbol is the **digraph** /t͡ʃ/. A digraph is a pair of

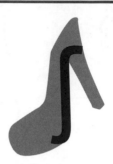

FIGURE 2–27. Mnemonic of *sh*oe for /ʃ/.

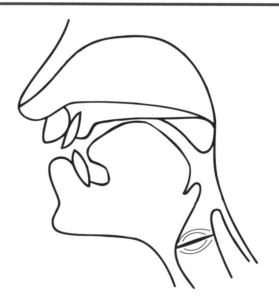

FIGURE 2–28. Articulation of [ʒ].

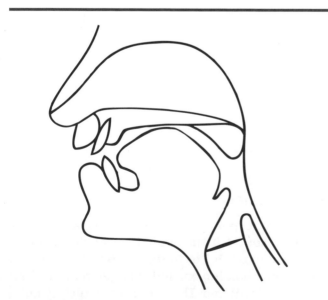

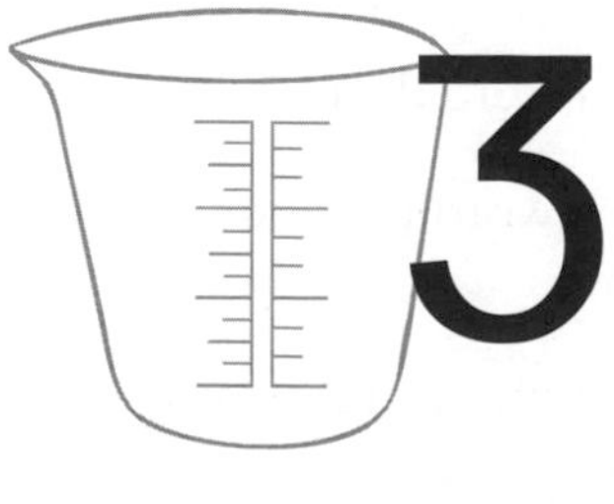

FIGURE 2–26. Articulation of [ʃ].

FIGURE 2–29. Mnemonic of measuring cup for /ʒ/.

symbols used to represent a single sound. We place a ligature, [͡], above /tʃ/ to indicate the combination of movements, as in [t͡ʃ]. The ligature also is called a **tie bar**. You can see the articulatory placement of [t͡ʃ] illustrated in Figure 2–30. We produce the cognate of [t͡ʃ] by adding voicing to our gestures, as shown in Figure 2–31. The resulting articulation is the sound we spell orthographically as "j" in the initial consonants in the words *jewelry* and *jury*. Its phonetic symbol is the digraph /d͡ʒ/.

To help you remember these two non-Latin alphabet phonetic symbols, see Figure 2–32 for a mnemonic of *ch*ime for /t͡ʃ/ and Figure 2–33 of *jug*gler for /d͡ʒ/.

<table>
<tr><td>?</td><td>2–9. Did You Get It?</td></tr>
</table>

1. Name a word that has /t͡ʃ/ in medial position.

2. Name a word that has /d͡ʒ/ in initial position.

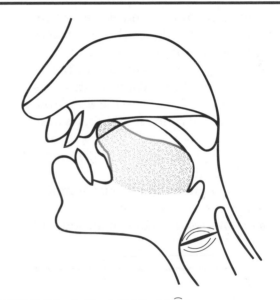

FIGURE 2–30. Articulation of [t͡ʃ].

FIGURE 2–31. Articulation of [d͡ʒ].

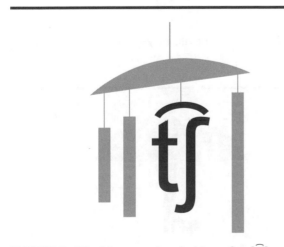

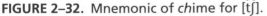

FIGURE 2–32. Mnemonic of *ch*ime for [t͡ʃ].

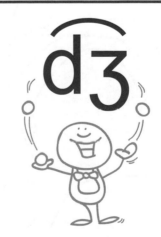

FIGURE 2–33. Mnemonic of *jug*gler for /d͡ʒ/.

Palatal

There are two sounds produced with the front of the tongue positioned close to the hard palate; these sounds are called palatals. One palatal consonant is the sound symbolized by the alphabet letter "y," as in *you*. You make it by raising the front of the tongue near, but not touching, the hard palate. The phonetic symbol for the consonant phoneme in the word *you* is /j/. So as not to be confused, try to remember that there is no "y" phonetic symbol in American English. Articulation of [j] is shown in Figure 2–34. To help you remember that /j/ phonetically represents the "y" sound in the alphabet, see the mnemonic of *yarn* in Figure 2–35.

The other palatal sound is the consonant "r" sound, as in the word *rue*. This is a voiced palatal sound symbolized phonetically by an upside down "r": /ɹ/. To help you remember that the "r" is written upside down phonetically, see the mnemonic of umbrella in Figure 2–36. This is a tricky sound—and not only because its phonetic symbol is upside down. The articulation of [ɹ] can vary by speaker and by dialect, making it misleading to designate one specific place of articulation.

The most common way consonantal [ɹ] is produced by speakers of American English is with the tongue tip lowered, the body of the tongue bunched inside the mouth and raised toward the hard palate, and the root of the tongue retracted in the pharynx; therefore, we will classify [ɹ] as a palatal production. This posture is called the **bunched-r**, as illustrated in Figure 2–37. The anterior and posterior tongue constrictions serve to create three cavities in the vocal tract, and you also can see that the lips are rounded slightly.

Another way that [ɹ] can be produced is by raising the tip of the tongue toward the alveolar ridge, while the back of the tongue is raised slightly toward the hard palate and the root of the tongue is retracted into the pharynx, as illustrated in Figure 2–38. This production of [ɹ] often is classified as post-alveolar. A third way to produce [ɹ] is by using a specific tongue gesture described as **retroflex-r**. A retroflex tongue gesture is when the tip of the tongue is curled up and back toward the alveolar ridge, as shown in Figure 2–39.

Many children acquiring speech have difficulty producing [ɹ], as do speakers learning English as a second language if /ɹ/ is not a phoneme in their first

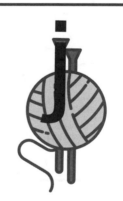

FIGURE 2–35. Mnemonic of *yarn* for /j/.

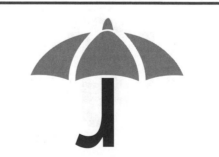

FIGURE 2–36. Mnemonic of umbrella for /ɹ/.

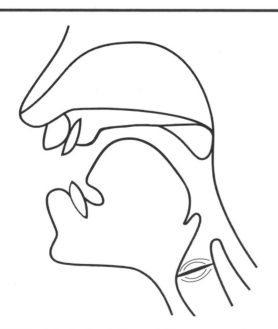

FIGURE 2–34. Articulation of [j].

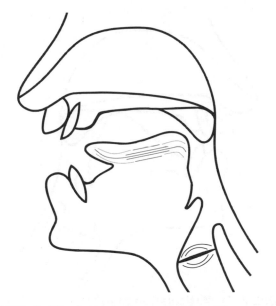

FIGURE 2–37. Articulation of [ɹ] with a palatal bunched tongue.

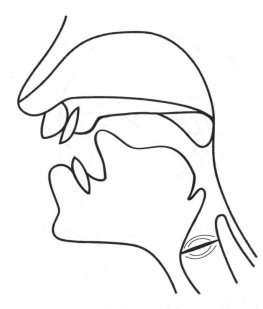

FIGURE 2–38. Articulation of [ɹ] as a post-alveolar consonant.

language. Given that [ɹ] is a difficult sound to learn to produce, it will help you clinically to be able to model these different productions so that you can help your clients discover which articulation is easiest for them to learn. Take some time now to figure out which type of production you use to articulate [ɹ] and practice producing the other types as well.

?	**2–10. Did You Get It?**

1. Name a word that has /j/ in initial position.

2. Name a word that has /ɹ/ in initial position.

Velar

There are three velar consonants in American English, including two cognates. We produce all three velar consonants by raising the back of the tongue to the velum, the soft palate. The velum is the place of articulation for the three velar consonants, and the tongue is the articulator as it raises to touch the velum. The velar cognates include the sounds we spell orthographically as "k," as in the word *kill*, and the sound we spell as "g," as in *gill*. We produce

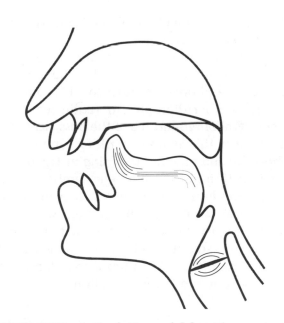

FIGURE 2–39. Articulation of [ɹ] with a retroflex tongue.

"k" without vocal fold vibration, making it voiceless, and "g" with vocal fold vibration, making it the voiced cognate. Both "k" and "g" are oral sounds; therefore, they are produced with the velum in a raised position. To see an illustration of the articulation of "k" and "g," refer to Figures 2–40 and 2–41.

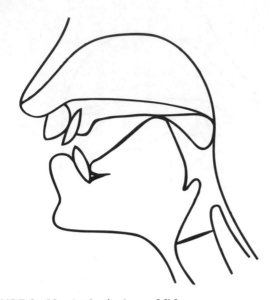

FIGURE 2–40. Articulation of [k].

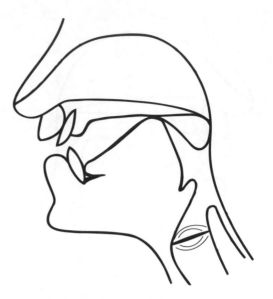

FIGURE 2–41. Articulation of [g]

Both sounds are symbolized phonetically using their Latin symbols: /k/ and /g/.

The other velar consonant is the voiced sound "ng," the single sound at the end of the words *ring* and *sing*. The phonetic symbol for this consonant sound is another digraph: /ŋ/ (Latin letter eng). The eng symbol reminds us of the bass clef (F clef). To remember this symbol think of a music note, as shown in the mnemonic of si*ng* in Figure 2–42. You might think of the phonetic symbol /ŋ/ as a written combination of the letter "n" with the tail of a "g." Like we produce [k] and [g], we produce [ŋ] by raising the back of our tongue to the velum and then releasing it, as illustrated in Figure 2–43. Unlike /k/ and /g/, /ŋ/ is a nasal sound, produced with our velum in a lowered position.

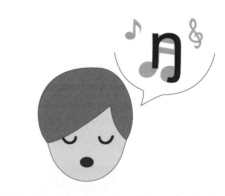

FIGURE 2–42. Mnemonic of si*ng* for /ŋ/.

?	2–11. Did You Get It?

1. Name a word that has /k/ in medial position.

2. Name a word that has /g/ in initial position.

3. Name a word that has /ŋ/ in final position.

Glottal

The most posterior place of articulation for consonant sounds is the glottis. Remember that the glottis is the space created when the vocal folds are not fully closed during speech. We produce one consonant sound at the glottis, the voiceless sound "h," as in the word *hi*. Its phonetic symbol is the Latin letter /h/. When we produce the phoneme [h], we adduct the vocal folds slightly and air passes through their lateral edges, as shown in Figure 2–44.

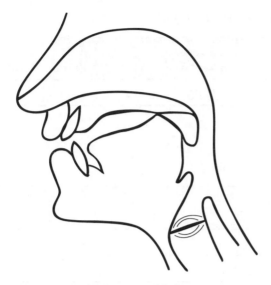

FIGURE 2–43. Articulation of [ŋ].

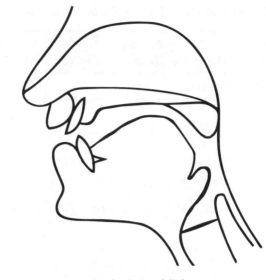

FIGURE 2–44. Articulation of [h].

? 2-12. Did You Get It?

1. Name a word that has /h/ in initial position.

2. Name a word that has /h/ in medial position.

Summary of Articulatory Place

There are 24 consonants in American English, and we produce them at nine different places in the vocal tract. When listing the nine places, it is conventional to begin with the most anterior place (i.e., bilabial) and work posteriorly (i.e., glottal). Table 2–2 provides a summary of the nine places of articulation and the consonants associated with each place for American English consonants.

Now that we have introduced the phonetic symbols for all 24 consonant phonemes in English, we urge you to start paying very close attention to how speech sounds *sound* in words; otherwise, you will be fooled into thinking alphabetically instead of phonetically. When you pay attention to alphabetic spellings, your phonetic transcriptions will be inaccurate. Try hard to remember that the ortho-graphic spelling of all the sounds are variable, and that what matters in phonetics is the actual sound that is made, not the alphabet letter used to represent it. For each given phone, the phonetic symbol always remains the same. Don't be fooled by multiple orthographic spellings of sounds. To see a sampling of the many different ways each speech sound can be spelled orthographically, refer to Table 2–3.

Consonant Manner Classes in American English

While articulatory place refers to *where* sounds are produced, articulatory manner refers to groupings of sounds based on *how* they are produced. Take for example the alveolar consonants /t/ and /s/. We can tell these two sounds apart from one another, even though both consonants are produced with the tongue tip (or blade) on or near the alveolar ridge. We produce [t] using one quick motion that results in a single burst of air, and we produce [s] by holding our tongue close to, but not touching, the alveolar ridge, while blowing out air. The result is that the [t] sound is composed of a short silence followed by a little burst of air, while [s] is a steady flow of turbulent air. Classifying sounds by manner class gives us another way to understand consonant articulation.

TABLE 2–2. Phonetic Chart of Place Classes for Consonants in American English

Place	Bilabial	Labio-dental	Inter-dental	Alveolar	Post-Alveolar	Alveo-palatal	Palatal	Velar	Glottal
Phone	p b m w	f v	θ ð	t d n s z l	ʃ ʒ	t͡ʃ d͡ʒ	j ɹ	k g ŋ	h

TABLE 2–3. Phonetic Symbols and Some Associated Alphabetic Spellings

Phonetic Symbol	Alphabetic Spellings and Examples in Words
p	p: *pen* pp: ha*pp*y gh: hiccou*gh*
b	b: *b*ox bb: bo*bb*er
t	t: *t*oe tt: a*tt*ack tw: *tw*o th: *th*yme d: ice*d*
d	d: *d*ad dd: da*dd*y dh: *dh*arma
k	k: *k*ite c: *c*at cc: a*cc*ount ch: a*ch*e ck: che*ck* q: *q*uay
g	g: *g*o gh: *gh*ost gg: ha*gg*ard
m	m: *m*agic mm: to*mm*y mb: la*mb* mn: hy*mn*
n	n: *n*o nn: bu*nn*y kn: *kn*ee mn: *mn*emonic gn: *gn*ome pn: *pn*eumonia
ŋ	ng: thi*ng* n: thi*n*k
w	w: *w*ay wh: *wh*ale u: pers*u*ade null: one
j	y: *y*es j: halleluja*h* ll: torti*ll*a null: use
f	f: *f*ull ph: *ph*oto ff: o*ff* gh: lau*gh* wh: *wh*ew pph: sa*pph*ire
v	v: *v*eer vv: sa*vv*y ph: Ste*ph*en f: o*f*
θ	th: *th*eater tth: Ma*tth*ew
ð	th: smoo*th* the: soo*the*
s	s: *s*een sc: *sc*ene c: *c*ity ss: me*ss*y cc: fla*cc*id ps: *ps*ychic sw: *sw*ord
z	z: *z*uiz s: i*s* zz: pizza*zz* ss: di*ss*olve x: *x*ylophone
ʃ	sh: ca*sh* ch: ca*ch*e s: *s*ugar c: o*c*ean t: ra*t*ion ss: ti*ss*ue
ʒ	z: sei*z*ure s: plea*s*ure t: equa*t*ion g: re*g*ime ge: bei*ge*
h	h: *h*ave wh: *wh*o j: *j*alapeño
t͡ʃ	ch: *ch*ick c: *c*ello cz: *Cz*ech tch: ma*tch* t: na*t*ure
d͡ʒ	j: *j*ury g: *g*erm dg: le*dg*e dj: a*dj*ective
l	l: *l*oose ll: ba*ll*et sl: ai*sl*e cl: mus*cl*e
ɹ	r: *r*oom rr: a*rr*ive wr: *wr*ong rh: *rh*yme

42

Several different manner class categorization systems exist in phonetics. We will categorize consonants in American English using six manner classes based on two factors: (1) how each consonant is articulated and (2) how each consonant is acquired by young children. Some types of consonants require only ballistic-type movements; others require more articulatory precision and finesse. The consonants that require less articulatory precision tend to be mastered by typically developing children at younger ages. For practical applications in speech-language pathology and audiology, it is helpful to learn which sounds are mastered earlier and which are mastered later by children, in addition to understanding how (and where) each consonant is articulated. The six manner classes include **stops**, **nasals**, **glides**, **fricatives**, **affricates**, and **liquids**. Generally speaking, the first three manner classes—stops, nasals, and glides—can be considered earlier-mastered sounds; whereas fricatives, affricates, and liquids can be considered later-mastered sounds. As you read about the manner classes for consonants, keep in mind that the information pertains specifically to consonants in American English, including how they are produced, as well as how they are used in words. A brief description of each of the manner classes can be found in Table 2–4.

Stops

The terms used to describe this manner class of consonants convey the way in which these sounds are produced. To produce a stop consonant, you use two articulators to temporarily, but completely, block the air flowing up from your lungs before releasing the obstruction. There are two types of stops: oral stops and nasal stops. Oral stops have air flowing through the oral cavity, while nasal stops have air flowing through the nasal cavity. As is common convention, we will use the term "stops" to refer exclusively to the oral stops. We will use the term "nasals" to refer exclusively to the nasal stops.

There are six stop phonemes in American English: /p, b, t, d, k, g/. When you produce these sounds, your velum is in a raised position, and for some of the phonemes, your vocal folds also will be vibrating. When you release the obstruction, air bursts from the mouth, making the actual consonant sound. Because of this burst of air, stops also can be called *plosives*. Before reading this information, did you know that you created bursts of air when producing certain sounds? Well, you can feel the bursts of air you create when you articulate stops. Let's try it. Begin by holding your fingertips from one hand

TABLE 2–4. Descriptions of Manner Classes for Consonants in American English

Manner Class	Description
Stops	Consonant sounds produced by two articulators touching and temporarily stopping airflow while the velum is raised, resulting in a sudden release of air that travels through the mouth
Nasals	Consonant sounds produced by two articulators touching and temporarily stopping airflow while the velum is lowered, so air travels through the nose
Glides	Consonant sounds produced with minimal friction by the smooth movement of the articulators
Fricatives	Consonant sounds produced by the partial obstruction of airflow by two articulators closely approximating one another to create turbulence
Affricates	Consonant sounds produced by rapidly sequencing a stop and a fricative produced in the same place
Liquids	Consonant sounds produced with minimal friction by the smooth movement of the articulators; variable types and places of articulation

in front of your mouth. Say the voiceless sound [p] a few times—you should be able to feel little bursts of air after each production. The air bursts through the mouth because your velum was raised, directing the air into your oral cavity. Now say the voiced sound [b] a few times—you still should be able to feel bursts of air after each production. However, the strength of the bursts between [p] and [b] should feel differently on your fingers. Do they feel differently to you? How so? Yes, the burst for [p] is stronger than the burst for [b]. And did you know that you also can *see* the difference in the strength of the bursts? Well, you can! To see the difference, loosely hold an edge of a piece of lightweight paper or a tissue up to your lips while articulating [p] and [b]. You will see the paper wave or bend from the bursts.

Try the same experiment articulating the phones [t], [d], [k], and [g]; be certain to try to feel *and* see the bursts for each of these stop consonants. Two of these phones have a stronger burst than the other two. Which ones had the stronger bursts? Yes, [t] and [k] productions had the stronger bursts. Can you identify the pattern for which consonants have stronger bursts and which have weaker bursts? The burst, or plosion, for the voiceless phones [p, t, k] is stronger than for the voiced stop consonants [b, d, g]. In addition, you now also have discovered that the stop manner class contains three pairs of cognates, /p, b/, /t, d/, and /k, g/, and that /p, t, k/ are voiceless and /b, d, g/ are voiced.

The actual obstruction of the airflow for the stop consonants is created by structures related to place of articulation. The stops /p, b/ are created by the lips blocking airflow; these phonemes are called bilabial stop consonants. The stop /p/ is described fully as a voiceless bilabial stop and /b/ is described as a voiced bilabial stop. The stops /t, d/ are created by the tongue placed on the alveolar ridge to temporarily stop the airflow; these phonemes are called alveolar stop consonants. The stops /k, g/ are created by the back of the tongue touching the velum to tem-porarily stop the airflow; these phonemes are called velar stop consonants. All six of these phonemes can occur in word-initial, -medial, and -final positions in American English. For example, the voiceless alveolar stop /t/ occurs in the words *toe, hotel,* and *oat,* and the voiced velar stop /g/ occurs in the words *go, ago,* and *log.* In addition to being represented alphabetically by the letter "k," /k/ also is represented alphabetically by the letter "c," called the "hard c sound," as in the words *cape* and *macaroni.*

Table 2–5 shows the six stop consonants organized by place and manner of articulation. Note also that the voicing feature is displayed in the chart by same-place consonants listed in voiceless-voiced pairs. As we proceed through this chapter, we will expand this chart by adding new consonants to it after each manner class is discussed.

? 2–13. Did You Get It?

1. Why are stop consonants called stops?

2. Why are oral stop consonants sometimes called plosives?

3. When you articulate the six stops, in what position is the velum?

4. Which stops are produced using the lips to temporarily block oral airflow?

5. Which articulator temporarily blocks oral airflow when producing /t/ and /d/?

6. Which articulator temporarily blocks oral airflow when producing /k/ and /g/?

7. Write the phonetic symbol for the voiced bilabial stop consonant.

8. Name a word that contains an initial-position voiced alveolar stop consonant.

9. Name a word that contains a medial-position voiceless velar stop consonant.

TABLE 2–5. Phonetic Chart of Place, Manner, and Voicing of Stop Consonants

Manner/ Place	Bilabial	Labio-dental	Inter-dental	Alveolar	Post-Alveolar	Alveo-palatal	Palatal	Velar	Glottal
Stops	p **b**			t **d**				k **g**	

Note. Voiced consonants are in bold.

Nasals

There are three nasal stop phonemes in American English, which we call nasals: /m, n, ŋ/. In contrast to the three nasal consonants, the other 21 consonants are called oral consonant phonemes. To produce the nasal consonants, you use one active articulator to temporarily block airflow from escaping out of your mouth while you keep your velum in a lowered position and your vocal folds vibrating, creating voicing. Your velum being lowered results in air flowing through the nasal cavity, as well as in the oral cavity. Here are two ways to help you hear that nasal resonance and see that nasal airflow. First, begin by prolonging the nasal consonant /m/, as in "mmmmmmmm." Place one finger on one side of your nose and push that nostril closed while you continue saying "mmmmmmmm"; you can hear and feel the nasal vibrations. One way to help you see the nasal airflow is to place a small mirror or a pen made of shiny metal under your nostrils while you say "mmmmmmmm." Quickly remove the mirror and you should see fogging on its surface, created by the warm air leaving your nostrils and hitting the cooler surface. You can practice doing this for all three nasal consonants. The nasals are the only consonants produced in American English with the velum lowered, resulting in nasal airflow. Consequently, sound resonates in the nasal cavity for the nasals.

The nasal [m] is shaped by bringing the lips together; this phoneme is classified as a bilabial nasal consonant. The nasal [n] is shaped by placing the tongue tip or blade on the alveolar ridge; this phoneme is classified as an alveolar nasal consonant. The nasal phone [ŋ] is shaped by the back of the tongue touching the velum; this phoneme is classified as a velar nasal consonant. Because all three of the nasals are voiced, it is unnecessary to include voicing as a descriptor. In American English, only two of these phonemes can occur in word-initial, -medial, and -final positions: /m/ and /n/. For example, the bilabial nasal /m/ occurs in the words *magic*, *image*, and *gym*, and the alveolar nasal /n/ occurs in the words *no*, *running*, and *loan*. The velar nasal /ŋ/ occurs only in word-medial and -final positions, as in *hanger* and *hang*. Refer to Table 2–6 to see the three nasal consonants added to our chart of consonant place, manner, and voicing.

? 2–14. Did You Get It?

1. Why are nasal consonants called nasals?

2. In what position is the velum during the articulation of the nasals?

3. Which nasal is shaped using the lips?

4. Which articulator shapes the resonance of /n/?

5. Which articulator shapes the resonance of /ŋ/?

6. Write the phonetic symbol for the velar nasal consonant.

7. Name a word that contains an initial-position bilabial nasal consonant.

8. Name a word that contains a medial-position alveolar nasal consonant.

9. Name a word that contains a final-position velar nasal consonant.

TABLE 2–6. Phonetic Chart of Place, Manner, and Voicing of Stop and Nasal Consonants

Manner/ Place	Bilabial	Labio-dental	Inter-dental	Alveolar	Post-Alveolar	Alveo-palatal	Palatal	Velar	Glottal
Stops	p **b**			t **d**				k **g**	
Nasals	**m**			**n**				**ŋ**	

Note. Voiced consonants are in bold.

Glides

There are two glide phonemes in American English: /w, j/. Like the two previous manner classes, the term "glide consonant" describes how speech sounds are produced. To produce a glide consonant, you move the articulators in a smooth gliding motion. Both glides in American English are voiced, so your vocal folds are vibrating during their articulation, and your velum is raised, directing airflow through your mouth.

The glide phone [w] is produced by rounding your upper and lower lips slightly and then opening your lips smoothly, while keeping the tongue body raised high in the back of your mouth. The /w/ phoneme is called the voiced bilabial glide consonant. You articulate the glide [j] by situating your tongue high and flat in your mouth, toward the hard palate. /j/ is called the voiced palatal glide consonant phoneme. Glides /w/ and /j/ sometimes are referred to as **onglides** because they occur only before vowels, leaving some phoneticians to consider them to be part of the vowels they precede and not separate consonants. Glides never occur before a consonant or in word-final position. Because they occur only before vowels, glides are found only in word-initial and -medial positions. For example, /w/ occurs in words such as *way* and *away*, and /j/ occurs in words such as *yak* and *kayak*.

You might sometimes hear a word ending in [w] or [j], especially if you say words very slowly—like you do when you are first learning to transcribe phonetically. Words ending with certain vowels may sound as though they end in one of the glide consonants. For [w] sounds, those vowels include the long "u" sound (as in *boo*) and the long "o" sound (as in *so*). If you exaggerate and use citation speech to articulate a word that ends in one of those vowel sounds, the final articulation can sound like the glide phone [w]; however, that gliding sound is part of the vowel and not a separate consonant. For example, say the word "boo" using citation-form speech. If you said it slowly enough, it could have sounded like "boo + w(uh)." For the glide [j], those vowels include the long "e" sound (as in *bee*) and the long "a" sound (as in *bait*). To hear this example, say the word "bee" slowly, and it might sound like "bee + y(uh)." Again, that final sound is part of the vowel and not a separate consonant. We will explain this phenomenon in detail when we discuss vowels in Chapter 3, and again in Chapter 8 when we discuss vowel variations.

Our chart of consonant place, manner, and voicing has now been expanded to include the two glides. Refer to Table 2–7 to see these categorizations of stops, nasals, and glides.

? 2–15. Did You Get It?

1. Why are glide consonants called glides?

2. In what position is the velum during the articulation of the glide consonants?

3. Which articulators are used to produce /w/?

4. Which articulator is used to produce /j/?

5. Write the alphabetic letter that often is used to represent /j/.

6. In which word position do /w/ and /j/ never occur?

7. Name a word that contains the initial-position bilabial glide consonant.

8. Name a word that contains the medial-position palatal glide consonant.

TABLE 2–7. Phonetic Chart of Place, Manner, and Voicing of Stop, Nasal, and Glide Consonants

Manner/ Place	Bilabial	Labio-dental	Inter-dental	Alveolar	Post-Alveolar	Alveo-palatal	Palatal	Velar	Glottal
Stops	p **b**			t **d**				k **g**	
Nasals	**m**			**n**				**ŋ**	
Glides	**w**						**j**		

Note. Voiced consonants are in bold.

Fricatives

There are nine fricative consonant phonemes in American English: /f, v, θ, ð, s, z, ʃ, ʒ, h/. To produce a fricative consonant, you position an articulator near an oral structure, so it is partially obstructing the air flowing up from your lungs. This partial obstruction creates a turbulent airstream that sounds like hissing. If you prolong saying the fricatives "sssssssss" and "zzzzzzzz" you will hear that hissing-like sound. When producing all the fricative consonants, your velum is in a raised position, and for some of the fricatives, your vocal folds also will be vibrating. There are four pairs of fricative cognates: /f, v/, /θ, ð/, /s, z/, and /ʃ, ʒ/; /h/ is voiceless and the only unpaired fricative. Four of the fricatives create a louder and more turbulent sound, called sibilance, than the other fricatives. These four sounds are called **sibilants**. Produce each fricative aloud to see if you can determine which four are the louder and more turbulent sibilants. Yes, the sibilants include [s, z, ʃ, ʒ].

The partial obstruction of airflow for the fricatives is created by structures related to place of articulation. The phonemes /f, v/ are called labiodental fricatives and are created by the lower lip and upper teeth partially obstructing airflow. The fricative /f/ is described fully as a voiceless labiodental fricative and /v/ is described as a voiced labiodental fricative. The fricative phones [θ, ð] are created by the tongue tip protruding slightly through the upper and lower teeth to partially obstruct airflow. The phonemes /θ, ð/ are called interdental fricatives. The fricative phones [s, z] are created most commonly by placing the tongue tip or blade close to the alveolar ridge to partially obstruct airflow; these phonemes are called alveolar fricatives. Remember also that some individuals produce the alveolar fricatives with the tongue tip lowered. The fricative phones [ʃ, ʒ] are created by raising the blade of the tongue toward the posterior portion of the alveolar ridge to partially obstruct airflow; these phonemes are called post-alveolar fricatives. There is a secondary articulation that involves the lips for production of the fricatives [ʃ, ʒ]. Take a moment to say [ʃ, ʒ], paying close attention to any movement of your lips. What did you feel? When producing [ʃ, ʒ], the lips typically are rounded. In American English, seven of these eight fricatives occur in word-initial, -medial, and -final positions. For example, the voiceless labiodental fricative /f/ occurs in the words *foot*, *awful*, and *hoof*, and the voiced labiodental fricative /v/ occurs in the words *very*, *heavy*, and *move*. The voiced post-alveolar fricative /ʒ/ occurs only very rarely in word-initial position in loanwords, and infrequently in word-medial and -final positions.

The last fricative phoneme in American English is /h/. You articulate this voiceless fricative by abducting and then pushing air through the vocal folds. You also hold the velum in a raised position so that the air flows out through your opened mouth. Say a prolonged "hhhhhhhh" sound. Practice periodically stopping the airflow by adducting your vocal folds and then opening them again. The phoneme /h/ occurs in word-initial position in words such as *how* and *half*, and in word-medial position in words such as *anyhow* and *behalf*, but does not occur in word-final position. To see the chart of consonant place, manner, and voicing expanded to include fricatives, refer to Table 2–8.

TABLE 2–8. Phonetic Chart of Place, Manner, and Voicing of Stop, Nasal, Glide, and Fricative Consonants

Manner/ Place	Bilabial	Labio- dental	Inter- dental	Alveolar	Post- Alveolar	Alveo- palatal	Palatal	Velar	Glottal
Stops	p **b**			t **d**				k **g**	
Nasals	**m**			**n**				**ŋ**	
Glides	**w**						**j**		
Fricatives		f **v**	θ **ð**	s **z**	ʃ **ʒ**				h

Note. Voiced consonants are in bold.

? 2–16. Did You Get It?

1. When you articulate the nine fricatives, in what position is the velum?

2. Which fricatives are produced using the lower lip touching the upper teeth?

3. Which fricatives are produced using the tongue tip between the upper and lower teeth?

4. Which fricatives are produced using the tongue tip or blade near the alveolar ridge?

5. Which fricatives are produced using the front of the tongue near the hard palate?

6. Write the phonetic symbols for the voiceless and voiced labiodental fricative consonants.

7. Name a word that contains a final-position voiceless alveolar fricative consonant.

8. Name a word that contains a medial-position voiced post-alveolar fricative consonant.

9. Name a word that contains a final-position voiceless interdental fricative consonant.

10. Name a word that ends in one of the sibilant fricatives.

Affricates

There are two affricate cognates: /t͡ʃ, d͡ʒ/. We produce the affricates by rapidly articulating a combination of articulatory gestures that result in a single consonant sound. The voiceless affricate [t͡ʃ] is articulated by producing a stop-like sound at the alveolar ridge before immediately moving the tongue to produce a palatal fricative. Try to articulate the phone [t͡ʃ] slowly, so you can feel its movement sequence. Begin by articulating a [t]-like sound and slowly move your tongue into producing a [ʃ]-like sound, which should result in the articulation of [t͡ʃ]. You can produce the cognate phone [d͡ʒ] by adding voicing. Even though there are two places of articulation for the phones [t͡ʃ, d͡ʒ], they are articulated rapidly, so they result in a single sound. The rapid articulation is captured by using the ligature, [͡], above the symbols. In American English, /t͡ʃ/ and /d͡ʒ/ can occur in word-initial, -medial, and -final positions, as in *chick*, *itching*, and *itch* for /t͡ʃ/, and as in *germ*, *major*, and *urge* for /d͡ʒ/. We now add affricates to our chart of consonants categorized by place, manner, and voicing, as displayed in Table 2–9.

Liquids

Consonant sounds that are produced with minimal friction by smoothly moving articulators are called liquids. There are two liquid phonemes in American

TABLE 2–9. Phonetic Chart of Place, Manner, and Voicing of Stop, Nasal, Glide, Fricative, and Affricate Consonants

Manner/ Place	Bilabial	Labio-dental	Inter-dental	Alveolar	Post-Alveolar	Alveo-palatal	Palatal	Velar	Glottal
Stops	p **b**			t **d**				k **g**	
Nasals	**m**			**n**				**ŋ**	
Glides	**w**						**j**		
Fricatives		f **v**	θ **ð**	s **z**	ʃ **ʒ**				h
Affricates						t͡ʃ **d͡ʒ**			

Note. Voiced consonants are in bold.

English: /l, ɹ/. Both [l] and [ɹ] can be produced using various articulatory gestures secondary to phonetic context and/or individual speaker differences. There are two ways to produce the liquid phone [l] depending on phonetic context. When /l/ occurs in syllable-initial position, you articulate it by parting your lips slightly and raising the tip and blade of your tongue to the alveolar ridge, keeping the back of the tongue lowered so air flows around one or both sides of the tongue. You also raise your velum and phonate throughout the production. Holding your tongue tip on the alveolar ridge while producing [l] results in air being blocked from flowing centrally. Instead, the air flows over the sides, the lateral portions, of the tongue. For this reason, /l/ is classified as the alveolar **lateral** liquid consonant. To feel the air flowing laterally, position your tongue for an [l] production and slowly inhale air, feeling the air flowing over the sides of your tongue. To heighten the sensation, it may help if you suck on a mint or an ice cube prior to trying this tactile experiment. The only lateral phoneme in American English is /l/. In contrast to the lateral /l/, the other 23 consonants in American English are called **central** consonants. When /l/ occurs in syllable-initial position, it is in **prevocalic** position, as in the words *let* and *loose*. This articulation is called clear-l or light-l, and its production is as described above, with the tongue tip and blade on the alveolar ridge.

However, when a vowel precedes /l/ in the same syllable, it is in **postvocalic** position, as in the words *bull* and *mall*. A postvocalic [l] phone is produced with the tongue tip lowered and the tongue body raised toward the hard and soft palates, with air flowing over the lateral portions of the tongue. Production of a postvocalic [l] is called dark-l or velarized-l. In American English, roughly half of all [l] productions are prevocalic and the other half are postvocalic.

Experiment now to determine which allophones of [l] you produce, particularly in postvocalic position. Say the words *Lee*, *low*, and *law*, paying attention to the placement of your tongue during articulation. Most people use an alveolar tongue placement, resulting in light-l productions. Did your productions follow this pattern? Now say the words *eel*, *old*, and *awl*. Was your tongue in the same place for the postvocalic [l] productions as it was in the prevocalic positions in the first set of words?

Most people produce a dark-l in postvocalic position. Last, say the multisyllabic words *ballot*, *silly*, and *allergy* using a casual register. Where was your tongue when you articulated the [l] phones? In multisyllabic words with word-medial /l/ phonemes, the lateral consonant can be ambisyllabic, that is, produced across both syllables, resulting in some individuals producing a dark-l, even though the vowel and lateral consonant are in different syllables. We will talk more about dark-l in Chapter 7, including when and how it is used in American English. It is important clinically for you to understand these articulatory variations of [l], so that you can model and teach them to individuals who are enrolled in intervention to address speech sound errors or dialect differences that they want to change.

The other liquid consonant phoneme is /ɹ/. While consonant /ɹ/ occurs frequently in American English, as in the words *run* and *rich*, it is rare in other languages. It is difficult to capture the place of articulation for the liquid consonant [ɹ] because of the three different ways it can be produced: (1) with the tongue tip down, the tongue body bunched below the hard palate, and the tongue root retracted; (2) with the tongue tip raised toward the alveolar ridge and the tongue root retracted; and (3) with the tongue tip curled up and back toward the alveolar ridge in a retroflex position. In all three productions, the lips are slightly rounded. Because [ɹ] is voiced, the vocal folds vibrate during its articulation, and air flows orally because the velum is raised. We will categorize /ɹ/ as a voiced palatal liquid.

Adding to the complexity of this consonant, there are two forms of /ɹ/: the consonant form and the vowel form. Both forms are called **rhotics**. We classify prevocalic /ɹ/, that is, /ɹ/ + vowel in the same syllable, as a rhotic consonant phoneme. Alternatively, when /ɹ/ occurs in postvocalic position in the same syllable, that is, vowel + /ɹ/, as in the words *her* and *star*, the vowel + /ɹ/ forms a rhotic vowel phoneme. For example, we would specify the word *her* as having a phonotactic structure of CV: /h/ + rhotic vowel. Likewise, we would specify the word *star* as having a structure of CCV: /st/ + rhotic vowel. You will learn more about rhotic vowels in Chapter 3.

Is vowel + /ɹ/ ever *not* in the same syllable, resulting in a consonant [ɹ] production? This situation arises in compound words, as well as in other multisyllabic words, so you need to listen carefully to be able to differentiate the two forms of rhotics. Consider the compound word *showroom*. *Showroom* is a two-syllable word that has five phones: [ʃ], long "o," [ɹ], long "u," and [m], with a phonotactic structure of CV.CVC. The long vowel sound "o" is in the first syllable, whereas /ɹ/ begins the second syllable. Therefore, /ɹ/ functions as a consonant in the word *showroom*. The disyllabic word *around* also has one consonant /ɹ/ phoneme, with /ɹ/ initiating in the second syllable. When /ɹ/ is in medial position in some words, however, it can be ambisyllabic, resulting in the production of a rhotic consonant and a rhotic vowel, as in the word *earring*. In *earring*, you can hear a rhotic vowel in the first syllable, with the second syllable beginning with a consonant rhotic.

Let us consider one final example, the word *square-root*, to help you differentiate the consonant and vowel rhotic phonemes. There are two rhotics in the compound word *square-root*. Take a moment to identify each /ɹ/, then try to determine if each rhotic functions as a vowel or a consonant. The phonotactic structure of *square-root* is CCCV.CVC. In *square-root*, /ɹ/ in the first syllable is a rhotic vowel and /ɹ/ in the second syllable is a rhotic consonant. In American English, the consonant /ɹ/ occurs primarily in words in initial position (e.g., *run*, *rich*), occasionally in words in medial position (e.g., *showroom*, *shrink-wrap*, *square-root*), and never in final position (in which cases we always consider it to be a rhotic vowel, as in *her* and *star*). In Chapter 3, we will explain rhotic vowels in more detail.

We now are finished categorizing all 24 consonants in American English by manner class, and have categorized each consonant by manner class in Table 2–10. Note that there are six stops, three nasals, two glides, nine fricatives, two affricates, and two liquids in American English.

There is one other superordinate manner classification. Liquid and glide consonants share some articulatory similarities, namely that their articulatory places vary based on the phonotactic structures of the other segments in the words containing them.

For this reason, and a few others, such as how they pattern similarly in words, glides and liquids also can be grouped phonetically into a single, superordinate manner class called **approximants**. For sounds in American English, the approximant manner class includes the consonant phonemes /w, j, l, ɹ/. However, for clinical reasons we find it helpful to separate these four sounds into the two separate manner classes we have presented: glides and liquids. Whereas it is common for children and individuals learning English as a second language to have difficulty learning how to produce liquids, it is rare to have someone misarticulate glides.

This completes our categorization of consonants by not only manner class, but also by place and voicing. For a comprehensive summary of place, manner, and voicing for the 24 consonants in American English, see Table 2–11.

? | 2–17. Did You Get It?

1. In what position is the velum during the articulation of the liquids?

2. Explain why /l/ is called a lateral sound.

3. Name a word that contains the initial-position palatal liquid consonant.

4. Name a word that contains the initial-position lateral alveolar liquid consonant.

5. Name a word that contains a light-l.

6. Name a word that contains a dark-l.

7. Write the alphabetic letter that is used to represent /ɹ/.

8. Explain one of the three ways American English speakers articulate /ɹ/.

9. List the four consonant sounds that make up the approximant manner class.

TABLE 2–10. Phonetic Chart of Manner Classes for Consonants in American English

Manner	Stops	Nasals	Glides	Fricatives	Affricates	Liquids
Phoneme	p b t d k g	m n ŋ	w j	f v θ ð s z ʃ ʒ h	t͡ʃ d͡ʒ	l ɹ

TABLE 2–11. Phonetic Chart of Place, Manner, and Voicing of Stop, Nasal, Glide, Fricative, Affricate, and Liquid Consonants

Manner/ Place	Bilabial	Labio-dental	Inter-dental	Alveolar	Post-Alveolar	Alveo-palatal	Palatal	Velar	Glottal
Stops	p **b**			t **d**				k **g**	
Nasals	**m**			**n**				**ŋ**	
Glides	**w**						**j**		
Fricatives		f **v**	θ **ð**	s **z**	ʃ **ʒ**				h
Affricates						t͡ʃ **d͡ʒ**			
Liquids				**l**			**ɹ**		

Note. Voiced consonants are in bold.

Summary of Articulatory Manner

We have discussed the manner classes for the 24 consonants in American English. We presented six consonant manner classes, grouped as such because of how the sounds are made, as well as when they are mastered by children developing speech. For clinical purposes, it can be helpful to think of the manner classes as two *sets* of consonants: the first set containing the earlier-mastered stops, nasals, and glides, and the second set containing the later-mastered fricatives, affricates, and liquids.

Putting It All Together

We have reviewed the articulation of the 24 consonant sounds in American English, as well as provided you with their phonetic symbols. There are nine places of articulation, six manners of articulation, and two types of voicing.

Learning how to phonetically transcribe is part art and part science, requiring both knowledge and skills. We recommend that you begin your journey into phonetic transcription by learning the different phonetic consonant symbols and the sound each one represents, and in which word positions each sound occurs. As a study guide, we have provided examples of each phoneme in words in initial, medial, and final positions in Table 2–12.

It also is important that you learn how to type phonetic symbols into your documents. There are several different ways to accomplish this feat. One way is to download a phonetic keyboard; an easy Internet search will yield several options. If you use Microsoft Word, then you can insert the non-Latin alphabet phonetic symbols by clicking on the "Insert" tab, then opening the "Symbol" dropdown window. From that window, you can click on "More Symbols" to access a wide variety of fonts under the "Symbols" tab. One popular phonetic font for Word documents is called Lucida Sans Unicode. You can type in that font name to get the character map. Perhaps a faster way is to directly type in the "Character code" from "Unicode (hex)" of the symbol you want. Table 2–13 displays all the non-Latin character codes for consonants. Open a document, follow the directions above, and practice typing the consonants in phonetic font. With practice, it will become second nature to you.

In addition to understanding articulatory place, manner, and voicing of consonants, it is important that you understand that the consonants in each place and manner class vary across languages. There are several other places of articulation that we have not yet discussed but that are used by speakers of languages other than English. Likewise, there also are other manner classes of consonants produced at the various articulatory places. It's exciting to learn how speakers of other languages use the same mechanisms to articulate different phonemes. You will learn more about how speakers of other languages use articulatory place and manner classes to produce speech sounds in Chapter 9.

TABLE 2–12. Phones in Words

Phonetic Symbol	Word Initial	Word Medial	Word Final
p	*p*en	o*p*en	pe*p*
b	*b*ox	ho*bb*y	ro*b*
t	*t*oe	ho*t*el	oa*t*
d	*d*ab	bo*d*y	ba*d*
k	*k*ite	bi*k*er	hi*k*e
g	*g*o	a*g*o	fo*g*
m	*m*agic	i*m*age	gy*m*
n	*n*o	du*nn*o	loa*n*
ŋ	—	ha*ng*er	ha*ng*
w	*w*ay	a*w*ay	—
j	*y*ak	ka*y*ak	—
f	*f*ull	aw*f*ul	o*ff*
v	*v*eer	e*v*er	e*v*e
θ	*th*eater	a*th*lete	wrea*th*
ð	*th*ey	ba*th*ing	ba*th*e
s	*s*ame	me*ss*y	me*ss*
z	*z*oo	ka*z*oo	oo*z*e
ʃ	*sh*e	wi*sh*y	wa*sh*
ʒ	*g*enre	mea*s*ure	bei*g*e
h	*h*ave	be*h*ave	—
t͡ʃ	*ch*ick	it*ch*ing	it*ch*
d͡ʒ	*g*erm	ma*j*or	ur*g*e
l	*l*augh	fo*ll*y	fa*ll*
ɹ	*r*oom	show*r*oom	—

Note. — indicates that the phone does not occur in that word position in American English.

TABLE 2–13. Character Codes and Unicode Names for Non-English Alphabetic Consonant Symbols

Phonetic Symbol	Character Code	Unicode Name
ŋ	14b	Latin small letter eng
θ	3b8	Greek small letter theta
ð	0f0	Latin small letter ethe
ʃ	283	Latin small letter esh
ʒ	292	Latin small letter ezh
t͡ʃ	2a7 + 311	Latin small letter tesh digraph + Combining inverted breve
d͡ʒ	2a4 + 311	Latin small letter dezh digraph + Combining inverted breve
ɹ	279	Latin small letter turned r

Applied Science: Revisited

Summary

In this chapter, you learned how to think about consonant production and how to phonetically transcribe consonants in American English. Let's see how this information is used to solve the questions.

One Step at a Time

1. Phonetically transcribe each set of words, as below. Then compare your transcriptions with ours and see if you can detect a pattern.

   Set 1. Transcribe the consonant sound(s) at the *beginning* of each word.

kit	_____	–	cat	_____
kwanza	_____	–	quick	_____
young	_____	–	Jung	_____
shell	_____	–	charade	_____
sycamore	_____	–	psyche	_____
hope	_____	–	who	_____
fast	_____	–	phase	_____
note	_____	–	knot	_____
not	_____	–	gnat	_____

   Set 1. Compare your transcriptions with ours. See if you can detect a pattern.

kit	/k/	–	cat	/k/
kwanza	/k/	–	quick	/kw/
young	/j/	–	Jung	/j/

   (remember, no capitalization in the IPA)

shell	/ʃ/	–	charade	/ʃ/
sycamore	/s/	–	psyche	/s/
hope	/h/	–	who	/h/
fast	/f/	–	phase	/f/
note	/n/	–	knot	/n/
not	/n/	–	gnat	/n/

   Set 2. Transcribe the consonant sound(s) at the *end* of each word.

gym	_____	–	hymn	_____
box	_____	–	socks	_____
bus	_____	–	fuss	_____
moose	_____	–	juice	_____
rough	_____	–	huff	_____
until	_____	–	sill	_____
bet	_____	–	debt	_____
lift	_____	–	laughed	_____
beak	_____	–	back	_____

   Set 2. Compare your consonant transcriptions with ours. See if you can detect a pattern.

gym	/m/	–	hymn	/m/
box	/ks/	–	socks	/ks/
bus	/s/	–	fuss	/s/
moose	/s/	–	juice	/s/
rough	/f/	–	huff	/f/
until	/l/	–	sill	/l/
bet	/t/	–	debt	/t/
lift	/ft/	–	laughed	/ft/
beak	/k/	–	back	/k/

   Set 3. Transcribe the consonant sound(s) at the *beginning* of each word.

carrot	_____	–	cereal	_____
thigh	_____	–	thy	_____
chase	_____	–	chaos	_____
chair	_____	–	chic	_____
mutt	_____	–	muse	_____
suit	_____	–	suite	_____
few	_____	–	food	_____
gum	_____	–	gem	_____
scene	_____	–	scare	_____

Set 3. Compare your consonant transcriptions with ours. See if you can detect a pattern.

carrot	/k/	–	cereal	/s/
thigh	/θ/	–	thy	/ð/
chase	/t͡ʃ/	–	chaos	/k/
chair	/t͡ʃ/	–	chic	/ʃ/
mutt	/m/	–	muse	/mj/
suit	/s/	–	suite	/sw/
few	/fj/	–	food	/f/
gum	/g/	–	gem	/d͡ʒ/
scene	/s/	–	scare	/sk/

Set 4. Transcribe the consonant sound(s) at the *end* of each word.

axis	_____	–	axes	_____
gas	_____	–	Arkansas	_____
cough	_____	–	bough	_____
rage	_____	–	beige	_____
smooth	_____	–	booth	_____
braise	_____	–	base	_____
Texas	_____	–	taxes	_____
epoch	_____	–	poach	_____
aced	_____	–	phased	_____

Set 4. Compare your consonant transcriptions with ours. See if you can detect a pattern.

axis	/s/	–	axes	/z/
gas	/s/	–	Arkansas	No final consonant!
cough	/f/	–	bough	No final consonant!
rage	/d͡ʒ/	–	beige	/ʒ/
smooth	/ð/	–	booth	/θ/
braise	/z/	–	base	/s/
Texas	/s/	–	taxes	/z/

epoch	/k/	–	poach	/t͡ʃ/
based	/st/	–	phased	/zd/

2. What patterns did you see in the sounds and spellings in each set? How can you relate the patterns you discovered to phonetics?

Answer

1. Set 1: The words in each of these pairs begin with the same sound, but the orthographic letters representing those sounds are different.

2. Set 2: The words in each pair end with the same sound, but the orthographic letters representing those sounds are different.

3. Set 3: When we look at the orthographic spelling of the beginning of the words in each of these word pairs, we see that the spelling is the same, unlike in the first set. However, even though the spelling is the same, those sounds are pronounced differently.

4. Set 4: When we look at the orthographic spelling of the end of the words in each of these word pairs, we see that the spelling is the same, unlike in the second set. However, even though the spelling is the same, those sounds are pronounced differently.

Science Applied

By applying your new knowledge of consonant production, we hope that you see how beneficial phonetic transcription is for capturing precisely how we speak. Using phonetic symbols disambiguates pronunciation. Think how much easier it would have been to learn how to read, write, and spell using a symbol set that had a one-to-one correspondence to the sound each symbol represented.

Interest Piqued?

Recommended materials to further your understanding of topics covered in this chapter.

Print Resources

Edwards, H. T. (2003). *Applied phonetics* (3rd ed.). Clifton Park, NY: Delmar Learning.

Ladefoged, P., & Disner, S. F. (2012). Making English consonants. In *Vowels and consonants* (3rd ed.) (pp. 114–122). Malden, MA: Blackwell.

McLeod, S., & Singh, S. (2009). *Seeing speech: A quick guide to speech sounds*. San Diego, CA: Plural.

Online Resources

http://www.internationalphoneticsassociation.org

The official website of the International Phonetic Association has a wealth of information for students and professionals.

http://ipa.typeit.org

For access to an online phonetic symbols keyboard.

http://smu-facweb.smu.ca/~s0949176/sammy

To experiment with articulatory positions related to consonant production.

Macmillan Education Apps: Sounds

A useful app for the iPhone that provides the full IPA chart, including the ability to click on a sound and hear it played. Provides quizzes to test your knowledge of phonetic symbols.

http://soundsofspeech.uiowa.edu/anatomy.html

Anatomy and physiology of speech sound production.

https://www.youtube.com/watch?v=-m-gudHhLxc

Anatomy and physiology of speech sound production.

? Did You Get It?

ANSWER KEY

2–1.

1. Voicing results because the vocal folds are <u>vibrating</u>.

2. Place of articulation refers to <u>where</u> a sound is produced.

3. Manner of articulation refers to <u>how</u> a sound is produced.

2–2.

1. Airflow that originates in the lungs is called <u>pulmonic</u> air.

2. All speech sounds in American English are produced on an <u>exhaled</u> airstream.

3. We <u>adduct</u> the vocal folds so they vibrate and produce sound.

4. We <u>abduct</u> the vocal folds to keep them from vibrating.

5. When the velum is in a raised position, where can air flow? <u>through the mouth</u>

6. When the velum is in a lowered position, where can air flow? <u>through the nose</u>

7. In what position is the velum when we are breathing quietly through our nose? <u>lowered</u>

8. Name a word that begins with a sound produced using each of the following anatomical structures.

both lips	words beginning with /p, b, m, w/
tongue tip or blade	words beginning with /t, d, n, θ, ð, ʃ, t͡ʃ, d͡ʒ/
upper teeth	words beginning with /f, v, θ, ð/
hard palate	words beginning with /j, ɪ/

2–3.

Circle the correct word and name the cognate of the following sounds to complete each sentence.

1. The voiceless/<u>voiced</u> cognate of the "t" sound is <u>"d."</u>

2. The <u>voiceless</u>/voiced cognate of the "v" sound is <u>"f."</u>

2–4.

1. Name a word that has /p/ in medial position. <u>examples will vary; happy, puppy, soapy, etc.</u>

2. Name a word that has /b/ in final position. <u>examples will vary; tub, stab, bib, etc.</u>

3. Name a word that has /m/ in both initial and medial positions. <u>examples will vary; mommy, moment, monument, etc.</u>

4. Name a word that has /w/ in initial position. <u>examples will vary; way, which, wag, etc.</u>

2–5.

1. Name a word that has /f/ in medial position. <u>examples will vary; laughing, buffalo, traffic, etc.</u>

2. Name a word that has /v/ in final position. <u>examples will vary; have, live, save, etc.</u>

2–6.

1. Name a word that has /θ/ in final position. <u>examples will vary; bath, teeth, moth, etc.</u>

2. Name a word that has /ð/ in medial position. <u>examples will vary; together, bathing, mother, etc.</u>

2–7.

1. Name a word that has /t/ in final position. <u>examples will vary; hate, mitt, light, etc.</u>

2. Name a word that has /d/ in final position. <u>examples will vary; shade, bid, mud, etc.</u>

3. Name a word that has /n/ in medial position. <u>examples will vary; running, lioness, honey, etc.</u>

4. Name a word that has /s/ in final position. <u>examples will vary; miss, bus, loss, etc.</u>

5. Name a word that has /z/ in initial position. <u>examples will vary; zipper, zoo, zest, etc.</u>

6. Name a word that has /l/ in medial position. <u>examples will vary; silo, ruling, hilly, etc.</u>

2–8.

1. Name a word that has /ʃ/ in final position. <u>examples will vary; hush, cache, mesh, etc.</u>

2. Name a word that has /ʒ/ in medial position. <u>examples will vary; measure, fissure, treasure, etc.</u>

2–9.

1. Name a word that has /t͡ʃ/ in medial position. <u>examples will vary; achoo, teacher, matches, etc.</u>

2. Name a word that has /d͡ʒ/ in initial position. <u>examples will vary; jury, joust, gel, etc.</u>

2–10.

1. Name a word that has /j/ in initial position. <u>examples will vary; young, yelp, you, etc.</u>

2. Name a word that has /ɹ/ in initial position. <u>examples will vary; rang, rich, write, etc.</u>

2–11.

1. Name a word that has /k/ in medial position. <u>examples will vary; leaky, tracking, joker, etc.</u>

2. Name a word that has /g/ in initial position. <u>examples will vary; got, give, guppy, etc.</u>

3. Name a word that has /ŋ/ in final position. <u>examples will vary; rang, wing, tongue, etc.</u>

2–12.

1. Name a word that has /h/ in initial position. <u>examples will vary; hear, hold, height, etc.</u>

2. Name a word that has /h/ in medial position. <u>examples will vary; ahead, yahoo, ahoy, etc.</u>

2–13.

1. Why are stop consonants called stops? <u>because the airstream is temporarily stopped during the production</u>

2. Why are oral stop consonants sometimes called plosives? <u>because a burst of air often results from the production</u>

3. When you articulate the six stops, in what position is the velum? <u>raised</u>

4. Which stops are produced using the lips to temporarily block airflow before it exits through the mouth? <u>/p, b/</u>

5. Which articulator temporarily blocks oral airflow when producing /t/ and /d/? <u>tip or blade of the tongue (raises to touch the alveolar ridge)</u>

6. Which articulator temporarily blocks oral airflow when producing /k/ and /g/? <u>back of the tongue (raises to touch the velum)</u>

7. Write the phonetic symbol for the voiced bilabial stop consonant. <u>/b/</u>

8. Name a word that contains an initial-position voiced alveolar stop consonant. <u>words beginning with /d/, such as dog, don't, donut, etc.</u>

9. Name a word that contains a medial-position voiceless velar stop consonant. <u>words that have /k/ in the middle, such as turkey, peacock, lucky, etc.</u>

2–14.

1. Why are nasal consonants called nasals? <u>because air flows into the nasal cavity during production</u>

2. In what position is the velum during the articulation of the nasals? <u>lowered</u>

3. Which nasal is shaped using the lips? <u>/m/</u>

4. Which articulator shapes the resonance of /n/? <u>tongue tip or blade (raised to touch the alveolar ridge) while the velum is raised</u>

5. Which articulator shapes the resonance of /ŋ/? <u>back of tongue (raised to touch the raised velum)</u>

6. Write the phonetic symbol for the velar nasal consonant. /ŋ/

7. Name a word that contains an initial-position bilabial nasal consonant. words beginning with /m/

8. Name a word that contains a medial-position alveolar nasal consonant. words with /n/ in the middle

9. Name a word that contains a final-position velar nasal consonant. words ending with /ŋ/

2–15.

1. Why are glide consonants called glides? because the articulators move slowly, as though "gliding" during production

2. In what position is the velum during the articulation of the glide consonants? raised

3. Which articulators are used to produce /w/? lips (and tongue body)

4. Which articulator is used to produce /j/? front of tongue (near the hard palate)

5. Write the alphabetic letter that often is used to represent /j/. "y"

6. In which word position do /w/ and /j/ never occur? in word-final position

7. Name a word that contains the initial-position bilabial glide consonant. words beginning with /w/

8. Name a word that contains the medial-position palatal glide consonant. words with /j/ in the middle

2–16.

1. When you articulate the nine fricatives, in what position is the velum? raised

2. Which fricatives are produced using the lower lip touching the upper teeth? /f, v/

3. Which fricatives are produced using the tongue tip between the upper and lower teeth? /θ, ð/

4. Which fricatives are produced using the tongue tip or blade near the alveolar ridge? /s, z/

5. Which fricatives are produced using the front of the tongue near the hard palate? /j, ɹ/

6. Write the phonetic symbols for the voiceless and voiced labiodental fricative consonants. /f, v/

7. Name a word that contains a final-position voiceless alveolar fricative consonant. words ending in /s/

8. Name a word that contains a medial-position voiced post-alveolar fricative consonant. words with /ʒ/ in the middle

9. Name a word that contains a final-position voiceless interdental fricative consonant. words ending in /θ/

10. Name a word that ends in one of the sibilant fricatives. words ending in /s, z ʃ, ʒ/

2–17.

1. In what position is the velum during the articulation of the liquids? the liquids, /l, ɹ/ are oral sounds, so the velum is raised, blocking air from entering the nasal cavity

2. Explain why [l] is called a lateral sound. because the air flows over the sides—the lateral portions—of the tongue

3. Name a word that contains the initial-position palatal liquid consonant. <u>examples will vary; racket, race, ribbon, etc.</u>

4. Name a word that contains the initial-position lateral alveolar liquid consonant. <u>examples will vary; like, llama, loop, etc.</u>

5. Name a word that contains a light-l. <u>words with /l/ + vowel in the same syllable</u>

6. Name a word that contains a dark-l. <u>words with vowel + /l/ in the same syllable</u>

7. Write the alphabetic letter that is used to represent /ɹ/. <u>"r"</u>

8. Explain one of the three ways American English speakers articulate /ɹ/.

9. List the four consonant sounds that make up the approximant manner class. <u>/w, j, l, ɹ/</u>

3

ARTICULATORY PHONETICS OF VOWELS

Learning Objectives

By reading this chapter, you will learn the:

1. similarities and differences between consonant and vowel production

2. anatomical structures we use to produce vowel sounds

3. four categories used to classify vowels

4. distinctions between monophthong, diphthong, and triphthong vowels

5. phonetic transcription of English vowels

6. concept and types of rhotic vowels

Applied Science

In English, words with the same vowel sound are spelled a variety of ways. The following excerpt from the poem, "I Take It You Already Know" (author unknown), highlights some of the different and often confusing ways we spell vowel sounds in English:

> Beware of heard, a dreadful word
>
> That looks like beard and sounds like bird.
>
> And dead; it's said like bed, not bead.
>
> For goodness sake, don't call it deed!
>
> Watch out for meat and great and threat,
>
> (They rhyme with suite and straight and debt).

This stanza includes four English vowel sounds spelled more than one way. Can you find them?

1. Group the words by the four English vowel sounds they represent.
2. Can you think of other ways to spell those four vowel sounds?

Introduction to Vowels

There are many different **dialects** of English: over 40 spoken in the British Isles, over 30 in North America, 10 or more in Australasia, at least 10 in India, and many other dialects in Asia and Africa. Most of these dialects of English are largely identifiable because of subtle and large phonetic and phonological vowel differences.

This chapter focuses on vowels of the General American English (GAE) dialect. From this point forward we will primarily refer to GAE as English, noting in the text if we are referring to a dialect different from GAE. GAE is purported to be the dialect of American English spoken without geographic, ethnic, or socioeconomic influences. It is not actually true that GAE has no external influences. GAE has been heavily influenced by Midland American English, Western American English, and Standard Canadian English. This dialect is thought to have gained in popularity when individuals from non-coastal New England areas spread the dialect as they moved west. During the mid-twentieth century, GAE was the preferred dialect in the US and was commonly called "the broadcaster dialect." Many individuals who wanted to work in the media strived for the GAE dialect as they attempted to switch between or even lose the English of their home and community environments.

English Vowels: Sounds Versus Spelling

If you ask a 6-year-old (and many adults) how many vowels there are in English, you are likely to be told there are five or six: "a, e, i, o, u, and sometimes y." This answer refers to the alphabetic symbols used to *spell* English vowels—English orthography—but does not reflect the vowel *sounds* of English. As we saw with consonants and in the introduction to this chapter, English has many ways to write out different spoken vowel sounds, with the letters *a, e, i, o, u* as well as some consonant symbols used in a variety of written combinations. English vowel spelling gets even more complicated because we use two consonant symbols—the *y* in *yes* and the *w* in *win*—as part of vowels in words like *day* and *cow*. But there are many more vowel sounds in English than are represented by these letters, and English has some creative ways of spelling vowels. For example, the letter *o* can represent at least seven different vowel sounds, as in the words *not, so, tough, through, people, power,* and *leopard*. Another example is the *er* vowel sound spelled multiple ways in *sure, burr, sir, her, vigor,* and *altar*. And the spelling *ough* can represent many different vowel sounds; compare *dough, bough, through, cough, rough,* and *bought*.

While how we spell vowels in English can seem quite confusing, vowel phonetic transcription is systematic and clear. Below we explore how vowels are articulated and then how they are transcribed.

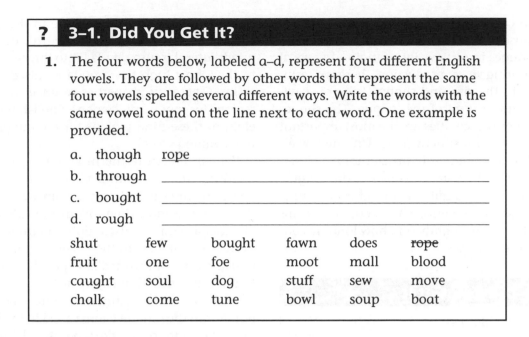

? 3–1. Did You Get It?

1. The four words below, labeled a–d, represent four different English vowels. They are followed by other words that represent the same four vowels spelled several different ways. Write the words with the same vowel sound on the line next to each word. One example is provided.

a. though   <u>rope</u>

b. through   _____

c. bought   _____

d. rough   _____

shut	few	bought	fawn	does	~~rope~~
fruit	one	foe	moot	mall	blood
caught	soul	dog	stuff	sew	move
chalk	come	tune	bowl	soup	boat

Consonants Versus Vowels

Consonants and vowels are divided into two categories because of their different functions in languages. Vowels are the center of and define syllables; consonants are added to vowels to provide word contrasts, allowing languages with few vowels (many have as few as three) to have countless distinct words.

Vowels serve as the nucleus of words and syllables. While consonants are critical for adding meaningful word contrasts in languages, adding vowel sounds is how we add syllables to words. For example, the word *at* is written with two letters and has a two-phoneme VC word shape. The word *bat* is written with three letters and has a three-phoneme CVC word shape. The word *scratched,* written with nine letters, is a six-phoneme word with a CCCVCC word shape. Despite the differing number of phonemes, all three of these words are one syllable in length and all of them have the vowel "a" as the syllable nucleus. It is only if we add another vowel sound, as in the word *batty*, that the word increases in syllable length, having a CV.CV word shape. Vowels can represent a syllable or a word by themselves (as in the V word shapes found in *a* or *eye*); with few exceptions consonants cannot represent a word or syllable alone.

Similarities and Differences in the Use of the Vocal Tract for Consonants and Vowels

In addition to functional differences, consonants and vowels are produced and defined differently. Consonants are defined by degrees and places of vocal tract obstruction; vowels are produced with limited vocal tract obstruction, with changes in sound arising mostly from changes in vocal tract shape.

While how we articulate vowels differs from consonants, other aspects of the speech system function in the same way during vowel and consonant production. English vowels and consonants are produced on exhalation—the outward flow of air from the lungs. This air goes through the vocal folds, creating vibration for many consonants and for all English vowels. English vowel phonemes are oral in the same way as most English consonants, with the velum raised, the nasal cavity obstructed, and airflow through the pharynx and the oral cavity manipulated to make vowel distinctions. Thus, vowels and consonants are produced with similar respiratory, phonatory, and oro-nasal action. To produce different vowels, we manipulate air flow in the pharynx and the oral cavity.

Differences between consonants and vowels result from differences in the articulatory systems of speech. While both vowels and consonants are produced by altering airflow, the means of doing so is quite different for each, and the resultant change in acoustic quality is what is perceived as a vowel or as a consonant by listeners in all languages. As you learned in Chapter 2, consonants rely on air obstruction for their distinct properties; vowels do not involve vocal tract obstruction, but different vocal tract shapes.

Similar to consonants, a listener hears different vowels because of distinct acoustic qualities resulting from changes in airflow. By changing the vocal tract shape during vowel production, there is a resultant change in the size and shape of the air cavities behind and in front of the tongue. The shapes and sizes of these air cavities are the most important properties in vowel distinctiveness. Unique vowels are made through changes in articulatory gestures, including how and where we constrict the tongue, whether or not the mandible is raised (in conjunction with tongue placement), whether or not the lips are rounded, and how tightly and how long we constrict vocal tract muscles.

? 3–2. Did You Get It?

1. Fill in the blanks

   Vowels and consonants are similar in their use of these three components of the speech system:

   a. _____

   b. _____

   c. _____

2. The production of vowels and consonants differs primarily in the amount of _____ during articulation.

Visualizing Place of Articulation: The Vowel Quadrilateral

The **vowel quadrilateral** provides a visual representation of vowels and is shown in Figure 3–1. While the vowel quadrilateral is simplistic and is only a partially accurate representation of vowel production, it is useful in understanding the articulatory differences and similarities among English vowels.

The principal factor in determining distinct vowels is where we raise our tongue in the oral cavity. If we superimpose the vowel quadrilateral on a sagittal (side) view of the vocal tract, we see the different possibilities for raised tongue position. Figure 3–1 demonstrates the vowel quadrilateral and its nine regions. The quadrilateral is divided into thirds on the x-axis to differentiate where in the oral cavity the tongue is raised: front, central, or back. The quadrilateral is also divided into thirds on the y-axis to show how high the tongue is raised: high, mid, or low. These six properties result in nine possible regions for tongue placement. English makes use of eight of these nine regions for meaningful distinctions among vowels.

We can illustrate the nine regions of the vowel quadrilateral on sagittal views of the vocal tract. There are three articulatory postures that result from the tongue being raised forward in the oral cavity. The tongue can be raised high and front, illustrated in the sagittal view of the vocal tract in Figure 3–2; mid and front, illustrated in Figure 3–3; and low and front, as illustrated in Figure 3–4.

There are three central articulatory postures that result from the tongue being raised in the oral cavity near the center of the hard palate. The tongue can be placed high and central, illustrated in the sagittal view of the vocal tract in Figure 3–5; mid and central, illustrated in Figure 3–6; and low and central, as illustrated in Figure 3–7.

The final three vowel quadrant possibilities involve the tongue raised in a posterior position in the oral cavity, toward the soft palate. These three postures are high and back, as illustrated in Figure 3–8; mid and back, as illustrated in Figure 3–9; and low and back, as illustrated in Figure 3–10.

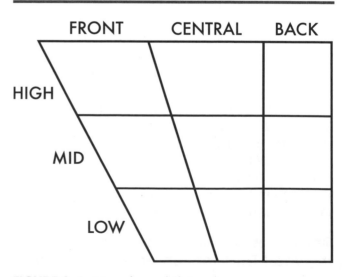

FIGURE 3–1. Vowel quadrilateral.

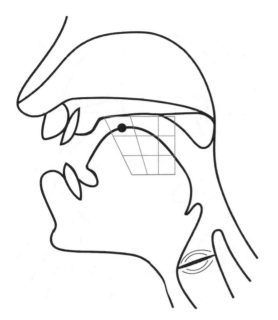

FIGURE 3–2. Vowel quadrilateral superimposed on sagittal view of a high front vowel.

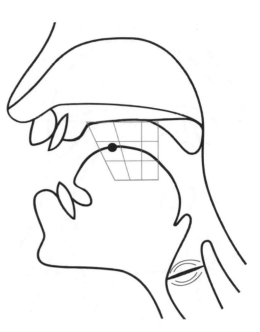

FIGURE 3–3. Vowel quadrilateral superimposed on sagittal view of a mid front vowel.

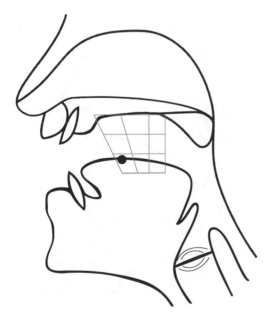

FIGURE 3–4. Vowel quadrilateral superimposed on sagittal view of a low front vowel.

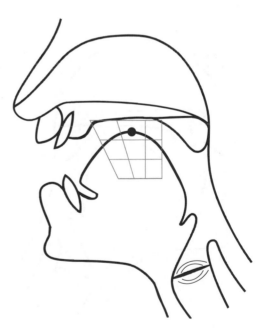

FIGURE 3–5. Vowel quadrilateral superimposed on sagittal view of a high central vowel.

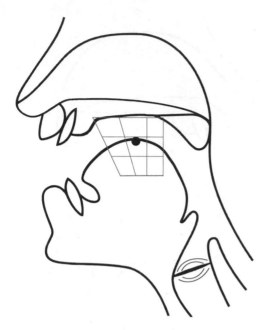

FIGURE 3–6. Vowel quadrilateral superimposed on sagittal view of a mid central vowel.

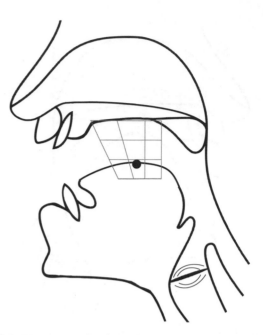

FIGURE 3–7. Vowel quadrilateral superimposed on sagittal view of a low central vowel.

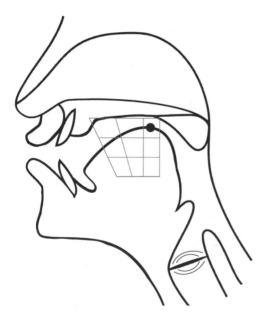

FIGURE 3–8. Vowel quadrilateral superimposed on sagittal view of a high back vowel.

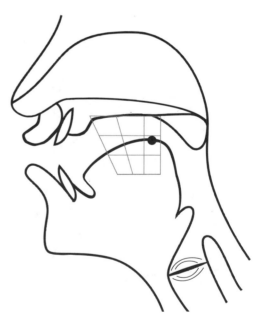

FIGURE 3–9. Vowel quadrilateral superimposed on sagittal view of a mid back vowel.

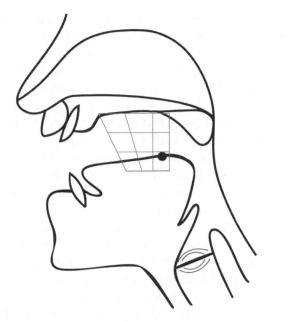

FIGURE 3–10. Vowel quadrilateral superimposed on sagittal view of a low back vowel.

Types of English Vowels

Monophthong Vowels: Steady-State Production

English vowel production can be divided into two categories: **steady-state vowels**, which require a single articulatory movement during their production, and **dynamic vowels**, which require multiple movements during their production. Vowels requiring a single articulatory movement are considered steady state vowels because there is little change in articulation during the vowel's production. Steady-state vowels are called **monophthongs**.

Diphthong Vowels: Dynamic Movement

For the second vowel category, our articulators—typically the tongue and lips—rapidly glide from one articulatory position to another during the vowel's production. Even though there are multiple movements, the result is a single vowel phoneme. These changing vowels are called diphthongs if there are two vowel qualities in the changing production and triphthongs if there are three vowel qualities in the changing production. GAE has three diphthong

phonemes, as well as two monophthong vowels that are produced as diphthong allophones. As we introduced in Chapter 1, allophones are non-meaning-based articulatory modifications of a sound.

Rhotic Vowels: Static Versus Dynamic Movement Involving R-Colorings

GAE is characterized by the high number of vowels that contain r-coloring. You will hear these vowels called rhotic vowels, r-colored vowels, and rhotacized vowels. Rhotic describes the "r" sound at the core of the monophthong vowel, as in the word *sir,* diphthong vowels where the vowel glides from a nonrhotic monophthong to the r-coloring, as in *for,* and triphthong vowels where we glide from a nonrhotic diphthong into the r-quality, as in *tire.* English has five rhotic diphthongs and two rhotic triphthongs.

Articulatory Dimension of Vowels

We use four categories to describe the different ways we alter our vocal tract to produce monophthong vowels. These four categories are **tongue height**, **tongue advancement** (or frontness), **tenseness**, and **lip rounding**. Because diphthong and triphthong vowels are defined by multiple movements during their production, we cannot use static vowel categories to define them. Instead, we use the same four categories of monophthongs to describe where the articulators are during initial and subsequent movements of the dynamic vowel production.

As mentioned, the primary way we make vowels distinct is by altering our tongue shape. These changes in tongue gestures affect the shape or geometry of the pharyngeal and oral cavities. The two most important categories for vowel production describe the highest point of the tongue body: tongue height and tongue advancement. These are the dimensions that are represented on the two axes of the vowel quadrilateral.

While we present tongue shape as two-dimensional to understand the basics of vowel production, remember that there also are changes in tongue shape such as narrowing and widening of the tongue that contribute to each vowel's unique acoustic properties.

Tongue Height

Can you detect differences in tongue height? Say the vowels "ee" (as in *heed*) and "a" (as in *hat*) right after each other multiple times: "ee/a/ee/a/ee/a." Try the same thing with "oo" (as in *boot*) and "ah" (*as in hot*): "oo/ah/oo/ah/oo/ah." What is your jaw doing during the two strings of vowels? What is your tongue doing? Notice that your jaw goes up and down during each vowel string, as does your tongue, with your tongue close to the roof of your mouth for "ee" and "oo" and lowered for "a" and "ah." The vowel pairs "ee/a" and "oo/ah" differ in tongue height.

Tongue height is defined by how near the tongue body is to the roof of the mouth. Altering how high the tongue is in the oral cavity thereby alters how large the air space is above the tongue. In reality, the up and down tongue movement is not that big. So tongue height, particularly in single words, is largely a matter of raising or lowering the lower mandible, or jaw. The higher the mandible is raised, the higher the tongue is in the oral cavity and the smaller the space through which air flows. The lower the mandible is, the lower the tongue is and the larger the space in the oral cavity becomes.

Tongue height differs on a three-step continuum of **high, mid,** and **low,** differences reflected in the vowel quadrilateral. We have introduced how these tongue body changes can be seen through two-dimensional sagittal views of the vocal tract showing articulatory placement. High vowels have the tongue raised close to the palate, as shown in Figure 3–11. Mid vowels have the tongue body and jaw in a more neutral position, as shown in Figure 3–12. Low vowels are produced when the tongue is low because of the lowered mandible, as shown in Figure 3–13. These tongue height gradations create a variety of vowel phoneme opportunities.

Try manipulating tongue (and mandibular) height to see how we change vowel phonemes. On exhalation, with air flowing through the vocal folds and the vocal folds vibrating, make an "ee" sound. Notice how your tongue is close to the roof of your mouth? Now, slowly—slowly—drop your jaw. Notice as your jaw lowers how the vowel quality changes. Instead of an "ee" you should hear a vowel more like the "ih" sound in *fish*. Keep lowering that jaw slowly. Do you hear the vowel "ay" *as in say*? And then "eh" as in *bed*? And as you further drop your jaw, do you hear "a" as in *bat*? The "ee" and "ih" are high vowels, "ay" and "eh" are mid vowels, and "a" is a low vowel. Try saying them a little faster: ee/ih/ay/eh/a.

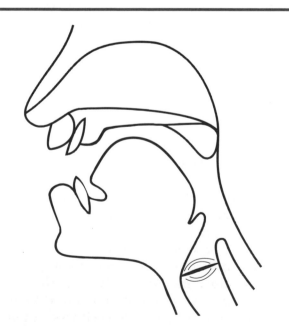

FIGURE 3–11. Sagittal view of a high vowel production.

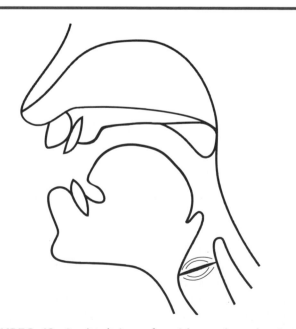

FIGURE 3–12. Sagittal view of a mid vowel production.

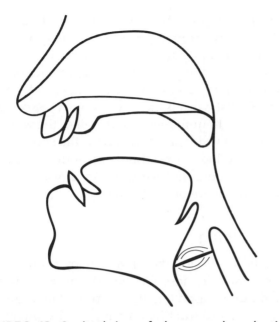

FIGURE 3–13. Sagittal view of a low vowel production.

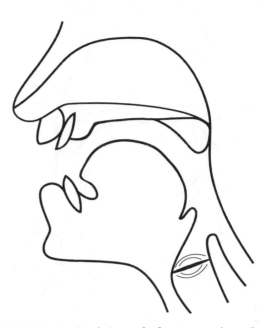

FIGURE 3–14. Sagittal view of a front vowel production.

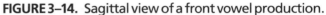

Tongue Advancement

In addition to tongue height, *where* the tongue is raised in the oral tract on an anterior/posterior (i.e., front/back) scale affects vowel quality. This category is called **tongue advancement**, also referred to as tongue anterior/posterior position, tongue frontness, and front/back tongue position.

To illustrate tongue advancement, say some new vowel pairs. Say the vowels "ee" (as in *beet*) and "oo" (as in *boot*) one right after the other multiple times: "ee/oo/ee/oo/ee/oo." What is your tongue body doing during these vowel pairs? You should notice that your tongue body is more forward in your mouth for the first vowel "ee" and farther back for the second vowel "oo."

Tongue advancement is divided into three categories: **front**, **central**, and **back**. Front vowels are those where the highest point in the tongue is raised anteriorly, toward the hard palate. Figure 3–14 shows the tongue body raised toward the front of the mouth. Central vowels are produced with the body of the tongue raised in a neutral position: in the center of the mouth or toward the back of the hard palate, as shown in Figure 3–15. Back vowels are produced with the highest point in the tongue raised posteriorly: toward the soft palate, as in Figure 3–16. The tongue

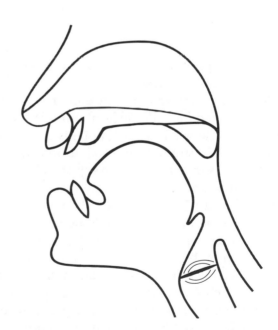

FIGURE 3–15. Sagittal view of a central vowel production.

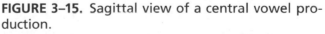

advancement category for vowels can be harder to identify in your mouth because where the tongue is raised does not have to be high, it only needs to be higher than other parts of the tongue. Nevertheless,

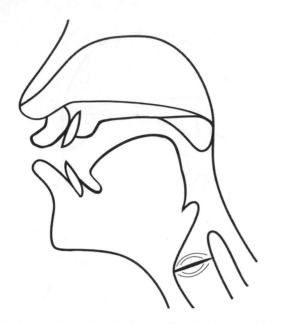

FIGURE 3–16. Sagittal view of a back vowel production.

where in the mouth the tongue is raised affects the vocal tract shape and dramatically affects the vowel phoneme that is perceived.

Now manipulate tongue placement to change low vowel categories. Produce a short "a" vowel (as in *hat*). Note where your tongue is as you prolong this "a." Go straight from "a" (as in *hat*) to the vowel "ah" (as in *hot*). No breaks, just "a" to "ah." Now go back and forth between the two vowels "a/ah/a/ah/a/ah." Your jaw should not be going up and down but your tongue should be moving from a front position for the "a" to a back posture for the "ah." As you probably guessed, "a" is a front vowel and "ah" is a back vowel. You might notice that the front to back change in these low vowels is not quite as big as the front-to-back change in "ee" and "oo," which are high vowels. There is more space in the high part of our mouth than there is in the low part of our mouth. This space difference is why the upper part of the vowel quadrilateral is drawn longer than the lower part of the quadrilateral.

In summary, if we combine how high the mandible is raised (tongue height) with where the body of the tongue is raised (tongue advancement) we have nine possible vocal tract shapes for vowel production, all of which were shown in Figures 3–2 to 3–10.

These nine tongue body positions are high front, mid front, low front, high central, mid central, low central, high back, mid back, and low back. So just by moving the tongue body forward or back and the jaw up and down slightly, we can make a lot of different English vowels. However, these two scales are not enough to uniquely describe all of the vowels of English. We will learn more about the specific vowels after we look at the final categories for vowels, providing additional ways to move articulators to create even more potential vowels.

Lip Rounding

In addition to classifying vowels by tongue body placement, we describe vowels as **rounded** or **unrounded** based on lip posture. Lip rounding results in vocal tract lengthening and significantly changes the acoustic quality (resonance) of vowels. Figure 3–17 shows a rounded vowel, which can be compared with an unrounded vowel in Figure 3–18.

In general, as English vowel production moves posteriorly and the tongue raises toward the palate, the lips become more rounded. Rounding of the lips in the production of back vowels increases the perceptual distinctiveness of these vowels from front vowel phoneme counterparts. Unrounded vowels can range from spread lips (as in the vowel "ee") to lips in a neutral position (as in the vowel "uh" as in *bud*). Rounded vowels range from tightly rounded, in "oo," to a slightly rounded posture, as in the vowel "uh" (as in *hook*).

In English, lip rounding is important for vowel production but it is not contrastive for vowel meaning. This is because lip rounding is not used to distinguish vowels that share the same tongue height and tongue advancement; back mid and back high vowels are rounded in English, while all other vowel phonemes are unrounded.

Try changing the shape of your lips to change vowel quality. Take a deep breath. On the exhale, say the "ee" sound with your lips spread as widely as possible. Start moving your lips slowly out and closer together, ending with them rounded and slightly protruded: "ee/oo." Keep vocalizing, and do not move anything but your lips. The rounded version of "ee" sounds a lot like "oo." Note that these changes in vowels were made without tongue movement; the only changes were in lip posture.

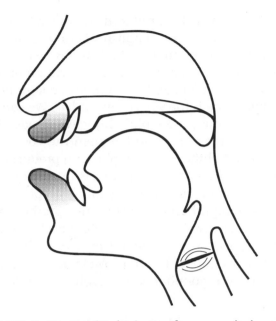

FIGURE 3–17. Sagittal view of a rounded vowel production.

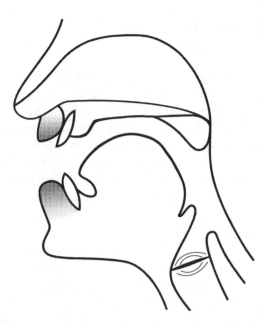

FIGURE 3–18. Sagittal view of an unrounded vowel production.

Tenseness

You learned about consonant cognates in Chapter 2, where two consonants share the same place and manner of articulation and differ only in voicing. Cognates also are used to describe four pairs of vowels that share tongue height, tongue advancement, and lip rounding categories, but differ in a fourth category: **tenseness** (also called the tense/lax distinction, or tension). For each cognate pair, one vowel is produced with the tongue body slightly more central in the oral cavity. This centralized vowel is defined as **lax**; the vowel that is produced with more extreme articulation (farther forward for front vowels and farther back for back vowels) is defined as **tense**. In addition to the more extreme tongue position, the tense vowel of each pair is produced with a more advanced tongue root and is longer in duration. Some phoneticians consider tense vowels to be produced with slightly more muscular tension than their lax vowel counterparts, although this view is not accepted by all. In Chapter 8 you will learn how tense and lax vowels function differently in English words.

Can you detect a difference in tenseness during vowel production? Place your hand on the fleshy part just under your chin and produce the vowels in the words *heat* and *hit*: "ee/ih." Do you feel a change? Which is tense? The production of "ee" and "ih" sounds is different for most speakers, with the "ee" produced with the tongue root more advanced than the "ih" vowel; therefore "ee" is the tense vowel. Note that these two vowels are produced with the same tongue blade placement and lip posture.

? 3–3. Did You Get It?

1. In this section, we introduced two types of vowels. These are steady-state vowels, called _____, and dynamic, changing vowels, called _____.

2. What do we call vowels that end with r-coloring? _____

3. A monophthong vowel can be described in four ways. These are tongue height, _____, _____, and _____.

Diphthong and Triphthong Vowel Categories

Together, tongue height, tongue advancement, lip rounding, and tenseness are sufficient to describe monophthong vowels because of their steady-state quality. Monophthongs are produced using a single articulatory gesture that can be produced indefinitely. In contrast, **diphthongs** and **triphthongs** are defined by dynamic articulator movement and a gradually changing vowel quality during their production. Diphthongs and triphthongs cannot be characterized in the static way of monophthongs.

It is easier to hear and feel the difference between monophthongs and diphthongs if you elongate a vowel's production. If we only produce the first half of the diphthong in *ride*, the word sounds like *rod*, changing the vowel and the word meaning. To compare a monophthong and diphthong, say the words *bee* and *bye* aloud. Start with *bee*. As soon as you let go of your lips from the "b," hold the "ee" vowel for a few seconds. Note that you can hold the vowel "ee" in *bee* for a long time. When you do, you are just making the monophthong "ee" longer—lengthening the whole vowel in *bee*. Now say *bye*. When you elongate the vowel in *bye,* you have to make a choice: either holding the first part or the second part of the vowel. You cannot say the whole vowel for a few seconds, though, because it is a dynamic vowel with two movements and is hence a diphthong. The "I" sound in *bye* is an example of a phonemic diphthong where there is a change in the vocal tract during its production that changes the meanings of words.

What does a nonphonemic diphthong sound like? Say the vowel in *bay* very slowly. Can you feel the shape of your vocal tract changing during the vowel production, your tongue moving slightly toward a *y* sound? That is the diphthong quality. Now say *bay* but this time do not let your tongue move during the vowel. You have produced this word with a steady-state monophthong. It still sounds like *bay,* just shorter, right? Both productions represent the same word, and meaning is retained, so "ay" is an example of a nonphonemic diphthong. Now say the vowel in the word *boat* slowly. For this diphthong, the most noticeable movement is a change in lip posture.

There are two different types of diphthongs in English. There are **phonemic** diphthongs, like the vowel in *bye*. For phonemic diphthongs, the entire diphthong must be produced to understand the meaning of the word. English also has two **nonphonemic** (or phonetic) diphthongs, which are nonphonemic variants of the underlying monophthong vowel phoneme. An example of a nonphonemic diphthong is the vowel "ay" in *bay*. We can say *bay* with a short, monophthong vowel production, but we are more likely to lengthen the vowel and produce a diphthong. The diphthong production is allophonic, where the allophone is the spoken production of an underlying phonemic concept. In nonphonemic diphthongs, if we do not produce both parts of the vowel allophone, the vowel meaning is still understood. The vowel in *boat* is the other example of a monophthong vowel phoneme that is produced as a nonphonemic allophone in GAE.

Rhotic Vowels: Monophthongs, Diphthongs, and Triphthongs

GAE has many rhotic vowels. The monophthong rhotic vowel is produced as a steady-state vowel, but with a more complex tongue posture than other monophthongs. This tongue posture is also the **offglide** for many rhotic diphthongs and rhotic triphthongs in English. Rhotic vowels are described with tongue advancement, height, and rounding categories and the additional dimension of **rhoticity** to give them their r-like auditory quality. The auditory quality of rhotic vowels can be produced in a number of ways, like the consonant "r." The tongue tip and bunched tongue gestures are the most common rhotic productions and will be used to describe rhotic vowel production.

To demonstrate rhoticity, contrast the English rhotic monophthong with another English monophthong. Try saying "uh" followed by "er" many times: "uh/er/uh/er/uh/er." Elongate each vowel so you really feel how they are produced. Do you notice more tongue and lip movement and more tension for "er"? Can you feel more of your tongue move for "er"? You should be able to feel the back of your tongue, the tip of your tongue, and the body of your tongue become tenser in "er" than "uh." Compare "er" to other monophthongs to become more aware of your tongue postures for vowels.

Rhotic diphthongs are also created by adding an r-like tongue movement to the end of some vowels. When the r sound follows a monophthong, we call the resulting vowel a rhotic diphthong. Examples of rhotic diphthongs include the vowels in the words *start, horse,* and *fair.* When the "r" sound follows a diphthong, we call the vowel a rhotic triphthong. Examples of rhotic triphthongs include the vowels in the words *fire* and *hour* if they are produced as single-syllable words.

If r-coloring comes after a vowel, it is still part of the vowel and <u>not</u> a consonant. This differs from many linguistic approaches to final "r." Thus the word *soar* has a CV word shape made up of /s/ and the vowel *oar.* For comparison, there are words like *robe,* which start with an initial consonant /ɹ/; words like *trip,* which start with an initial consonant cluster containing /ɹ/; words like *her* that have two sounds: the consonant /h/ and a rhotic vowel; and words like *bore* that end with a vocalic "r" in the form of a rhotic diphthong. Like diphthongs, these rhotic vowels that end with an "r" quality have two or three movements to their production: a monophthong or diphthong vowel that glides into the "r" quality in the same syllable.

Rhotic vowels have greater importance in a clinical phonetics textbook than they do in a linguistics phonetics textbook. This is because rhotic vowels have clinical relevance for clinical scientists. Consonant and vowel "r" sounds are often produced in error in individuals with speech sound disorders. Reasons for errors in "r" production can be articulatory, acoustic, and linguistic. Most pediatric speech-language pathologists will treat "r" errors in children with speech sound disorders. And some speech-language pathologists will teach rhotic vowels because they provide accent instruction to people learning English as a second language. Therapists will often treat rhotic vowels before they treat the consonant /ɹ/. There are also error patterns for rhotic vowels that differ from consonant /ɹ/ error patterns. For all of these reasons, it is essential that you understand rhotic consonant and vowel production.

Description of English Vowel Phonemes: Monophthongs and Diphthongs

We have defined vowels by the movements of the articulators and the placement of the tongue during the vowel productions and have seen the many ways the same vowel sound can be spelled in English. Now that you have the tools to define English vowel phonemes, we turn to learning the unique characteristics of each English vowel. You will learn transcription of English monophthong, diphthong, and rhotic vowels using phonetic symbols, most of them from the International Phonetic Alphabet (IPA), but some adapted to represent the phonemes of GAE. For each vowel, you will learn its phonetic symbol, how the vowel is described and articulated, and the name(s) for these phonetic symbols. And we will then combine vowel and consonant symbols to start transcribing whole English words.

Describing Monophthongs
Below we will first introduce monophthong vowels, their phonemic categories, and the phonetic symbols for them. Remember, monophthong vowels are produced with one steady-state articulation and are transcribed with a single symbol, as shown below. The vowel properties of English monophthong vowel phonemes are typically described in the following order: tongue height, tongue advancement, rounding, and tenseness. You should learn the phonetic symbol and the articulatory properties of each vowel phoneme at the same time. In the future, you will need to know how to transcribe words and how sounds are produced to be able to teach someone how to make these sounds correctly.

Two English vowels have stressed and unstressed counterparts. For these two vowels, we will present the vowel phoneme, its articulatory categories, and its phonetic symbol. We then will introduce the unstressed allophone and its phonetic symbol.

Describing Diphthongs
Below we also describe diphthong vowel productions and phonetic symbols. Diphthongs are written with two phonetic symbols, with the first symbol representing the onglide, or the starting articulatory position for the diphthong. The second symbol is the offglide and represents the direction and ending position of the articulators during the diphthong production. All English diphthongs are rising diphthongs; that is, the offglide for English diphthongs has a higher tongue height than the onglide.

To emphasize that the two symbols in a diphthong are part of the same phoneme, as you learn to transcribe and as you learn to count the number of sounds in words, we suggest that you connect the diphthong onglide and the offglide with a ligature over the two phonetic symbols. Where you place (or even whether you use) the ligature differs among phoneticians. What does matter is that you recognize diphthongs as one vowel, noting that words with diphthongs, like *mouse*, have a CVC (and not a CVVC) word shape. In the diphthong drawings that follow, the sagittal views of each diphthong show the vowel's dynamic movement through shading.

As noted earlier, two English monophthongs are typically produced as diphthong allophones. For these two vowels, we first present the monophthong symbol and the phonemic categories, then introduce the allophonic productions of these vowels and the diphthong phonetic symbol that are common in GAE. The diphthong allophones will be used for the remainder of the textbook.

Monophthong Vowels: Articulation, Phonetic Symbols, and Key Words

Front Vowels

English has five front vowel phonemes: two high front vowels, two mid front vowels, and one low front vowel. The high and mid front vowels have cognate pairs and therefore their phonemic description requires tongue height, advancement, and tenseness properties. All front English vowels are unrounded. In GAE, four of the front vowels are produced as monophthongs and one is typically produced as its diphthong allophone.

/i/   The monophthong vowel in *tree*, transcribed /tɹi/, is illustrated in Figure 3–19. It is also the vowel in *chief, key,* and *reed.* /i/ is a high front unrounded tense vowel. [i] is produced with the highest part of the tongue raised high and forward in the oral cavity. The lips are spread. The symbol is called Latin small letter i.

/ɪ/   The monophthong vowel in *fish*, transcribed /fɪʃ/, is illustrated in Figure 3–20. It is also the vowel in *hit, switch,* and *rips.* /ɪ/ is a high front unrounded lax vowel. [ɪ] is produced with the highest part of the tongue raised high and forward in the oral cavity. The symbol is called Latin letter small capital i.

Figure 3–21 is a sagittal view of the oral cavity showing production of both high front vowels. The sagittal view does not distinguish between the lax and tense high front vowels.

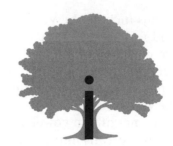

FIGURE 3–19. Mnemonic visualization of the vowel /i/.

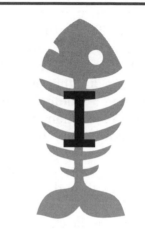

FIGURE 3–20. Mnemonic visualization of the vowel /ɪ/.

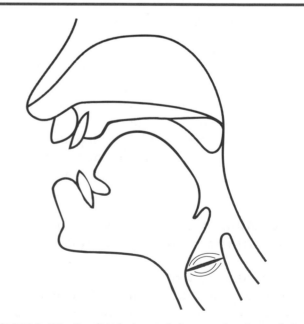

FIGURE 3–21. Sagittal view of the production of the high front unrounded vowels.

/e/ The monophthong vowel phoneme in *train,* transcribed phonemically as /tɹen/. This vowel is a mid front unrounded tense vowel.

In GAE, the monophthong phoneme /e/ is produced as the diphthong allophone [eɪ] more frequently than as [e]. From this point forward, /e/ will be presented as its GAE allophonic production [eɪ]. *Train,* transcribed [tɹeɪn], is illustrated in Figure 3–22. It is also the vowel in *say, rake,* and *beige.* When the diphthong [eɪ] is produced, the highest part of the tongue is raised midway in the front of the mouth for the onglide. The jaw is partially raised and the lips are in a neutral position. The tongue body raises and moves forward slightly in the offglide. This symbol is called Latin small letter e.

Figure 3–23 is a sagittal view of the oral cavity showing production of the mid front unrounded nonphonemic diphthong, illustrating the tongue movement during the diphthong production.

/ɛ/ The monophthong vowel in *bread,* transcribed /bɹɛd/, is illustrated in Figure 3–24. Also the vowel in *chest, friend,* and *left.* /ɛ/ is a mid front unrounded lax vowel. [ɛ] is produced with the highest part of the tongue raised midway in the mouth and forward in the oral cavity. The lips are in a relaxed, unrounded position and the vowel is lax. The symbol is called Greek small letter epsilon.

Figure 3–25 is a sagittal view of the oral cavity showing production of a mid front vowel.

/æ/ The monophthong vowel in *cat,* transcribed /kæt/, is illustrated in Figure 3–26. It is also the vowel in *wrapped, hatch,* and *bag.* /æ/ is a low front unrounded lax vowel. [æ] is produced with the highest part of the tongue low and forward in the mouth; the open jaw results in its low vowel property. [æ] is made with the lips unrounded. The symbol is called ash or referred to by saying the vowel sound. Although /æ/ looks like it is the letter "a"

followed by the letter "e," it is important to remember that ash is one symbol, not two, reflecting the fact that the /æ/ is a monophthong—a single, steady-state sound—and not a diphthong.

Figure 3–27 is a sagittal view of the oral cavity showing production of the low front vowel.

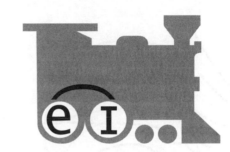

FIGURE 3–22. Mnemonic visualization of the diphthong /eɪ/.

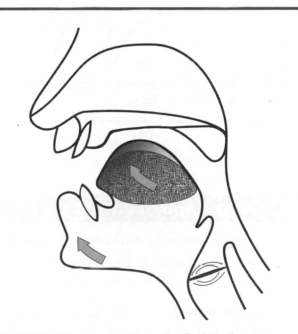

FIGURE 3–23. Sagittal view of the dynamic production of the nonphonemic mid front unrounded diphthong.

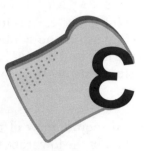

FIGURE 3–24. Mnemonic visualization of the vowel /ɛ/.

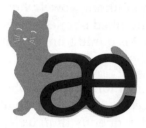

FIGURE 3–26. Mnemonic visualization of the vowel /æ/.

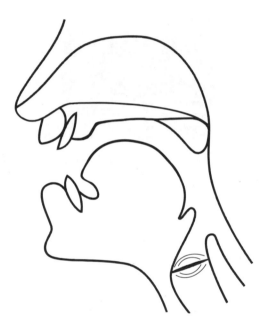

FIGURE 3–25. Sagittal view of the production of the mid front unrounded vowels.

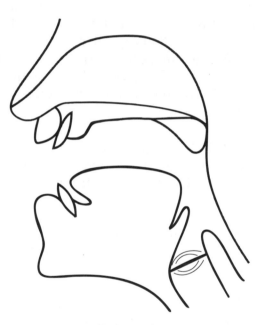

FIGURE 3–27. Sagittal view of the production of the low front unrounded vowel.

?   3–4. Did You Get It?

1. All front vowels are made with the highest part of the tongue raised toward the _____ part of the oral cavity.

2. Front vowels differ in tongue height and tension but share _____ and _____.

3. Which words below contain front vowels?
   bake   book   bee   best   boot   bat

4. Cross out the words that do not contain front vowels.
   kept   ship   rope   swerve   knack   thief

Central Monophthongs

There are two central monophthong vowels in English. One of them is a rhotic vowel that will be discussed in detail with other rhotic vowels later in this chapter.

/ʌ/ The monophthong vowel in *up*, transcribed /ʌp/, is illustrated in Figure 3–28. It is also the vowel in *duck, nut,* and *hush.* /ʌ/ is a mid central unrounded lax vowel. [ʌ] is produced with the highest part of the tongue in a neutral position. The jaw is lowered slightly and the highest part of the tongue is raised midway toward the center of the mouth or the hard palate. [ʌ] is made with the lips unrounded. The symbol is called caret, wedge, or inverted v.

The **schwa** is the unstressed allophone of the central monophthong /ʌ/ and is transcribed [ə]. [ə] is a common allophonic production of vowel phonemes in English and appears frequently, occurring in most two-syllable English words and often occurring multiple times in words that are three syllables or longer. [ə], like /ʌ/, is a mid central unrounded lax vowel. It is produced with the tongue, mandible, and lips in a neutral resting position, with the lips slightly parted. The production of [ə] is as central as a vowel can be: the tongue is not front or back or high or low—the lips are not rounded, nor are they spread. From an articulatory perspective, [ə] and [ʌ] are produced similarly, although the wedge is made with the jaw slightly lower in the mouth. If you say the word *above,* you can hear the difference between [ʌ] and [ə]; this word is typically said with stress on the second vowel and is transcribed [ə.bʌv]. Two other words produced with the schwa in their unstressed syllables are *rises* and *enough,* transcribed [ɹaɪ.zəz] and [ə.nʌf].

Figure 3–29 is a sagittal view of the oral cavity showing production of the mid central unrounded vowel, reflecting the stressed and unstressed production.

> **? 3–5. Did You Get It?**
>
> 1. Central vowels are made with the highest part of the tongue raised toward the _____ part of the oral cavity.
>
> 2. Which words below contain central vowels?
>   hut   tough   book   ball   dove   flood
>
> 3. Cross out the words that do not contain the mid central unrounded nonrhotic lax vowel.
>   suit   suds   could   plush   con   love
>
> 4. Say the words below aloud. Differentiate the stressed and unstressed central vowel that is in boldface in the two-syllable words below. To do so, circle stressed [ʌ] and underline unstressed [ə].
>   c**u**tting   **a**gain   min**u**te
>   s**u**nny   b**e**lieve   beg**u**n

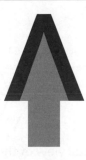

FIGURE 3–28. Mnemonic visualization of the vowel /ʌ/.

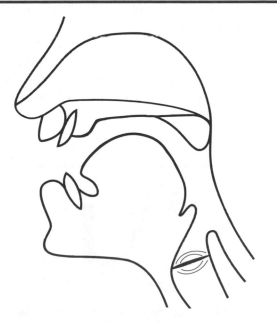

FIGURE 3–29. Sagittal view of the production of the mid central unrounded vowel.

Back Monophthongs

English has five back vowel phonemes: two high back vowels, two mid back vowels, and one low back vowel. In GAE, four back vowel phonemes are produced as monophthongs and one is produced as a nonphonemic back diphthong. The two high and two mid back vowels have cognate pairs. Therefore their phonemic description requires tongue height, advancement, and tenseness properties. The high and mid back vowels in English are rounded. The low back vowel is unrounded. In GAE, four of the back vowels are produced as monophthongs and one is typically produced as its diphthong allophone.

/u/   The monophthong vowel in *boot*, transcribed /but/, is illustrated in Figure 3–30. It is also the vowel in *juice, loop,* and *sue*. /u/ is a high back rounded tense vowel. [u] is produced with the highest part of the tongue raised high at the back of the oral cavity. The lips are rounded and it is tense. The symbol is called Latin small letter u.

/ʊ/   The monophthong vowel in *bull,* transcribed /bʊl/, is illustrated in Figure 3–31. It is also the vowel in *push, good,* and *foot*. /ʊ/ is a high back rounded lax vowel. Like [u], in producing [ʊ] the tongue is high in the oral cavity toward the soft palate and the lips are rounded. The symbol is called Latin small letter upsilon, or hook u.

Figure 3–32 is a sagittal view of the oral cavity showing production of both high back vowels. The sagittal view does not distinguish between the lax and tense high back vowels.

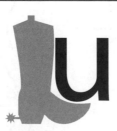

FIGURE 3–30. Mnemonic visualization of the vowel /u/.

/o/   The monophthong vowel phoneme in *phone,* transcribed phonemically as /fon/. This vowel is a mid back rounded tense vowel.

In GAE, the monophthong phoneme /o/ is produced as the diphthong allophone [oʊ] more frequently than as [o]. From this point forward, /o/ will be presented as its GAE allophonic production [oʊ]. *Phone,* transcribed /foʊn/, is illustrated in Figure 3–33. It is also the vowel in *though, nope,* and *rose*. When the diphthong [oʊ] is produced, the articulatory

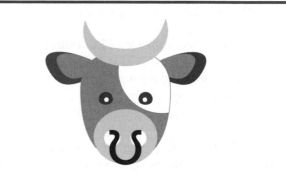

FIGURE 3–31. Mnemonic visualization of the vowel /ʊ/.

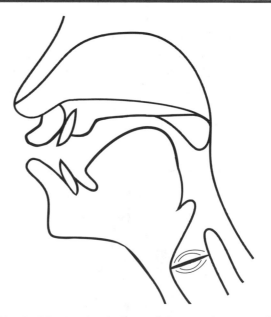

FIGURE 3–32. Sagittal view of the production of the high back rounded vowels.

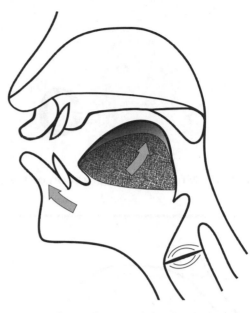

FIGURE 3–34. Sagittal view of the dynamic production of the nonphonemic mid back rounded diphthong.

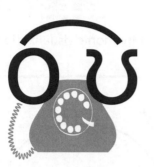

FIGURE 3–33. Mnemonic visualization of the diphthong /o͡ʊ/.

movement is slight and both the onglide and offglide are produced with the tongue body raised at the back of the oral cavity. The onglide is produced with the highest part of the tongue raised midway in the back of the oral cavity with the jaw partially raised. The lips are rounded. The tongue body raises and moves back slightly and the lips are rounded more in the offglide. This symbol is called Latin small letter o.

Figure 3–34 is a sagittal view of the oral cavity showing production of the mid back rounded nonphonemic diphthong, illustrating the movement from the onglide to the offglide during the diphthong production.

/ɔ/   This vowel is a phoneme for about half of GAE speakers; others do not make a meaningful distinction between /ɔ/ and /ɑ/. If you produce the words *cot* and *caught* differently, /ɔ/ is the rounded vowel in *caught*, transcribed [kɔt] and illustrated in Figure 3–35. It is also the vowel in *thought*, *dog*, and *raw*. /ɔ/ is a mid back rounded lax

vowel. [ɔ] is produced with the highest point of the tongue raised toward the soft palate at a mid-range level with the lips slightly rounded. The symbol is called Latin small letter open o.

Figure 3–36 is a sagittal view of the oral cavity showing production of mid back rounded vowels.

/ɑ/   The monophthong vowel in *stop*, transcribed /stɑp/, is illustrated in Figure 3–37. It is also in the words *tot, clock,* and *mop.* If you do not produce *cot* and *caught* differently, it is the vowel in both, transcribed /kɑt/; if you do pronounce these words differently, /ɑ/ is the vowel in *cot.* /ɑ/ is a low back unrounded tense vowel. [ɑ] is produced with the highest/bunched part of the tongue raised posteriorly in the mouth with the mandible lowered. It is made with the lips unrounded. The symbol is called Latin small letter alpha.

Figure 3–38 is a sagittal view of the oral cavity showing production of the low back unrounded vowel.

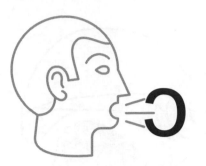

FIGURE 3–35. Mnemonic visualization of the vowel /ɔ/.

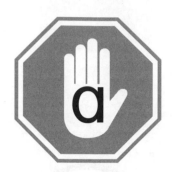

FIGURE 3–37. Mnemonic visualization of the vowel /ɑ/.

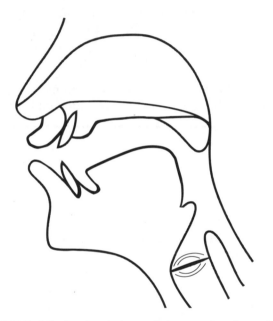

FIGURE 3–36. Sagittal view of the production of the mid back rounded vowels.

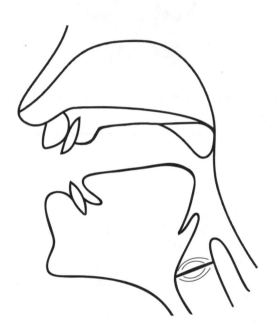

FIGURE 3–38. Sagittal view of the production of the low back unrounded vowel.

? 3–6. Did You Get It?

1. All back vowels are made with the highest part of the tongue raised toward the _____ part of the oral cavity.

2. In English all high back and mid back vowels share the category of _____.

3. Which words below contain back vowels?
   push   stoop   flute   coke   though   shop

4. Cross out the words that do not contain back vowels.
   stool   sat   rope   bog   taught   fun

Phonemic Diphthongs

GAE has three phonemic diphthongs. These diphthongs cannot be produced as monophthong allophones. Phonemic diphthongs also differ from nonphonemic diphthongs by requiring a larger movement from the onglide to the offglide portion of the vowel.

/aɪ/ The phonemic diphthong in *bike,* transcribed /baɪk/, is illustrated in Figure 3–39. It is also the vowel in *lie, shy,* and *file.* The /aɪ/ diphthong starts as a low central unrounded lax vowel and ends as a high front unrounded vowel. The onglide [a] is produced with the tongue body low and central and the lips unrounded. There is a smooth and rapid movement of the tongue body forward and upward. The offglide is made with the tongue body raised toward the front of the mouth and close to the palate. The lips are unrounded throughout this diphthong. The offglide of [aɪ] is usually lax in running speech but can be produced tense as well. This vowel is referred to as long i or by the sound it represents.

For the diphthong /aɪ/, note that the first symbol [a] represents its low central starting point; it is not transcribed [ɑ]. /a/ is a low central vowel in some dialects of English but is not a phoneme in GAE. This symbol is used in the phonemic diphthong /aɪ/ because of that diphthong's starting position, which is low central, not low back. To demonstrate, start to say the word *hot,* elongating the [ɑ]. While still phonating, change to the word *height.* Do you feel how you moved your tongue forward for the onglide? If so, you have changed to the low central [a] to make the diphthong [aɪ].

Figure 3–40 is a sagittal view of the oral cavity showing production of the [aɪ] diphthong, illustrating the movement from the onglide to the offglide during the diphthong production.

/ɔɪ/ The phonemic diphthong in *coin,* transcribed /kɔɪn/, is illustrated in Figure 3–41. It is also found in *soy, choice,* and *noise.* /ɔɪ/ starts as a mid back rounded vowel and ends as a high front unrounded lax vowel. The onglide for [ɔɪ] starts with the highest part of the tongue in a mid position toward the back of the mouth with the lips rounded. During the vowel production, the highest part of the tongue moves anteriorly and raises toward the front of the hard palate. In this textbook, the onglide for the diphthong is written with an open o, [ɔ], and not the long o (although some phoneticians transcribe this diphthong [oɪ]). These differing transcriptions represent differences in convention, not production.

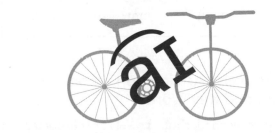

FIGURE 3–39. Mnemonic visualization of the diphthong /aɪ/.

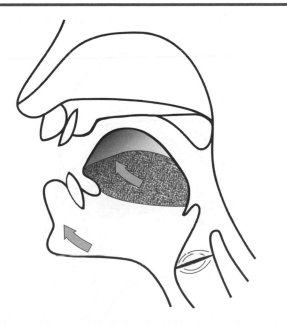

FIGURE 3–40. Sagittal view of the dynamic production of the phonemic low central unrounded to high front unrounded diphthong.

This vowel is typically referred to by the sound it represents.

Figure 3–42 is a sagittal view of the oral cavity showing production of the /ɔɪ/ diphthong, illustrating the movement from the onglide to the offglide position.

/aʊ/ The phonemic diphthong in *owl,* transcribed /aʊl/, is illustrated in Figure 3–43. It is also in the words *how, shout,* and *bough*. /aʊ/ begins as a low central unrounded vowel and ends as a high back rounded lax vowel. The onglide [a] is produced with the tongue body

low and raised toward the center of the hard palate, with the lips unrounded. From this position the tongue body moves rapidly up and back while the lips are simultaneously rounded for the offglide, ending with the tongue body raised toward the back of the mouth and close to the palate. The offglide of [aʊ] is usually lax in casual speech. As with /aɪ/, the first symbol in /aʊ/ is an [a] to represent its low central starting point; it is not a script *a*. This vowel is referred to by the sound it represents.

Figure 3–44 is a sagittal view of the oral cavity showing production of the [aʊ] diphthong, illustrating the movement from the onglide to the offglide position.

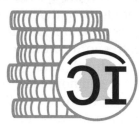

FIGURE 3–41. Mnemonic visualization of the diphthong /ɔɪ/.

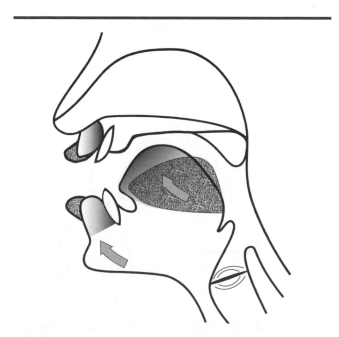

FIGURE 3–42. Sagittal view of the dynamic production of the phonemic mid back rounded to high front unrounded diphthong.

? 3–7. Did You Get It?

1. Monophthong vowels are produced with a steady state production. Diphthong vowels are produced with a

   _____.

2. If a diphthong vowel does not change meaning if you produce only the onglide, it is called a _____ diphthong.

3. The two parts of the diphthong are called the _____ and the

   _____.

4. Cross out the words that do not contain diphthong vowels.

   sound   ploy   cake   fawn   blow   seep

5. Below are words containing phonemic and nonphonemic diphthongs. Underline the phonemic diphthongs.

   raise   couch   fly   mow   moist   might

Rhotic Vowels: Articulation, Phonetic Symbols, and Key Words

As you have learned, rhotic vowels are characterized by an r-quality. Rhotics contain the orthographic "r" when spelled. There are a variety of rhotic vowels. The steady-state rhotic monophthong is produced with the articulatory gesture that results in the acoustic quality associated with the English "r." Rhotic diphthongs are produced with two articulatory gestures: an onglide monophthong and the offglide rhotic. Rhotic triphthongs are produced with three articulatory gestures: an onglide diphthong (two gestures) and the offglide rhotic (one gesture). The articulatory description of rhotic diphthongs and triphthongs involves the onglide vowel followed by the rhotic or r-colored offglide.

Phonetic transcription of rhotics differs depending on whether the rhotic is a steady-state or dynamic vowel. The monophthong rhotic "er" sound is transcribed with a single symbol specific to the stressed rhotic vowel. Rhotics made with multiple movements are transcribed with two symbols. The first symbol represents the monophthong onglide starting position for the vowel followed by the symbol for the unstressed rhotic vowel offglide. Rhotic triphthong vowels are transcribed with three symbols. Triphthong rhotics, which start with the phonetic symbol for the onglide portion of the diphthong, are followed by the symbol for the second part of the diphthong. They end with the unstressed rhotic vowel symbol to reflect the offglide rhotic production. To emphasize that diphthong and triphthong rhotics are one vowel, we connect the two or three components with a ligature. The ligature in *far*, transcribed /fɑɚ/, will help you remember that *far* has a CV word shape. In English, there is one monophthong rhotic, five diphthong rhotics, and two triphthong rhotics.

Rhotic Monophthong

/ɝ/   The monophthong rhotic vowel in *girl*, transcribed /gɝl/, is illustrated in Figure 3–45. It is also in the words *heard, word,* and *sir.* /ɝ/ is categorized as a mid central rounded tense rhotic vowel. [ɝ] is produced the same way as the consonant /ɹ/, but when it functions as a vowel we use vowel terminology to categorize it. Most speakers of English produce the r-colored monophthong as a bunched rhotic with the tongue tip down and the highest point of the tongue raised in a mid position toward the center of the mouth or the hard palate. The back edges of the tongue touch the back molars. The alternative tongue tip rhotic has the tongue raised midway toward the back of the hard palate and the back edges of the tongue touching the back molars. The lips are rounded. However, some speakers of English produce [ɝ] using a retroflex

FIGURE 3–43. Mnemonic visualization of the diphthong /aʊ/.

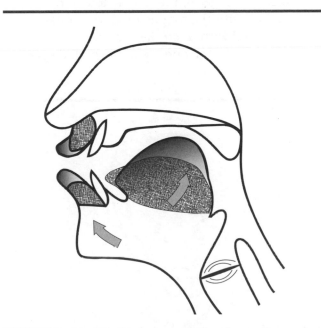

FIGURE 3–44. Sagittal view of the dynamic production of the phonemic low central unrounded to high back rounded diphthong.

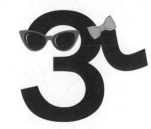

FIGURE 3–45. Mnemonic visualization of the rhotic /ɝ/.

tongue gesture, that is, with the tongue tip curled up and back. The symbol is called a reverse hooked epsilon or stressed **schwar**.

The rhotic monophthong /ɝ/ has stressed and unstressed allophonic variations. The unstressed allophone of /ɝ/ is [ɚ]. The stressed /ɝ/ is a mid central rounded tense vowel; the unstressed [ɚ] is its unrounded lax counterpart. Lip rounding differences are very slight; in fact, some speakers do not make a distinction in vowel rounding between the two productions. There are parallel distinctions between the stressed and unstressed rhotic monophthongs and the stressed [ʌ] and unstressed [ə]. Examples of words containing the unstressed [ɚ] include *teacher* and *butter*, transcribed [ti.t͡ʃɚ] and [bʌ.ɾɚ].

As you learned in Chapter 2, there are different articulatory gestures for producing rhotics. Figure 3–46 is a sagittal view of the oral cavity showing the mid central [ɝ] produced with a retroflex tongue.

Rhotic Diphthongs

Rhotic diphthongs start with differing onglide vowels but all end with the same rhotic offglide schwar. The phonetic symbol for the rhotic diphthong and a key word are provided. Rhotic vowels do not have tense and lax contrasts; for transcription consistency we present rhotic diphthongs with a lax vowel onset if there is a lax/tense contrast in English. For each rhotic diphthong, the onglide vowel is described, followed by descriptions of both the tongue tip and bunched [ɚ] offglide possibilities for each.

/ɪɚ/ The rhotic diphthong in *ear*, transcribed /ɪɚ/, is illustrated in Figure 3–47. It is also in the words *sneer, here*, and *fierce*. The onglide is high front unrounded and the offglide is a mid central rounded rhotic. There are a few possibilities for production of this rhotic vowel. If [ɪɚ] is produced with an alveolar rhotic, the onglide is produced with the highest part of the tongue raised and forward in the oral cavity. The offglide is produced by lowering the tongue slightly and moving the tongue posteriorly so it is raised toward the back of the hard palate. The sides of the tongue come close to the molars and the tongue tip raises slightly toward the alveolar ridge. If [ɪɚ] is produced with a tongue bunched rhotic, the tongue moves from the onglide to the offglide position by lowering the highest part of the tongue slightly and raising it toward the back of the hard palate: the back edges of the tongue touch the molars with the tongue tip down. If [ɪɚ] is produced with a retroflex rhotic, the tongue moves from the onglide to the offglide posi-

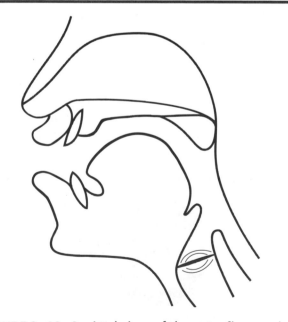

FIGURE 3–46. Sagittal view of the retroflex production of the mid central rounded vowel /ɝ/.

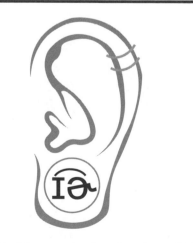

FIGURE 3–47. Mnemonic visualization of the rhotic diphthong /ɪɚ/.

tion by raising the underside of the tip of the tongue toward the post-alveolar region and raising the back of the tongue toward the back of the hard palate: the back edges of the tongue touch the molars with the tongue tip down. For all [ɪɚ] productions, the lips move from slightly spread during the onglide to a slightly rounded posture for the offglide.

Figure 3–48 is a sagittal view of the oral cavity during the production of [ɪɚ] with a retroflex rhotic. Figure 3–49 is a sagittal view of the oral cavity showing the production of [ɪɚ] with a bunched tongue rhotic. Both illustrate the movement from the onglide to the offglide rhotic position. Other rhotic diphthongs and triphthongs will show the same pattern of onglide vowel to the tongue tip or bunched tongue rhotic.

/ɛɚ/ The rhotic diphthong in *bear*, transcribed /bɛɚ/, is illustrated in Figure 3–50. It is also in the words *chairs, hare*, and *air*. The onglide for /ɛɚ/ is mid front unrounded; the offglide is mid central rounded rhotic. The onglide for [ɛɚ] is produced with the highest part of the tongue raised slightly toward the front of the hard palate. For a tongue tip rhotic offglide, the tongue moves back toward the hard

palate, with the sides of the tongue touching the molars and with the tongue tip raised slightly toward the alveolar ridge. If [ɛɚ] is produced with a tongue bunched rhotic, the tongue moves from the onglide to the offglide position, which involves moving the highest part of the tongue posteriorly so it is below the hard palate while raising the back edges of the tongue toward the molars. For both [ɛɚ] productions, the lips move from slightly spread during the onglide to a slightly rounded posture for the offglide.

/ʊɚ/ The rhotic diphthong in *tour,* transcribed /tʊɚ/, is illustrated in Figure 3–51. It is

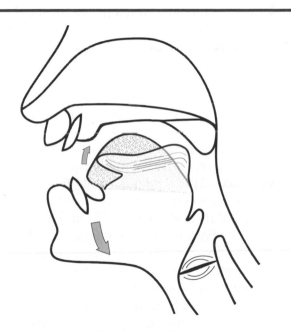

FIGURE 3–49. Sagittal view of the dynamic production of the high front unrounded to the tongue bunched rhotic diphthong.

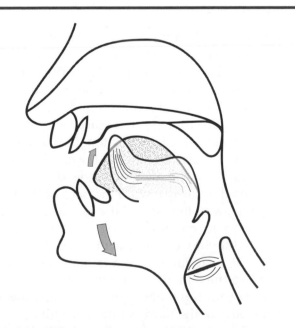

FIGURE 3–48. Sagittal view of the dynamic production of the high front unrounded to the tongue tip rhotic diphthong.

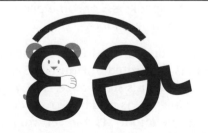

FIGURE 3–50. Mnemonic visualization of the rhotic diphthong /ɛɚ/.

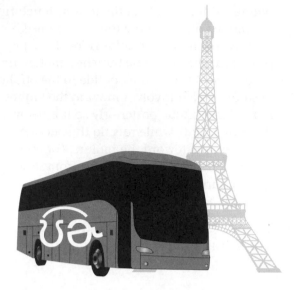

FIGURE 3–51. Mnemonic visualization of the rhotic diphthong /ʊ͡ɚ/.

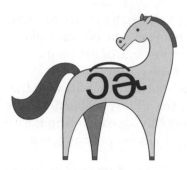

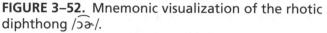

FIGURE 3–52. Mnemonic visualization of the rhotic diphthong /ɔ͡ɚ/.

also in the words *lured, pure,* and *cure.* The onglide for /ʊ͡ɚ/ is high back and rounded; the offglide is mid central rounded rhotic. The onglide for [ʊ͡ɚ] is produced with the highest part of the tongue raised near the soft palate. For a tongue tip offglide, the tongue moves anteriorly to the back of the hard palate and is lowered to mid height, with the back edges of the tongue touching the molars; the tongue tip is raised slightly toward the alveolar ridge. If [ʊ͡ɚ] is produced with a tongue bunched rhotic, the movement from the onglide to the offglide position involves moving the highest part of the tongue forward slightly toward the back of the hard palate with the back edges of the tongue touching the molars. The lips are rounded throughout both [ʊ͡ɚ] productions. Note that /ʊ͡ɚ/ doesn't exist in the dialect of some GAE speakers. For some people, *tour* is homonymous with *tore.*

/ɔ͡ɚ/ The rhotic diphthong in *horse,* transcribed /hɔ͡ɚs/, is illustrated in Figure 3–52. It is also in the words *sport, force,* and *gorge.* The onglide for /ɔ͡ɚ/ is mid back rounded and lax and the offglide is mid central rounded rhotic and tense. The onglide for [ɔ͡ɚ] is

produced with the highest part of the tongue raised slightly toward the soft palate. For a tongue tip offglide, the highest point of the tongue moves anteriorly toward the back of the hard palate, with the back edges of the tongue touching the molars and the tongue tip raised slightly toward the alveolar ridge. If [ɔ͡ɚ] is produced with a tongue bunched rhotic, the offglide is produced with the tongue shifted slightly forward so it is raised toward the back of the hard palate. The back edges of the tongue touch the molars and the tongue tip is down. The lips move from rounded to slightly rounded during the [ɔ͡ɚ] production.

/ɑ͡ɚ/ The rhotic diphthong in *art,* transcribed /ɑ͡ɚt/, is illustrated in Figure 3–53. It is also in the words *shark, party,* and *farm.* The onglide for /ɑ͡ɚ/ is low back and unrounded and the offglide is mid central rounded rhotic. The onglide for [ɑ͡ɚ] is produced with the mandible lowered and the tongue low but with the highest part of it raised toward the soft palate. For a tongue tip offglide, the tongue is raised midway toward the back of the hard palate, with the sides of the tongue coming close to the molars and with the tongue tip raised slightly toward the alveolar ridge. If [ɑ͡ɚ] is produced with a tongue bunched rhotic, the offglide is produced with the tongue raising midway and anteriorly toward the back of the hard palate and with the back edges of the tongue touching the back molars. For both [ɑ͡ɚ] productions, the lips

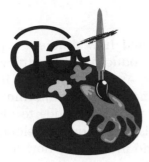

FIGURE 3–53. Mnemonic visualization of the rhotic diphthong /ɑɚ/.

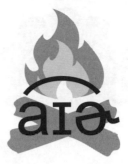

FIGURE 3–54. Mnemonic visualization of the rhotic triphthong /aɪɚ/.

move from unrounded during the onglide to a slightly rounded posture for the offglide.

Rhotic Triphthongs

Rhotic triphthongs are phonemic diphthongs followed by the offglide schwar, represented by the phonetic symbol [ɚ]. The onglide diphthong and the offglide are connected with a ligature to emphasize their single vowel property. In addition to phonetic symbols and key words, the articulation of each of the rhotic triphthongs is described below, including the onglide diphthong and the [ɚ] offglide.

/aɪɚ/ The rhotic triphthong in *fire*, transcribed /faɪɚ/, is illustrated in Figure 3–54. It is also in the words *higher, liar,* and *choir.* The onglide for /aɪɚ/ starts low central and unrounded, glides to a high front unrounded position, and then ends with the mid back rounded rhotic offglide. The triphthong [aɪɚ] is produced with the highest part of the tongue low in the mouth below the center of the hard palate, with the mandible slightly lowered. The onglide is followed by movement of the tongue body forward and upward in the oral cavity. For a tongue tip offglide, the tongue is lowered slightly and moves posteriorly toward the hard palate, with the sides of the tongue touching the molars and with the tongue tip raised slightly toward the alveolar ridge. If [aɪɚ] is produced with a tongue bunched rhotic, the offglide is produced with the highest part of the tongue moving posteriorly and lowering

slightly beneath the back of the hard palate. The back edges of the tongue touch the back molars. For both [aɪɚ] productions, the lips move from unrounded to spread through the first two positions to a slightly rounded posture for the offglide rhotic. Note that we transcribe the rhotic triphthong [aɪɚ] if a word is spoken as one syllable. If a word like *fire* is said as two syllables, it would be transcribed as the CV.V word [faɪ.ɚ].

/aʊɚ/ The rhotic triphthong in *flower*, transcribed /flaʊɚ/, is illustrated in Figure 3–55. It is also in the words *showers, power,* and *hour.* The onglide for /aʊɚ/ is low central and unrounded, then glides to a high back rounded position and ends as a mid central rounded rhotic offglide. The triphthong [aʊɚ] starts with the highest part of the tongue low in the mouth below the back of the hard palate, with the mandible slightly lowered. This posture is followed by raising the tongue body posteriorly to below the soft palate. For a tongue tip offglide, the tongue is lowered slightly and moves toward the back of the hard palate, with the back edges of the tongue touching the molars and with the tongue tip raised slightly toward the alveolar ridge. If [aʊɚ] is produced with a tongue bunched rhotic, the offglide is produced with the highest part of the tongue moving slightly forward and lowered, so the highest point in the tongue is below the back of the hard palate. The back edges of the tongue

FIGURE 3–55. Mnemonic visualization of the rhotic triphthong /aʊ&/.

touch the back molars. For both [aʊ&] productions, the lips move from unrounded through the onglide to a rounded position and to a less rounded posture for the offglide rhotic. Note that a word is produced with the rhotic triphthong [aʊ&] if spoken as one syllable. If a word like *shower* is said as two syllables, it would be transcribed as the CV.V word [ʃaʊ.&], with a diphthong followed by an unstressed schwar rather than a triphthong rhotic.

? | 3–8. Did You Get It?

1. The difference between rhotic vowels and other vowels is _____.

2. There are three types of rhotic vowels. These include one _____, five _____, and two _____.

3. A unique quality of rhotic vowels is the touching of the _____ of the tongue to the _____.

4. Cross out the words that do not contain a monophthong rhotic.

   churn   scour   word   flair   hire   purred

Summary

We have covered how different types of vowels are defined, produced, and written phonetically in this chapter. As a clinician, it is important that you not only memorize this information, but learn how to apply your knowledge to identifying and transcribing disordered and developmental speech and to teaching individuals how to produce these vowels.

Early in this chapter, we introduced you to vowel production by superimposing a vowel quadrilateral on a sagittal view of the vocal tract to illustrate tongue postures during vowel production. When not placed over the sagittal view, the vowel quadrilateral serves as a schematic depicting approximate tongue positions during vowel production, with high/mid/low phonetic symbols placed top to bottom and front/central/back phonetic symbols placed left to right. We can also depict lip rounding on a vowel quadrilateral via shading. In sections where more than one vowel is represented, the more centralized vowel is the lax vowel phoneme, whereas the vowels presented on the outer edges of the quadrilateral are the tense cognates. This schematic is useful for learning vowel properties.

Figure 3–56 is a vowel quadrilateral of English monophthongs. It provides you a visual representation of English phonemes and their tongue height, tongue advancement, lip rounding, and tension for these steady state vowels.

The vowel quadrilateral in Figure 3–57 shows production of diphthongs using arrows to depict the movement from the onglide to the offglide positions. Note that the nonphonemic diphthongs are also shown here.

Figure 3–58 is a vowel quadrilateral for the English rhotic diphthongs and triphthongs. Note that all rhotics in Figure 3–58 end in approximately the same place on the vowel quadrilateral, because all of them end with r-coloring.

Table 3–1 displays the non-Latin alphabetic symbols needed to transcribe English vowel phonemes. These symbols parallel those in Table 2–8 for consonants. For diphthongs, you can insert a code for each symbol in the diphthong, ending with the combining diacritic marker "inverted breve" to connect the symbols.

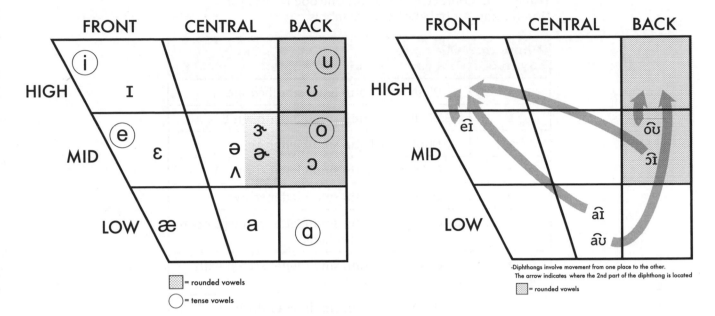

FIGURE 3–56. Vowel quadrilateral for English monophthongs.

FIGURE 3–57. Vowel quadrilateral for English diphthongs, with arrows indicating the moving articulation.

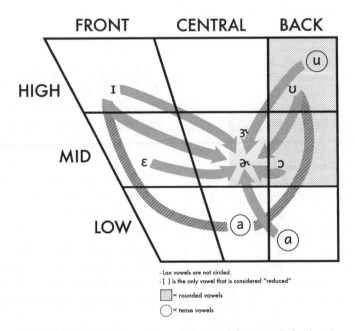

FIGURE 3–58. Vowel quadrilateral for English rhotic diphthongs and triphthongs, with arrows indicating the moving articulation during their production

TABLE 3–1. Character Codes and Unicode Names for Non-Roman Alphabetic Vowel Symbols

Phonetic Symbol	Character Code	Unicode Name
ɪ	026A	Latin letter small capital I
ɛ	025B	Latin small letter open E
æ	00E6	Latin small letter Ae
ʌ	028C	Latin small letter turned V
ə	0259	Latin small letter schwa
ɝ	025D	Latin small letter reversed open E with hook
ɚ	025A	Latin small letter schwa with hook
ʊ	028A	Latin small letter upsilon
ɔ	0254	Latin small letter open O
ɑ	0251	Latin small letter alpha
◌̑	0311	Combining inverted breve

Putting It All Together

As we saw at the beginning of this chapter, there are lots of ways to spell English vowels orthographically, and English spelling is not completely systematic. In this chapter, you learned a one-to-one symbol-to-sound system of transcribing English vowels phonetically. This single sound-symbol system makes it easy to capture spoken speech as a speech-language pathologist and to communicate speech errors to other professionals. Replacing the English alphabet with an internationally recognized phonetic system might make spelling easier to learn. Many phoneticians in the past few centuries have advocated for English to move to a phonetic spelling system, but to no avail.

You have learned a lot about vowel articulation for English in this chapter. It may feel overwhelming, but take the time to learn the information. It is critical that you memorize how to produce, define, and transcribe all of these vowels. You also need extensive practice transcribing written and spoken English. You can start by transcribing the written word as shown in this textbook. However, as a clinical scientist, you will need lots of practice transcribing English as spoken by monolingual English-speaking adults, individuals who have learned English as a second language, children who are still developing their speech sound system, and children and adults who have speech sound disorders.

? 3-9. Did You Get It?

1. Using the vowel quadrilateral, define the following monophthong vowels by tongue height, tongue advancement, lip rounding, and tenseness, if needed.

/i/ _____

/u/ _____

/ʌ/ _____

/ɑ/ _____

/ɝ/ _____

/æ/ _____

2. Which diphthongs are described below?

a. Low central unrounded onglide to high front unrounded offglide:

   _____

b. Mid central back rounded onglide to high front unrounded offglide:

   _____

Applied Science: Revisited

Summary

Now that you know how to transcribe English vowels, let's revisit the poem stanza we began our chapter with.

Beware of heard, a dreadful word

That looks like beard and sounds like bird.

And dead; it's said like bed, not bead.

For goodness sake, don't call it deed!

Watch out for meat and great and threat,

(They rhyme with suite and straight and debt).

One Step at a Time

Did you find the four vowel sounds that are spelled numerous ways in this poem? And other ways of spelling the vowel sounds in English? Now that you can transcribe these sounds, spell each word with the phonetic symbol that represents it.

#1:   Vowel:

   /ɝ/

   Spelled Differently in the Words:

   h**ear**d, w**or**d, b**ir**d

Examples of Other Spellings of /ɝ/:

   c**ure**d, st**ir**red

Phonetic Transcription of /ɝ/ Words:

   heard: /hɝd/

   word: /wɝd/

   bird: /bɝd/

   cured: /kjɝd/

   stirred: /stɝd/

#2:   Vowel:

   /ɛ/

Spelled Differently in the Words:

   d**ea**d, b**e**d, thr**ea**t, d**e**bt

Examples of Other Spellings of /ɛ/:

   j**eo**pardy, m**a**ny, fri**e**nd, h**ei**fer, s**ai**d

Phonetic Transcription of /ɛ/ Words:

   dead: /dɛd/

   bed: /bɛd/

   threat: /θɹɛt/

   debt: /dɛt/

   jeopardy: /dʒɛ.pɚ.di/

many: /mɛ.ni/
friend: /fɹɛnd/
heifer: /hɛ.fɚ/
said: /sɛd/

#3:   Vowel

/i/

Spelled Differently in the Words:
bead, deed, meat, suite

Examples of Other Spellings of /i/:
receipt, we, gene, field, baby, key

Phonetic Transcription of /i/ Words:

bead: /bid/
deed: /did/
meat: /mit/
suite: /swit/
receipt: /ɹi.sit/
we: /wi/
gene: /dʒin/
piece: /pis/
baby: /beɪ.bi/
key: /ki/

#4:   Vowel

/e/ (described below as produced with
the diphthong [eɪ])

Spelled Differently in the Words:
great, straight

Examples of Other Spellings of [eɪ]:
fate, day, lei, main, weigh

Phonetic Transcription of [eɪ] Words:

great: [gɹeɪt]
straight: [stɹeɪt]
fate: [feɪt]
day: [deɪ]
lei: [leɪ]
main: [meɪn]
weigh: [weɪ]

Science Applied

You just experienced that English spelling is as varied for vowel sounds as it is for consonant sounds. Luckily, you now know how to capture all of the different English vowel sounds using phonetic symbols that are unambiguous. Study the information regarding the production of vowels, as well as the phonetic symbols that represent them so that you can become adept at the skill of transcribing. We promise that this knowledge and skill will serve you well in your clinical and research work as a speech-language pathologist or audiologist.

Interest Piqued?

Recommended materials to further your understanding of topics covered in this chapter.

Print Resources

Ladefoged, P., & Disner, S. F. (2012). *Vowels and consonants* (3rd ed.). Malden, MA: Blackwell.

McLeod, S., & Singh, S. (2009). *Seeing speech: A quick guide to speech sounds*. San Diego, CA: Plural.

Online Resources

http://www.academic.muohio.edu/ipaarcade/learning.htm
Some IPA games for the phone.

http://ipa.typeit.org

Be sure to use the IPA symbols keyboard to make it easier to type phonetic symbols.

http://soundsofspeech.uiowa.edu/english/english.html

Use this website to select the properties of a vowel and then its phonetic symbol to see and hear its production.

http://web.uvic.ca/ling/resources/ipa/charts/IPAlab/IPAlab.htm

This website connects phonetic symbols from the IPA chart to an audiofile of what the phonetic symbol sounds like.

http://www.youtube.com/watch?v=TyPGfBM9nNM&feature=youtu.be

A short video honoring the schwa!

? Did You Get It?

ANSWER KEY

3–1.

1. The four words below, labeled a–d, represent four different English vowels. Underneath the words are the words that represent the vowels spelled a number of different ways.

   a. though
      rope, foe, soul, sew, bowl, boat

   b. through
      few, fruit, moot, tune, move, soup

   c. bought
      fawn, mall, caught, dog, chalk

   d. rough
      shut, does, one, blood, stuff, come

3–2.

1. Vowels and consonants are similar in their use of these three components of the speech system: respiratory, oro-nasal, phonatory

2. The production of vowels and consonants differ primarily in the amount of obstruction during articulation.

3–3.

1. In this section, we introduced two types of vowels. These are steady-state vowels, called monophthongs, and dynamic, changing vowels, called diphthongs.

2. What do we call vowels that end with r-coloring? Rhotics

3. A monophthong vowel can be described in four ways. These are tongue height, tongue advancement, lip rounding, tenseness.

3–4.

1. All front vowels are made with the highest part of the tongue raised toward the anterior part of the oral cavity.

2. Front vowels differ in tongue height and tension but share lip rounding and tongue advancement.

3. Which words below contain front vowels?
   bake   book   bee   best   boot   bat

4. Cross out the words that do not contain front vowels.
   kept   ship   ~~rope~~   ~~swerve~~   knack   thief

3–5.

1. Central vowels are made with the highest part of the tongue raised toward the <u>mid central</u> part of the oral cavity.

2. Which words below contain central vowels?

   <u>hut</u> <u>tough</u> book ball <u>dove</u> <u>flood</u>

3. Cross out the words that do not contain the mid central unrounded nonrhotic lax vowel:

   ~~suit~~ suds ~~could~~ plush ~~con~~ love

4. Say the words below aloud. Differentiate the stressed and unstressed central vowel that is in boldface in the two-syllable words below. To do so, circle stressed [ʌ] and underline unstressed [u].

   c(u)tting   <u>a</u>gain   min<u>u</u>te

   s(u)nny   b<u>e</u>lieve   beg(u)n

3–6.

1. All back vowels are made with the highest part of the tongue raised toward the <u>posterior</u> part of the oral cavity.

2. In English all high back and mid back vowels share the category of <u>roundness</u>.

3. Underline the words below that contain back vowels.

   <u>push</u> <u>stoop</u> <u>flute</u> <u>coke</u> <u>though</u> <u>shop</u>

4. Cross out the words that do not contain back vowels.

   stool ~~sat~~ rope bog taught ~~fun~~

3–7.

1. Monophthong vowels are produced with a steady-state production. Diphthong vowels are produced with a <u>dynamic state</u>.

2. If a diphthong vowel does not change meaning if you produce only the onglide, it is called a <u>nonphonemic</u> diphthong.

3. The two parts of the diphthong are called the <u>onglide</u> and the <u>offglide</u>.

4. Cross out the words that do not contain diphthong vowels.

   sound ploy cake ~~fawn~~ blow ~~seep~~

5. Below are words containing phonemic and nonphonemic diphthongs. Circle the phonemic diphthongs.

   raise <u>couch</u> <u>fly</u> mow <u>moist</u> <u>might</u>

3–8.

1. The difference between rhotic vowels and other vowels is <u>r-coloring</u>.

2. There are three types of rhotic vowels. These include one <u>monophthong</u>, five <u>diphthongs</u>, and two <u>triphthongs</u>.

3. A unique quality of rhotic vowels is the touching of the back edges of the tongue to the back molars.

4. Cross out the words that do not contain a monophthong rhotic.

   churn ~~scour~~ word ~~flair~~ ~~hire~~ purred

3–9.

1. Using the vowel quadrilateral, define the following monophthong vowels by tongue height, tongue advancement, lip rounding, and tenseness, if needed.

   /i/ high, front, unrounded, tense

   /u/ high, back, rounded, tense

   /ʌ/ mid, central, unrounded, lax

   /ɑ/ low, back, unrounded, tense

   /ɝ/ mid, central, rounded, tense

   /æ/ low, front, unrounded, lax

2. Which diphthongs are described below?

   a. Low central unrounded onglide to high front unrounded offglide: [aɪ]

   b. Mid central back rounded onglide to high front unrounded offglide: [ɔɪ]

4

BROAD AND NARROW PHONETIC TRANSCRIPTION

Learning Objectives

By reading this chapter, you will learn:

1. the meaning of listener- and speaker-oriented approaches to phonetic transcription

2. different types and systems of phonetic transcription

3. how to complete a broad phonetic transcription

4. strategies for increasing your transcription proficiency

5. how to complete a narrow phonetic transcription using diacritical symbols

6. diacritical symbols for transcribing disordered speech

Applied Science

You are a speech-language pathologist who for three years has been treating a five-year-old boy with a moderate speech sound disorder. The boy's mother approaches you with concerns about a possible speech disorder in her 2½-year-old daughter. When you question the mother about her concerns, she reports that her daughter "is not saying the final consonants on words." The mother cites examples of her daughter saying "ca" for *cat*, "my" for *mine*, and "ju" for *juice*. The mother is worried because her son produced those kinds of errors when he was younger, and she is fearful that her daughter may be showing signs of having a speech sound disorder.

You offer to see the child for a speech screening. During the screening, you have a wide variety of toys for the child to play with that have names with final consonants. The daughter is easy to engage in play and you obtain a speech sam-

ple that the mother says is representative of her speech and language. When you phonetically transcribe the sample, you note that the child produces developmentally appropriate speech sounds and uses them correctly, except in word-final position. Examples include the child saying [hæ] for /hæt/, [tʌ] for /tʌb/, [bʊ] for /bʊk/, [ma] for /mam/, and [bu] for /bum/. You also heard something different in the vowel sounds that you cannot quite explain. You show the complete list of misarticulated words to a colleague for a second opinion and she requests to listen to the audiotaped speech sample. After listening to the sample, your colleague confidently tells you not to be overly concerned about the child's misarticulations, because she predicts that the daughter soon should be producing word-final consonants. What could your colleague have heard that you did not, to predict this outcome?

Phonetic Transcription: Approaches, Types, and Systems of Representation

Congratulations, you are armed now with valuable knowledge of the phonetic symbols for the consonants and vowels in American English—in other words, you possess the basic tools to phonetically transcribe speech. But before you grab a pencil (with a good eraser) and set off to transcribe a speech sample, you want to first identify your purpose for transcribing that particular speech sample. You will be on your way to understanding the range of possible purposes after you have read this chapter, because you will learn different approaches to phonetic transcription, as well as different types of transcription

and when to use each one. You also will learn the different representation systems that are available to help you achieve your transcription goals.

Approaches to Phonetic Transcription

The first question you want to ask yourself prior to beginning to transcribe is, "What is the purpose of this transcription?" As shown in Figure 4–1, there are two possible responses to this question. One reason to transcribe a speech sample is to capture on paper the words you heard said by transcribing the phonemes in the words. This is known as taking a listener-orientation. The listener-oriented approach is used to transcribe the words the speaker pro-

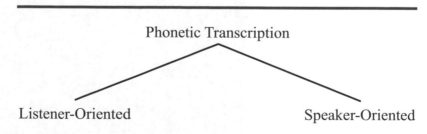

FIGURE 4–1. Approaches to phonetic transcription.

duced, with a focus on the meaning of the message. Another approach is to try to capture the articulatory movements of the speaker; this is known as taking a speaker-orientation. A speaker-orientation is used when you want to know how the person used his or her respiratory, phonatory, resonatory, and/or articulatory systems to produce speech. As a speaker-oriented transcriber, you are trying to figure out how the individual articulated the speech sounds in the words that were produced, sometimes down to the tiniest phonetic details. When would a speech-language pathologist choose to use one approach over the other?

You typically would employ the listener-orientation approach when you want to record the words produced by a speaker for whom you have no prior reason to be concerned about articulation and/or when you want to use a transcription to assess the speaker's language skills. In these cases, it is not even necessary that the sample be phonetically transcribed; however, you may do this to derive cursory information about the individual's speech sound system, in addition to the language system. This approach would not be time-effective for individuals referred with speech concerns.

Another time that you might employ a listener-oriented approach to transcription is when a client struggles to achieve the precise articulation of a particular speech sound after being in intervention for a prolonged period of time. In such cases, you may decide to focus on how the productions sound, rather than how they are articulated. If a phone sounds "close enough" to the target sound, then you may not worry about the articulatory dimensions of the production, instead, you may focus on the perceptual aspects of it. In our experience, this situation happens most commonly when clients exhibit persistent errors on later-mastered sounds that can be articulated using different places and gestures of articulation, such as for the phones [s] and [ɹ].

Alternatively, you likely would employ the speaker-orientation approach when you transcribe disordered speech. A speech-language pathologist's goal is to figure out exactly how an individual is articulating speech to understand and help correct misarticulations. A speech-language pathologist phonetically transcribes a speech sample and then analyzes it in several ways. The speech-language pathologist first wants to identify all the consonants, vowels, and word shapes a client produced. The speech-language pathologist then compares target word productions to the client's productions, noting errors in consonants, vowels, and word shapes, and tries to identify patterns to those errors. The level of detail that you seek can differ from client to client; therefore, you need to ask yourself how much phonetic detail you need in your transcriptions to be able to treat a client with a speech sound disorder. In the listener-oriented approach, only surface-level phonetic information is needed, while in the speaker-oriented approach, gradations of phonetic information are needed. You will employ different types of phonetic transcription to achieve the goal of each transcription.

Types of Phonetic Transcription

The type of phonetic transcription you utilize is dependent in part on the type of sample you are transcribing. If you are transcribing the phonemes of a word, that is, the mental representation of the word, then you will complete a **systematic transcription**. In contrast, if you are transcribing someone's actual speech, that is, the way in which a person articulated a word, then you will complete an **impressionistic transcription**. Remember from Chapter 1 that when you complete a phonemic transcription, you place your transcriptions in-between virgules (i.e., / /), resulting in a phonemic transcription of the word *hat*, for example, as /hæt/. Alternatively, when you transcribe utterances as spoken, you place your transcriptions in-between brackets (i.e., [ ]), resulting in, for example, an infant's babbling transcribed as [ba.ba.ba].

Transcribing the speech of clients with moderate and severe speech sound disorders can be challenging for speech-language pathologists because those clients often misarticulate sounds in unique ways. Speech-language pathologists often try to capture as much articulatory detail as they can in their attempt to understand how a client produces speech. When a speech-language pathologist is interested in capturing articulatory detail across phonetic dimensions, he or she makes small marks on, above, under, and to the side of consonant and vowel phonetic symbols. These small marks are called **diacritics**. You will learn about diacritical marks for typical and disordered speech, as well as their uses, later in this chapter.

Up to this point, we have discussed the types of transcription completed on utterances in a language that we understand. There are times, though, when we may need to transcribe utterances produced by a speaker of a language we do not know or by an infant in the pre-verbal stage. In these instances, we would complete an impressionistic transcription. Think for a moment about the amount of phonetic detail you would need to capture in these types of utterances. Do you think you would need to pay a little or a lot of attention to phonetic detail? If you do not know which sounds are phonemes, which are allophones, and which are extraneous nonspeech sounds, then you would need to transcribe all the sounds you hear. Impressionistic transcriptions are filled with articulatory detail so you can figure out which sounds and sound variations are and are not linguistically important.

Do speech-language pathologists ever use impressionistic transcriptions, and if so, when? The short answer to this question is yes. Many speech-language pathologists generate phonetically detailed impressionistic transcriptions. Speech-language pathologists transcribing a foreign language or English influenced by a second language in a client who is bilingual, or those working with high-risk infants and toddlers, benefit from knowing how to complete highly detailed transcriptions. From our own clinical experiences, we have used our impressionistic transcription skills when a new baby is born into a family that has a child already diagnosed with a particular type of speech sound disorder called childhood apraxia of speech (CAS), a severe and persistent type of speech sound disorder. As speech-language pathologists, we periodically transcribe the infant's early vocal development in fine phonetic detail to monitor his or her development. In these cases, it is vital not only to know how to capture the infant's consonant-like and vowel-like productions, but also to know how to capture the infant's use of the respiratory, phonatory, and resonatory systems for vocal production, as these components of the speech system also are affected by CAS. If early signs of CAS are present, we can intervene early to stimulate vocal and verbal productions.

Systems of Phonetic Representation

To make a final determination of the type of phonetic transcription you will complete on a speech sample, you will need to decide which aspects of the speech system you are interested in learning about and capturing using phonetic symbols. As shown in Figure 4–2, there are two areas of the speech system that we will consider: **segmental** and **suprasegmental**. When we are interested in understanding an individual's production and use of consonants, vowels, and sequences of consonants and vowels, we need to know the segmental symbol sets. These sets include the phonetic symbols for consonants and vowels, as well as the symbols specifying various ways to articulate consonants and vowels. When we need to understand an individual's production and use of suprasegmentals, including pitch, intonation, stress, loudness, and rate of speech, among others, we need to know the suprasegmental symbol sets. You already have learned the symbol to note the edges of syllables (i.e., [.]), so you are off to a good start. While there are other symbol sets to mark suprasegmentals (e.g., Voice Quality Symbols), no single symbol set has been widely adopted; therefore, you may find yourself improvising notations to be able to mark those aspects of the speech system that concern you. For children with certain types of speech sound disorders, suprasegmental aspects of speech production can be highly informative and differentially diagnostic.

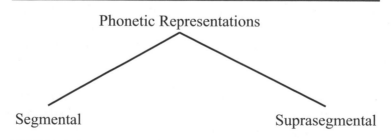

FIGURE 4–2. Systems of phonetic representations.

? 4–1. Did You Get It?

1. A speech-language pathologist interested in capturing a client's tongue placement and precise movements during articulation of words containing /s/ would employ a _____-oriented approach to transcribing.

2. A speech-language pathologist who wants to determine how many of a client's spoken words he or she can understand would employ a _____-oriented approach to transcribing.

Circle the correct word in the following sentences.

3. When transcribing a speech sample in a language you do not speak or understand, your transcription will be impressionistic/systematic in nature.

4. When transcribing the target words included on a test of articulation, your transcription will be impressionistic/systematic in nature.

Circle the type of phonetic representation system you would use for each of the following scenarios.

5. A teacher reports that a student in his class speaks with a monotone voice. You need to note intonation when you transcribe the student's speech. You would use a segmental/suprasegmental representation system.

6. You want to transcribe how a child articulated each consonant phoneme in a list of words. You would use a segmental/suprasegmental representation system.

Broad Segmental Phonetic Transcription

In this section, we will provide strategies so you can successfully transcribe words of increasing length and complexity. Your initial goal should be focused on accurately capturing the consonants and vowels as spoken by a speaker. To help you achieve this goal, we first will increase your ability to accurately transcribe segments in words as you pronounce them. You will use these skills when you complete more detailed transcriptions of your own and others' speech later in this chapter.

To become an accurate phonetic transcriber, you will need to apply the fundamental information that was covered in the first three chapters of this textbook. Those fundamental skills include correctly counting the number of syllables and sounds in words; identifying each consonant by its place, manner, and voicing classifications; reading and writing each consonant phonetic symbol; identifying each vowel by its height, advancement, and rounding classifications; and reading and writing each vowel phonetic symbol. Do not wait to learn this information—do it now. A commitment to learning the information thoroughly will make acquiring the skill of phonetic transcription easier. To aid in this effort, we will share strategies that our students have found helpful, as well as list orthographic combinations that frequently confuse them.

Strategies to Employ

1. As a beginning transcriber, make it a habit to count the number of sounds in a word and jot that number down next to the word *before* you transcribe it. Also, jot down the number of syllables the word has. After you have transcribed the word, look to see if the number of phonetic symbols matches the number of segments you said were in the word. Then see if the number of vowel phonetic symbols matches the number of syllables you said were in the word. If you have a discrepancy between any pair of numbers, double-check your transcription. It will be time well spent, and you will be amazed at how many errors you catch by employing this simple strategy.

2. After you have transcribed a word, compare the number of vowel symbols with the number of syllables in the word. These two numbers should match.

3. Hone your ability to hear speech sounds, as opposed to seeing letters. The orthographic spellings will confuse and confound you—so conquer any tendency to focus on the spelling of a word. For example, when transcribing a list of written words, read a word and then cover it up before you transcribe it, repeating the word silently or aloud as you transcribe. And then resist the urge to look at the written word again; instead, read your own phonetic transcriptions to recall each word.

4. Try hard to say each word as naturally as you can. Beginning transcribers tend to exaggerate and stretch out each word's pronunciation, which can lead to incorrect transcriptions. Take for example a word ending in a rounded vowel. When you stretch out the articulation of a rounded vowel, often you hear a glide consonant at the end, which could result, for example, in you incorrectly transcribing the word *who* as [ˈhu.wə].

5. Make lists of rhyming words to help increase your focus on the vowel rather than the vowel's spelling. Some strings of rhyming words all look and sound similar, such as *bat-cat-hat-mat*, all containing [æ], and *did-hid-kid-lid*, all containing [ɪ]. However, many strings look very different, such as *mate-bait-weight-straight*, all containing [eɪ], and *beau-go-glow-sew-whoa*, all containing [oʊ]. Pairing the vowels [eɪ] and [oʊ], for example, with all their different spellings, will help increase your auditory skills, which in turn will help your phonetic transcription skills.

6. Make lists of one-syllable words that are spelled with more letters than the words have sounds. For example, the words *push*, *still*, *back*, *hymn*, *comb*, *sneeze*, and *who* all have more letters than sounds. Practice transcribing them.

7. Make lists of words that have sounds without the expected orthographic spelling. Examples include *one, beauty, ax, few,* and *candle.* Practice transcribing them.

8. Practice transcribing every day. Write your to-do lists phonetically. Practice writing your own and others' names phonetically. Take class notes using phonetic symbols. Transcribe the things that you see while waiting in lines or for an appointment. Read letters and transcribe the sounds they make. Download a phonetics game app and play often. Download a phonetics keyboard and write your texts phonetically, tossing in an emoji ☺ so your recipients can get the gist of your messages!

9. When beginning to transcribe words, it can be beneficial to recall some of the spelling and reading rules you learned in grade school or in your English as a Second Language course, as simplistic as they were. The problem is, of course, that spelling and reading are not simplistic to learn at all, because there are too many exceptions to those rules. Nonetheless, just as those phonics rules were helpful when you were first learning to spell and read in English, it can help to recall some of those rules when you first start to transcribe. The phonics rules remind us to think about the sounds in words and not the letters. A few examples follow.

   ■ When a word has two consecutive vowels, the second vowel is often silent. Examples include *beat, wait,* and *boat.*
   To help you remember that even though two vowels are in the spelling of the word, typically only one vowel sound—the first one—is articulated; therefore, only one vowel is transcribed.

   ■ When one or more vowels is paired with "r," a new vowel sound is created. Examples include *deer, dare,* and *door.*
   To help you remember that a post-vocalic "r" typically is part of the vowel sound and is not a separate consonant sound.

   ■ When "c" and "g" are followed by "e," "i," and "y," they make soft sounds. Examples include *celery, city,* and *cycle,* and *gem, giraffe,* and *gym.*
   To help you remember that the letter "c" can represent the phoneme /s/ or /k/ and the letter "g" can represent /dʒ/ or /g/.

■ When "e" is the last letter in a syllable that has only one other vowel, the "e" is silent.

Examples include *ate*, *woke*, and *incite*.

To help you remember that even though you see two vowels in a word, you articulate only one; therefore, you transcribe only one.

Errors to Avoid

There are several phonetic transcription "tricky spots" where beginning students often struggle. Eight of these tricky spots include transcribing: (1) letters that are not phonetic symbols; (2) letters that do not represent a phoneme in one language but represent a phoneme in another language; (3) words spelled with capital letters; (4) morphosyntactic word endings for regular past tense verbs; (5) morphosyntactic word endings for regular plurals, possessives, and verbs; (6) words that end with the letters "s" and "z"; (7) consonant digraphs and clusters; and (8) vowel digraphs and diphthongs. Below are ideas for how to avoid making these common transcription errors.

1. There is a short list of only four consonant letters that are not used as phonetic symbols in American English. Memorize this list and check your transcriptions to be certain that you did not use any of them. If you did, then transcribe those sounds using the correct phonetic symbols. Can you think of which four letters they are? The consonant letters that are not used are "c," "q," "x," and "y."

2. Be mindful that a letter that does not represent a phoneme in one language may represent a phoneme in another language. For example, the letter "y" is not a phonetic symbol in American English; however, it is a phonetic symbol in languages such as French, where it represents a high front rounded vowel. Even slight variations to phonetic symbols can indicate a different phone or phoneme, so write them carefully.

3. Capitalization rules are not used in the phonetic alphabet. When transcribing

a word that begins with a capital letter, do not capitalize its phonetic symbol. For example, the words *brook*, as in a stream, and *Brooke*, as in someone's name, both would be transcribed as /bɹʊk/. Transcribing the name *Brooke* as /ʙʊk/ would be incorrect. (Interestingly, in this particular example, capitalizing the phoneme /b/ as /B/ could be confused for the phonetic symbol called bilabial trill, /ʙ/, or the phonetic symbol called bilabial fricative, /β/; both of these symbols represent phonemes in other languages. This is another reminder that so far you have learned only a subset of the international phonetic symbols, so be mindful when using and writing them.)

4. When a verb ends with the regular past tense "ed" morphosyntactic morpheme (i.e., the "ed" suffix is relevant to grammar), there are rules for pronouncing it as [t] or [d]. When the phoneme immediately preceding the suffix "ed" is /t/ or /d/, as in the verbs *wait* (/wct/) and *wade* (/wed/), we create a second syllable, as in *waited* and *waded*, and pronounce the words as disyllables. The suffix "ed" will be produced as [əd], as in ['weɪ.təd] and ['weɪ.dəd], respectively. When the phoneme before the "ed" morpheme is voiceless, the "ed" will be produced as voiceless [t]. For example, to make the verbs *clap* and *watch* past tense, we add "ed" to the end of each word, creating *clapped* and *watched*. Because the [p] in *clap* and the [t͡ʃ] in *watch* are voiceless phones, both words are pronounced with word-final [t], as in [klæpt] and [wat͡ʃt]. On the other hand, when the sound preceding the morpheme "ed" is voiced, then "ed" will be pronounced as [d]. For example, to make the verbs *hum* and *grab* past tense, we create *hummed* and *grabbed*. The phones [m] and [b] that precede the morpheme "ed" are both voiced; therefore, the pronunciations are [hʌmd] and [gɹæbd].

5. Like words ending with regular past tense "ed," when a word ends with an "s" morphosyntactic morpheme, there also

are pronunciation rules. This is true if the morpheme "s" marks plurality (e.g., *cats*), possession (e.g., *Bob's*), or verb tense (e.g., *swims*). When the sound immediately preceding the morpheme "s" is voiceless, the "s" will be produced as voiceless [s]. For example, to make the words *bat* and *cliff* plural, we add an "s" to the end of both words, creating *bats* and *cliffs*. Both words are pronounced with word-final [s], because "t" in *bat* and "f" in *cliff* are voiceless sounds. However, when the sound preceding the morpheme "s" is voiced, then the letter "s" will be pronounced as [z]. For example, the verbs *run* and *hide* in third person present tense are *runs* and *hides*. The phones [n] and [d] that precede the suffix "s" are both voiced; therefore, the pronunciations are [ɹʌnz] and [haɪdz]. There also are times when the morpheme "s" creates an additional final syllable, as in the words *buses*, *Mitch's*, and *fizzes*. These are words that end in a sibilant fricative or an affricate. In these cases, the final sound always is pronounced as [z], because a vowel, which is voiced, precedes the final fricative, as in ['bʌ.sɪz], ['mɪ.t͡ʃɪz], and ['fɪ.zɪz].

6. For words ending in nonmorphosyntactic "s" (e.g., *bus*), "ss" (e.g., *bass*), or "s" + silent "e" (e.g., *base*), there is no way to know from the orthographic spelling of the word if "s" is typically pronounced as [s] or [z], which often results in errors in transcription. The only way to know if [s] or [z] is the word-final target is to say the word using both productions. For example, is the word *hearse* articulated with final [s] or [z]? To help you determine the accurate pronunciation, say the word both ways, once with word-final [s] and once with word-final [z]. In this example, productions would be [hɝs] and [hɝz]. Listen carefully to both productions as you say the two versions. In cases where the word meaning actually changes with the different productions, as in the word pair [hɝs] (i.e., *hearse*) and [hɝz] (i.e., *hers*), it will be easier to differentiate that final sound. Some other

word pairs that create two different words that you could use to practice include *bus-buzz, peace-peas, hiss-his, Miss-Ms., mace-maze, police-please, lice-lies, dice-dies, loose-lose, pace-pays, fleece-fleas, lease-Lee's,* and *face-phase*. The second word in each of these word pairs is articulated with a final [z]. One clever example of this confusion can be found on the bumper sticker that reads, "Give Peas a Chance," which is a sound play on two words, one ending in [s] and the other in [z].

Once you have become skilled at hearing the "s-z" difference in the above word pairs, try to determine the final sound in the words *was, because, tis, has, is, tease, whose, cause, does, hose,* and *fuse*. What is the final sound in these words? All these words end in [z]. Last, listen carefully to your articulation of the italicized word in these two sentences: *A pencil is put to good <u>use</u> when transcribing* and *It's good to <u>use</u> a pencil when transcribing*. Can you hear the difference between [jus] in the first sentence and [juz] in the second sentence? If so, good job! If not, keep working at it and with practice, it will become easier to hear. Importantly, stay tuned: there is a reason why the final alveolar fricative [z] is difficult to differentiate from [s] at the ends of words. It is part of a phenomenon that we will discuss in Chapter 7.

7. Transcribing sequences of abutting consonants can also be tricky. Sometimes these sequences create consonant digraphs and other times they create consonant clusters. A consonant digraph is when two abutting consonants are produced as a single phoneme, as in the digraphs "wr" in *wreck* (i.e., [ɹɛk]) and "ss" in *mess* (i.e., [mɛs]). There also are **trigraphs** when three abutting consonants are articulated as one phoneme, as in "tch" in *watch* (i.e., [wat͡ʃ]). These consonants can be difficult to transcribe and again, your best strategy is to listen carefully and begin by counting the sounds you hear in a word. Do not be fooled by seeing multiple abutting letters and thinking that those letters represent multiple sounds.

Digraphs and trigraphs also are difficult for beginning transcribers when a consonant sequence represents a sound that is different from its actual letters. Examples include "sh" as in *ship*, "th" as in *think* and *that*, "ch" as in *chip*, "ph" as in *photo*, "gh" as in *rough*, "ng" as in *ring*, and "tch" as in *itch*. These letter combinations represent the single phones [ʃ], [θ], [ð], [t͡ʃ], [f], [f], [ŋ], and [t͡ʃ], respectively. The good news is that the above consonant combinations are used frequently, so learn those combinations and you will improve the overall accuracy of your transcriptions. The bad news is that this helpful hint does not always apply when the letter sequences are in the middle of words, such as in the words *mishap*, [ˈmɪs.hæp], "*anthill*," [ˈænt.hɪl], "*uphold*," [əp.ˈho͡ʊld], and "*ginger*," [ˈd͡ʒɪn.d͡ʒɚ], because the correct pronunciation requires that you articulate each of the abutting consonant sounds.

Differentiating voicing in a diagraph cognate pair can be difficult for beginning transcribers as well. Take, for example, the interdental fricative cognates /θ/ and /ð/. The best suggestions we have for helping you determine which phoneme is voiced and which is voiceless is to place your fingertips lightly on your larynx when you articulate each sound. If you feel vibrations, you know it is the voiced [ð] phone. The other suggestion is one we have suggested already, but it is worth repeating. Try saying the word you are transcribing one time with each of the different interdental phonemes inserted. For example, if you are having a difficult time deciding whether the word *thumb* begins with the voiceless or voiced interdental fricative, say the word both ways, as [θʌm] and [ðʌm]. You should be able to hear that the first production is correct when you contrast the productions. Another useful strategy for accurately transcribing the interdental cognates when they occur in word-initial position is related to their syntactic function. The phoneme /θ/ occurs in word-initial position in content words (such as nouns, verbs, and adjectives), whereas the phoneme /ð/ occurs in word-initial position in function words, such as *this*, *that*, and *the*.

There are other consonant sequences for which you articulate all the letters. These are called consonant clusters, as discussed in Chapter 2. There are many, many different clusters and they can occur in initial, medial, and final positions in words. Examples include "pl" in *play*, "st" in *mister*, and "mp" in bump. Clusters tend to be easier than digraphs for beginners to transcribe because each of the phonemes in clusters is usually represented by a phonetic symbol.

8. In addition to abutting consonants in words, there also are abutting vowels. Similar to some types of consonant strings, some of these vowel strings also create digraphs. In addition, vowel digraphs typically are articulated as single phonemes, and it typically is the first vowel in the sequence that is articulated. Take, for example, the words *meat*, *rain*, and *float*. The single vowel phone articulated in each of these words is the first vowel in each sequence, "ea" ([i]), "ai" ([e] or [e͡ɪ]), and "oa" ([o] or [o͡ʊ]); remember that diphthongs represent a single vowel sound. Of course, exceptions also apply to vowel digraphs, so try not to be fooled by vowel sequences that require that both vowels be articulated. For example, even though only one vowel phoneme is produced in the words *beat*, *mean*, and *seat*, those same sequences in the words *beatitude*, ([bi.ˈæ.tə.tud]), *meander*, ([mi.ˈæn.dɚ]), and *Seattle* ([si.ˈæ.təl]) require both vowels in the sequence to be articulated. Your strategy is to count the number of syllables and be certain that you have transcribed the same number of vowels as there are syllables.

Vowel strings also create diphthongs. As discussed in Chapter 3, diphthongs result when we rapidly sequence two vowel sounds to produce a single vowel phoneme, as in the words *shout* and *soil*. Review these vowel sequences to round out your practice sessions.

? 4–2. Did You Get It?

1. The words *seize, key, believe, meat* all contain which vowel? _____

2. Orthographically, write one word that has more alphabet letters than phonemes.

   _____

3. List one situation or routine that you take advantage of to practice transcribing every day.

   _____

   _____

4. The four consonants in the English alphabet that are not also phonetic symbols in English include _____, _____, _____, and _____.

5. The words *tries, dog's, buns* all end with the morpheme "s." How do you know that the morpheme "s" is produced as [z] in these words?

   _____

   _____

6. Is the final sound in these words typically produced as [s] or [z]?

   taxis _____ taxes _____ Texas _____

   axis _____ axes _____ access _____

7. Next to each of the following words, write whether the word contains a consonant digraph or a cluster.

   Example: echo <u>consonant digraph</u>

   a. shut _____

   b. skip _____

   c. cheese _____

   d. sound _____

8. Next to each of the following words, write whether the word contains a vowel digraph or a diphthong.

   Example: soil <u>vowel diphthong</u>

   a. beat _____

   b. caught _____

   c. height _____

   d. sound _____

Narrow Segmental Phonetic Transcription

It is at this point in the teaching of phonetics that we begin to turn many of the concepts we previously presented as black and white into shades of gray. We will start to shift away from basic ways of *describing* speech sound articulation and move toward complex and interactive ways of *understanding* it. Even though we presented the introductory and background information in Chapters 1 to 3 as being rudimentary in nature, we now will try to get you to see how complex these topics can be. For example, while you thought you understood the definition of a syllable, you soon will see that it is a little more complex than we initially led you to understand. Use the knowledge you already have built as a foundation for moving with us into the complexities of phonetics.

Hopefully you are seeing a noticeable improvement in your broad transcription skills by employing the strategies described earlier in this chapter, because we are increasing the difficulty by moving to narrow phonetic transcription next. You will complete a narrow phonetic transcription when you want to capture articulatory details, so you will love this practice if you thrive on detail. If you do not, then you will enjoy learning even more about the fascinating topic of how speech sounds can be produced, while maybe not enjoying learning all the additional symbols! We will first introduce two new phonetic symbols that are allophones in almost all the dialects of American English. We then will introduce a special set of symbols used to specify the articulation of a phoneme—either as the intended target production or as a speaker actually articulated the sound; we call these symbols diacritical marks.

Two Frequently Produced Consonant Allophones

As we begin to discuss subtle articulatory differences and how to capture those differences in your phonetic transcriptions, it is a good time to introduce you to two new consonant phonetic symbols that are used in American English: the **alveolar tap**, an allophone of /t/ and /d/, and the **glottal stop**, a sound that typically functions as an allophone of voiceless stops.

The alveolar tap phonetic symbol is the fish hook [ɾ] (Unicode character code 27e). We produce this sound by striking our tongue tip one time against our upper alveolar ridge. Articulation of a tap does not include a full obstruction and no burst of air accompanies its production as it does for the obstruents "t" and "d"; therefore, the tap is considered a sonorant sound. The alveolar tap occurs only in place of "t" or "d" when two conditions are met: (1) when /t/ or /d/ occurs in-between two vowels and (2) when the second vowel in the pair is unstressed. Examples of words meeting these two criteria include *lettuce, hottest, leading,* and *maiden.* Pause for a moment and say those four words aloud, using citation speech to clearly articulate the word-medial phonemes /t/ and /d/. Now say the words as you would in casual conversation. If the medial stop consonant in these words were produced with a tap motion, then we would transcribe the words as ['lɛ.ɾɪs], ['hɑ.ɾɪst], ['li.ɾɪŋ], and ['meɪ.ɾɪn], respectively. Next, practice saying the words in pairs, as in ['lɛ.tɪs]–['lɛ.ɾɪs], ['hɑ.tɪst]–['hɑ.ɾɪst], ['li.dɪŋ]–['li.ɾɪŋ], and ['meɪ.dɪn]–['meɪ.ɾɪn]. Keep in mind that we can articulate words such as *lettuce* and *leading* using either [t] or [ɾ], because the tap [ɾ] is an allophone of [t] and [d], and as such, does not change word meaning.

Words that do not fit the tap allophone pattern include *hotel* and *bending.* Why can a tap not replace the phone [t] in *hotel*? Because the second syllable is stressed; therefore, we need to articulate a strong [t] in the second syllable, which we would narrowly transcribe as [hoʊ.'tʰɛl], using a diacritical mark after the [t] that we will describe below. Why can a tap not replace [d] in *bending*? Because the

consonant "d" does not occur in-between two vowels but instead is between a consonant and a vowel. There are rules for how the alveolar tap is used in American English, which we will discuss in greater detail in Chapter 7.

The second new consonant symbol is called the glottal stop. As its name implies, this consonant is in the stop manner class and is produced using the vocal folds. You already learned one other sound that is produced using the vocal folds. What is it? Yes, it is [h], as in *house.* The glottal stop is produced by forcefully and quickly closing and then opening the vocal folds. It is the sound you make when you cough quietly. To practice producing a glottal stop, begin by prolonging [h], as in [h::::::]. Then intermittently interrupt the airflow by adducting the vocal folds momentarily before continuing to prolong it. The glottal stop sounds you will be making are like a string of very quiet coughs. In some dialects, when individuals articulate an isolated vowel sound or when a word begins with a vowel sound, a glottal stop proceeds the production of the vowels. However, because those glottal stop productions do not represent phonemes, we do not transcribe them unless they were produced with excessive force. The glottal stop phonetic symbol looks like a question mark without the dot underneath: [ʔ] (Unicode character code 294). The complete chart of American English consonant phones and allophones used in typical speech can be found in Table 4–1.

The glottal stop as an allophone occurs frequently, and is easily recognizable, in the Cockney dialect of British English. It also is recognizable in a New York dialect of American English, with speakers substituting glottal stops for voiceless stops in words such as *bottle* (e.g., ['bɑ.ʔəl]). The prevalence of glottal stop usage varies significantly from one American English dialect to another. Try to think of some words in which you personally substitute the glottal stop for phones [t] and [d]. Speakers of various dialects may say, for example, the words *important* and *football* using medial glottal stops, as in [ɪm.'pɔɚ.ʔənt] and ['fʊʔ.bɔl]. Once you tune into listening for glottal stops, we think you will be amazed at how often, and how differently, they are used in American English.

To help you better understand how the glottal stop is produced, pause to list the different ways you

TABLE 4–1. Phonetic Chart of Place, Manner, and Voicing Classes of American English Consonant Phones and Allophones

Manner/ Place	Bilabial	Labio-dental	Inter-dental	Alveolar	Post-Alveolar	Alveo-palatal	Palatal	Velar	Glottal
Stops	p **b**			t **d**				k **g**	ʔ
Nasals	**m**			**n**				**ŋ**	
Glides	**w**						**j**		
Tap				**ɾ**					
Fricatives		f **v**	θ **ð**	s **z**	ʃ **ʒ**				h
Affricates					tʃ **dʒ**				
Liquids				**l**			**ɹ**		

Note. Voiced consonants are in bold.

verbally can express *yes* and *no*. You can say the words *yes* and *no*, as well as variations of those words, such as *yea* and *naw*. But how else can you express those words? Can you think of how you would say *yes* and *no* without even opening your mouth while you voice sounds? You could say something such as *mhm* for *yes* and *m-m* for *no*. Take a moment to say those two forms. In which of those forms did you produce two strong glottal stops: in *mhm* or *m-m*? We produce glottal stops in the negative response, and we often also could find ourselves shaking our heads *no* as we say *m-m*. We could transcribe that production as [ʔm̩.ʔm̩] (notice the syllabic diacritic under the [m] phones, too, designating that *m-m* has two syllables, something else we will talk about soon). Now take a moment to say a form of *yes* and *no* that is produced with your mouth open: *uhuh* and *uh-uh*. We articulate two glottal stops when we express *no* in the utterance *uh-uh*, which is transcribed as [ʔʌ.ʔʌ]. (Listen carefully to your production of *uh-uh* and you will hear nasalized vowels, which we also will discuss later in this chapter.) It is interesting that we use glottal stops to express *no* but not *yes*. Why might that be? It may have something to do with the fact that the glottal stop sound is quite abrupt and forceful, serving us well when expressing the negative. One other word that we frequently produce using the glottal stop is the exclamation *uh-oh*, which is transcribed as [ʔʌ.ʔoʊ]. In Chapter 7, we will discuss patterns of glottal stop usage in American English.

? 4–3. Did You Get It?

Write "yes" or "no" next to each word to indicate if the medial "t" or "tt" can be replaced with a tap.

high-tops   _____

butter   _____

filter   _____

little   _____

letter   _____

listen   _____

attach   _____

city   _____

Introduction to Diacritical Marks

The symbols used to specify the articulation of speech sounds are called diacritical marks. In speech-language pathology, we commonly abbreviate this term as diacritics. In phonetic transcription, diacritics are small marks placed above, below, next to, or within consonant and vowel phonetic symbols. Each mark identifies a specific aspect of the way a sound was articulated or a specific aspect of how a sound typically is produced. A consonant or vowel with a diacritical mark does not indicate a new phoneme, but rather, a specific way the phoneme was produced. Speech-language pathologists frequently use diacritics to detail a client's productions when sounds are misarticulated. Understanding exactly how a client incorrectly produced a particular sound provides valuable information that is used in intervention. Once a speech-language pathologist knows which sounds an individual misarticulates, the speech-language pathologist then can move toward trying to understand why certain sounds are misarticulated. Intervention often is focused on correcting the underlying problem. Speech-language pathologists typically do not use diacritics when an individual's articulation matches the target articulation, because completing a narrow phonetic transcription is very time consuming. In the remainder of this chapter, we will learn how to capture a speaker's production using diacritics. In Chapters 7 and 8, we will learn about the patterns that underlie typical articulation of speech sounds in a wide variety of linguistic contexts. All of this information combines to inform decision making in clinical assessment and intervention.

To paraphrase the renouned linguist Roman Jakobson again, we speak to be heard to be understood. Pause for another moment to consider that thought: we speak to be heard to be understood. In other words, to even have a chance of being understood—our ultimate goal—we first must ensure that our listener(s) can hear us. As speakers, we could talk excessively loudly and clearly all the time, but we do not. What we do instead is balance those competing demands. As we discussed in Chapter 1, one demand is to make our speech loud and clear enough to be heard, hoping ultimately that we will be understood. The other demand is our desire to produce speech using minimal articulatory effort, a concept we termed ease of articulation. Our desire to be heard so that we may be understood drives us to articulate our speech loudly and carefully, but only as loudly and clearly as is necessary for each speaking situation. Clear articulation affords listeners the ability to differentiate one sound from another from another, the concept we termed perceptual separation. Diacritical marks help to capture those subtle differences in the articulation of speech sounds.

Some good news is that you already are familiar with diacritical marks as applied to alphabet letters, because a few **loanwords** (i.e., words adopted into English from other languages) continue to be spelled using them. Pause for a moment. Can you think of any written words that contain symbols other than alphabet letters? One diacritical mark you may be familiar with already is the acute accent mark [´], as in the words rosé, résumé, lamé, saké, and café. Does that accent mark tell us anything? Yes, it tells us to pronounce that final vowel; otherwise, the silent-e rule would apply. Four of these five words are different words when the acute accent mark is omitted. We have the word pairs rose and rosé, the first a flower, the second a pink wine, as well as resume and résumé, lame and lamé, and sake and saké. Another mark you may be familiar with is the diaeresis [¨], a mark placed above a vowel letter, as in the word naïve. What does the diaeresis specify? It tells you to pronounce both abutting vowels instead of producing them as a vowel digraph or diphthong. Hopefully you are realizing that you already have some familiarity with diacritics and are seeing how diacritics specify a sound's articulation, even when applied to alphabet letters.

There are many different diacritic classification systems available for phonetic transcription, ranging from symbol sets containing only common marks specific to a particular language to sets containing a wide array of marks that can be used to describe any language, any dialect, and/or disordered speech. No one language employs every one of the diacritics available; instead, smaller subsets of diacritics apply to different languages. It is also important to understand that there is not a single standard symbol set or placement of diacritical marks, so you may come across diacritic classifications that vary from the ones we will present in this textbook.

In this chapter, we will discuss some of the diacritics that can be applied to speech production in American English, including the various dialects of American English that result in speakers pronouncing some sounds and words differently than other speakers. Dialectal differences are not considered to be incorrect productions, but rather, different productions. Speech-language pathologists also can use diacritics to capture the articulation of individuals with speech sound disorders. A speech production is classified as a misarticulation if it does not fit the patterns of the speaker's language and/or dialect.

Overall, diacritics can provide information regarding a phoneme's place of articulation, manner of articulation, voicing, resonance quality, tongue position, airflow, release, or duration. There are diacritics specific to consonant articulation and diacritics specific to vowel articulation, as well as diacritics that can be used to describe both consonants and vowels. We turn now to describing the most commonly used diacritics in the typical pronunciation of words in American English, beginning with those that apply to consonant articulation.

Diacritical Marks Applied to Consonants

There are several ways to capture articulatory detail in consonant production. Consonant production can involve variations in the activity of the vocal folds, airstream mechanism, primary and secondary articulatory placements, and articulatory manner. All the diacritics that we will discuss were developed to describe the typical articulation of phonemes in languages.

Consonant Diacritics for States of the Glottis

Variations in vocal fold activity are referred to as **states of the glottis**. If you remember from Chapter 2, the glottis is the space in-between the open vocal folds. We can think of the different amounts of vocal fold opening—states of the glottis—as being on a continuum from wide open to moving toward midline to closed. Perceptually, as the states of the glottis change, listeners perceive voicing differently. When the vocal folds are abducted, there is no voicing; when they move slightly toward midline, there is breathy voicing. As the vocal folds approximate midline, resonant voicing, called modal voice, is produced. As the vocal folds are pulled tightly together

on one end, strained voicing is produced, and when the vocal folds are closed tightly, no sound results (unless they are opened quickly to produce a voiceless glottal stop, [ʔ]). The effects of the states of the glottis on sound quality will be discussed in additional detail in Chapter 9.

When a speech sound is produced in a word with a different degree of voicing than its citation-form target would suggest, diacritics are available to detail those articulatory modifications. A summary of the consonant diacritics for states of the glottis is in Table 4–2. Voiced consonants are fully voiced when we say them in isolation, as in, for example, [b], [m], and [z]. Likewise, voiceless consonants are unvoiced in isolation, as in [p] and [s]. If you articulated a voiced consonant without full voicing, then we could use the voiceless diacritic to describe that production as being only partially voiced. The voiceless diacritic is a small letter "o" placed under the consonant symbol, as in [b̥], indicating that the [b] phone was whispered. However, [b̥] indicates that some voicing was produced; otherwise, the word would have sounded like it was produced with [p]. Alternately, when a voiceless consonant is articulated with some degree of voicing, as is sometimes done by speakers of other languages, such as Hindi, the voicing diacritic is used. The symbol for voicing is the caron, or wedge, which is placed below the consonant, as in [pɪɡ̌]. The voicing diacritic specifies that the word was produced as a distorted version of the word.

When a consonant is produced with voicing described as **murmured** or **breathy**, then the diacritic for breathy voice is used. That diacritic is called the diaeresis below (i.e., [̈]), placed under the consonant, as in [ˈb̈ʌ.b̈əl], to indicate that both of the /b/ phonemes were articulated with the vocal folds

TABLE 4–2. Consonant Diacritics for States of the Glottis

Name	Diacritic	Explanation
Voiceless	x̥	Consonant produced without voicing from vocal fold vibrations
Breathy voice	x̤	Consonant produced with soft, murmured voicing
Voiced	x̌	Consonant produced with voicing from vocal fold vibrations
Creaky voice	x̰	Consonant produced with low, gravelly voicing

Note. x represents a consonant phonetic symbol.

loosely vibrating, resulting in a breathy voice. There are no breathy phonemes in English; however, there are in other languages, such as Hindi and Sanskrit. In the US, the use of a breathy voice characterizes the speech of some actors, perhaps the most famous being Marilyn Monroe. To hear an example of breathy voice, look online for an audio or video clip of Ms. Monroe singing "Happy Birthday" to President John F. Kennedy.

A very different type of voicing is produced when the anterior portion of the vocal folds is tightly closed, permitting only the posterior edges to vibrate; the sound that results has been described as the sound that a door makes when opening or closing on rusty hinges: **creaky**. The diacritic for creaky voice is a tilde placed under the consonant, as in ['b̰ʌ.bəl]. There are no creaky phonemes in English, although creaky phones appear to be on the rise (creaky voice also occurs on vowels in English, as we will discuss in an upcoming section). In the US, creaky voice recently has become the focus of media and research attention as more and more young Americans adopt this style of speaking, commonly called vocal fry. Perhaps the most famous examples of vocal fry can be heard in the speech of the three Kardashian sisters, who frequently use creaky voice, especially at the end of many utterances. In Chapter 9, we will discuss breathy and creaky voice as used phonemically in other languages.

Consonant Diacritics for Airstream Mechanisms

In addition to varying the degree of voicing, stop consonants can be articulated with changes in the airstream mechanism, specifically with varying degrees of aspiration. If a stop is produced with a burst of air following its production, we use the superscript [ʰ] diacritic, as in the word *pop* produced with aspirated stop consonants, resulting in [pʰapʰ], as displayed in Table 4–3. As a reminder, a way to check for aspiration is to articulate [pʰ] while holding up a light piece of paper, watching the corner of the paper bend when you say an airy [pʰ].

Consonant Diacritics for Primary Articulatory Place

There are three different diacritical marks that describe primary articulator placement during consonant production: **dental**, **apical**, and **laminal**, as displayed in Table 4–4. The dental diacritic technically is called a bridge; however, we tend to call it a tooth because it not only looks like a tooth, but calling it a tooth helps to remind us that it represents a dentalized placement. Whatever you decide to call it, it is the mark [ˌ], which is placed under a consonant symbol when the sound is produced with the tongue tip or blade on the upper teeth. A good example of a dental placement is in some dialects of Spanish, when production of the stop phonemes /t/ and /d/ are produced with the tongue more forward

TABLE 4–3. Consonant Diacritic for Airstream Mechanisms

Name	Diacritic	Explanation
Aspirated	xʰ	Consonant produced with a burst of air

Note. x represents a consonant phonetic symbol.

TABLE 4–4. Consonant Diacritics for Primary Articulatory Place

Name	Diacritic	Explanation
Dental	x̪	Consonant produced with the tongue tip/blade on the upper teeth
Apical	x̺	Consonant produced using the tip of the tongue
Laminal	x̻	Consonant produced using the blade of the tongue

Note. x represents a consonant phonetic symbol.

than in English, that is, touching the inside of the upper teeth rather than the alveolar ridge, as in English. Those Spanish stop phonemes can be transcribed as [t̪] and [d̪], as in ['t̪i.ə] (*aunt*) and [d̪os] (*two*).

When the tongue tip is used in the primary placement of a consonant, we call it an apical consonant and note it using the apical diacritic [◌̺]. The apical diacritic is called an inverted bridge and is placed under the consonant symbol. Apical consonants include dental phonemes and rare linguolabial (i.e., sounds produced with the tongue tip touching the bottom of the upper lip) stop, nasal, and fricative phonemes in some languages other than English. When the tongue blade, which is posterior to the tongue tip, is used in the production of a consonant, we use the laminal diacritic [◌̻], a small square placed under the consonant. Laminal consonants primarily include interdentals, alveolars, and alveopalatals. Interestingly, alveolars are produced as apical in some languages, but as laminal in other languages. Remember, we do not typically include diacritical marks if they are expected in the language we are transcribing.

Consonant Diacritics for Secondary Articulatory Place

The coarticulation of speech sounds in words creates secondary articulations, where one sound affects the production place and/or manner of another sound, creating a sound that has two places of articulation. This phenomenon occurs because our articulations can be affected by the surrounding sounds, creating overlapping gestures. These secondary articulations are phonetically motivated; however, they are learned by speakers of a language or dialect as being either acceptable or unacceptable pronuncia-

tions. Secondary coarticulatory effects can be specified using diacritical marks, which are displayed in Table 4–5. In speech-language pathology, four of the most commonly used secondary articulatory placement diacritics include those to capture nasalization, labialization, palatalization, and velarization.

Nasalization is when an oral consonant is produced with the velum in a lowered position, permitting sound to resonate in a second chamber—the nasal cavity—to create a nasalized sound. The nasalized diacritic is a tilde symbol placed over the affected consonant. If a speaker nasalized the /d/ phoneme in the word, for example, "*mad*," it would be transcribed narrowly as [mæd̃] and it would sound in-between [mæd] and [mæn].

The other common secondary articulations involve the lips (i.e., labialization), hard palate (i.e., palatalization), and soft palate (i.e., velarization). Labialization occurs when the lips also are used to produce a consonant that otherwise is produced elsewhere in the mouth. In English, several consonants typically are articulated with lip rounding as a second place of articulation. The following consonants typically are produced with lip rounding, even though they have another primary place of articulation: [ʃ, ʒ, t͡ʃ, d͡ʒ, ɹ]. When these or other consonants are produced with lip rounding, we can place the labialized diacritic [ʷ] on the upper right-hand side of the consonant symbol to capture that detail, as in the production [ʃʷu] for *shoe*, although it is rare that we would do so.

When a consonant is produced with the second place of articulation at the front of the tongue near the hard palate, like the articulatory place for palatal glide [j], we say that the consonant is palatalized. A palatalized consonant is different than a palatal

TABLE 4–5. Consonant Diacritics for Secondary Articulatory Place

Name	Diacritic	Explanation
Nasalized	x̃	Consonant produced with nasal resonance
Labialized	xʷ	Consonant produced with lip rounding
Palatalized	xʲ	Consonant produced with center of tongue near the hard palate
Velarized	x̴	Consonant produced with back of tongue near the soft palate

Note. x represents a consonant phonetic symbol.

consonant in that a palatal consonant (such as [j]) is produced with a single palatal articulatory place, whereas a palatalized consonant is produced with two places of articulation, one being palatal. The palatalized diacritic is a superscript mark [ʲ], which is placed on the upper right-hand side of the consonant. Try to produce the word *keep* with a palatalized articulation of [k]. If you were successful, you would be able to transcribe that production as [kʲip], which would sound like "kyeep."

When a consonant is produced with the back of the tongue pulled back toward the velum as a second place of articulation, we say that the consonant is velarized. A velarized consonant is different than a velar consonant in that a velar consonant (e.g., [k, g, ŋ]) is produced with the back of the tongue touching the soft palate as the single place of articulation. A velarized consonant is a produced with two places of articulation, one being tongue retraction toward the velum. The velarized diacritic is a tilde placed within the consonant symbol. In American English, the most commonly produced velarized consonant is [l] in post-vocalic position when the vowel and [l] are in the same syllable. For example, the words *highlight* and *hilltop* each have two syllables: /ˈhaɪ.laɪt/ and /ˈhɪl.tap/. In the first word, *highlight*, the first syllable ends in a vowel and /l/ begins the second syllable, so the vowel and /l/ are separated by a syllable boundary. In the second word, *hilltop*, /l/ is in the same syllable as the vowel preceding it, and /l/ often is articulated as velarized, as in [ˈhɪɫ.tap]. Hopefully you remember from Chapter 2 that a velarized-l also is called dark-l, with its alveolar-

only counterpoint occurring in pre-vocalic position and called light-l. Velarized-l is more common in some dialects of American English than others; however, most English speakers produce velarized-l in at least some words in postvocalic position. A narrow transcription of the words *elbow*, *fool*, and *talc* produced with a velarized-l would be [ˈɛɫ.boʊ], [fuɫ], and [tæɫk]. Some English speakers produce [l] in syllable-final position with velar as the primary place of articulation. Although the IPA includes a velar-l symbol /ʟ/, both the velar and velarized-l are typically transcribed using [ɫ].

Consonant Diacritics for Articulatory Manner

The manner in which consonants are articulated also can be specified using diacritical marks, which are displayed in Table 4–6. Three of the most commonly used diacritics capture how a consonant was released. If a stop consonant is released while the velum is lowering, a nasal consonant will result. For example, say the phoneme /d/ aloud—be sure to say it as a strong stop. Next, say it strongly again, but while holding your tongue tip on your alveolar ridge, lower your velum during its production. You will know you have lowered your velum when air escapes through your nose. You should hear a production that sounds like [d] + [n], with some sound coming through your nose at the release of the production. We capture that production phonetically as [dⁿ]. Similarly, if a stop consonant is produced by lowering the sides of the tongue instead of lowering the center of the tongue, then the resulting consonant sounds like the stop phone + [l], with air

TABLE 4–6. Consonant Diacritics for Articulatory Manner

Name	Diacritic	Explanation
Nasal release	xⁿ	Stop consonant released by lowering the velum
Lateral release	xˡ	Stop consonant released by lowering the sides of the tongue
Unreleased	x⁻	Stop consonant produced without the anticipated burst of air
Long	x:	Consonant produced with a longer than typical duration
Extra short	x̆	Consonant produced with a shorter than typical duration
Syllabic	x̩	Consonant produced as a syllable

Note. x represents a consonant phonetic symbol.

flowing over the sides of the tongue at the release of the sound. Take a moment now to produce [d] with a **lateral release**. We would capture your production phonetically as [dˡ]. Another type of consonant release is to not fully release it, which is called unreleased or no audible release. In English, stop consonants at the end of a word can be articulated as either fully released or unreleased. When fully released, a voiceless stop phoneme would be narrowly transcribed with the aspiration diacritic. For example, the word "mop" produced with a fully released word-final stop would be transcribed as [map*h*]. However, that same voiceless stop phoneme produced as an unreleased stop would be narrowly transcribed as [map˞], with the unreleased diacritic [˞] applied. Practice saying the following word pairs aloud until you understand the concept of unreleased: [hap*h*]–[hap˞], [sæt*h*]–[sæt˞], and [wik*h*]–[wik˞]. Note also that while we can fully release voiced stop phonemes, we typically do so without producing aspiration, as in [hɪd]–[hɪd˞].

The duration of sounds that we make also can be captured using diacritical marks. For our purposes, we will introduce only two duration-based diacritics: one for sounds held for a longer than typical amount of time, called long, and one for sounds held for a shorter than typical amount of time, called extra short. The diacritic for long is the symbol [ː], which is called a triangular colon. This diacritic modifies the sound it follows. For example, if I said, *Hhhhhi!*, we could narrowly transcribe it as [hːaɪ]. The longer a sound is produced, the more triangular colons we add. Contrastively, we use the diacritic [˘], called breve, to modify a sound that has been produced with a shorter than typical duration. If I produced the utterance *hi* using shortened frication, it could be narrowly transcribed as [ȟaɪ].

The last diacritic for consonants that we will discuss is the syllabic mark that denotes a syllable without a vowel, but one that contains a consonant with significant vowel-like quality. If you remember, we previously explained that every syllable had to contain a vowel. We now need to revise that previous statement by saying that every syllable must contain a vowel *or a* **syllabic consonant**. The syllabic diacritic is the small vertical line [̩], a mark placed under the vowel-like consonant. For practice, say the following two forms of the words *chasm* and *prison* as narrowly transcribed: ['kæ.zɪm]–['kæ.zm̩]

and ['pɹɪ.zɪn]–['pɹɪ.zn̩]. Can you articulate the differences? In each of the first words, the second vowel is produced fully. In each of the second variations, the weak vowels are omitted. In English, /m, n/, as well as /l/ can function as syllabic consonants, the latter as in the word "buckle," ['bʌ.kl̩].

A summary of all the diacritics we discussed is displayed in Table 4–7. In addition, a chart containing the consonant diacritic symbols and their character codes from Unicode are displayed in Table 4–8.

Diacritical Marks Applied to Vowels

We can modify vowel sounds similarly to how we modify consonant sounds. Vowel modifications can include variations in the state of the glottis, articulatory manner, and primary and secondary articulatory placement. A summary of vowel diacritics can be found in Table 4–9.

Vowel Diacritics for States of the Glottis

Like consonants, vowels also can be produced using a breathy or creaky voice and the diacritical marks are the same. For example, the vowel in the word *bus* that is produced with a breathy voice, such as when whispering, is narrowly transcribed as [bʌ̤s]. Producing the same word with a creaky vowel would be transcribed as [bʌ̰s]. Again, these glottal-based variations are not phonemic in English, but they are contrastive in other languages, which we will discuss in Chapter 9.

Vowel Diacritics for Primary Articulatory Place

There are times when we vary our primary tongue placement for vowel production. We typically modify vowel production because of changing coarticulatory demands as the sounds around a particular vowel vary. There are diacritics that can be used to detail four of the more basic tongue variations, including raising, lowering, advancing, and retracting the tongue from its idealized target place of articulation. These primary place modifications are not so extreme as to designate a brand-new vowel, but rather, they sound as though they are close to the target sound, but not quite the same. If a vowel sound is produced with a slightly higher than standard tongue position, we could use the up tack diacritic, [̝], to capture that articulation. For example, the word "pen" has a generalized American English

TABLE 4–7. Diacritical Symbols for Consonants

Name	Diacritic	Explanation
States of the Glottis		
Voiceless	x̥	Consonant produced without voicing from vocal fold vibrations
Breathy voice	x̤	Consonant produced with soft, murmured voicing
Voiced	x̬	Consonant produced with voicing from vocal fold vibrations
Creaky voice	x̰	Consonant produced with low, gravelly voicing
Airstream Mechanism		
Aspirated	x^h	Consonant produced with a burst of air
Primary Articulatory Placement		
Dental	x̪	Consonant produced with the tongue tip or blade on the upper teeth
Apical	x̺	Consonant produced using the tip of the tongue
Laminal	x̻	Consonant produced using the blade of the tongue
Secondary Articulatory Placement		
Nasalized	x̃	Consonant produced with nasal resonance
Labialized	x^w	Consonant produced with lip rounding
Palatalized	x^j	Consonant produced with center of tongue near the hard palate
Velarized	x̴	Consonant produced with back of tongue near the soft palate
Articulatory Manner		
Nasal release	x^n	Stop consonant released by lowering the velum
Lateral release	x^l	Stop consonant released by lowering the sides of the tongue
Unreleased	x⁻	Stop consonant produced without the anticipated burst of air
Long	xː	Consonant produced with a longer than typical duration
Extra short	x̆	Consonant produced with a shorter than typical duration
Syllabic	x̩	Consonant produced as a syllable

Note. x represents a consonant phonetic symbol.

TABLE 4–8. Character Codes and Unicode Names for Diacritical Symbols for Consonants

Name	Diacritic	Character Code	Unicode Name
Voiceless	x̥	325	Combining ring below
Breathy voice	x̤	324	Combining diaeresis below
Voiced	x̬	32c	Combining caron below
Creaky voice	x̰	330	Combining tilde below
Aspirated	xʰ	2b0	Modifier letter small h
Dental	x̪	32a	Combining bridge below
Apical	x̺	33a	Combining inverted bridge below
Laminal	x̻	33b	Combining square below
Nasalized	x̃	303	Combining tilde
Labialized	xʷ	2b7	Modifier letter small w
Palatalized	xʲ	2b2	Modifier letter small j
Velarized	x̵	334	Combining tilde overlay
Nasal release	xⁿ	207f	Superscript latin small letter n
Lateral release	xˡ	2e1	Modifier letter small l
Unreleased	x̚	31a	Combining left angle above
Long	xː	2d0	Modifier letter triangular colon
Extra short	x̆	306	Combining breve
Syllabic	x̩	329	Combining vertical line below

vowel target of [ɛ]. However, if a speaker with a Southern dialect articulated the word *pen*, the vowel likely would be raised, as in [ɪ̝], making it difficult for non-Southern dialect speakers to differentiate between the spoken words *pen* and *pin*. Similarly, if a speaker produced a vowel sound with a slightly lower than standard tongue position, we could use the down tack diacritic, [̞], to capture that articulation. For example, the word *Hamilton* has a generalized American English vowel target of [æ]. If a speaker with a New York City dialect articulated that word, the vowel would be lowered, narrowly transcribed as [æ̞]. A vowel production that is slightly advanced, such as in words containing a vowel following an alveolar consonant—for example, the word *tea*—would be transcribed narrowly using the plus sign diacritic, as [ti̟]. A production that is slightly retracted, such as in words containing a vowel

TABLE 4–9. Diacritical Symbols for Vowels

Name	Diacritic	Explanation
States of the Glottis		
Breathy voice	x̤	Vowel produced with soft, murmured voicing
Creaky voice	x̰	Vowel produced with low, gravelly voicing
Primary Articulatory Placement		
Raised	x̝	Vowel produced with the tongue higher than typical on the vertical plane
Lowered	x̞	Vowel produced with the tongue lower than typical on the vertical plane
Advanced	x̟	Vowel produced with the tongue more forward than typical on the horizontal plane
Retracted	x̠	Vowel produced with the tongue more back than typical on the horizontal plane
Secondary Articulatory Placement		
Nasalized	x̃	Vowel produced with nasal resonance
More rounded	x̹	Vowel produced with lip rounding or extra lip rounding
Less rounded	x̜	Vowel produced without lip rounding
Rhoticity	x˞	Vowel produced with /ɹ/ coloring
Articulatory Manner		
Long	x:	Vowel produced with a longer than typical duration
Extra short	x̆	Sound produced with a shorter than typical duration

Note. x represents a vowel phonetic symbol.

before and/or after a velar consonant—for example, the word *kick*—would be transcribed narrowly using the minus sign diacritic, as [kɪ̠k].

Vowel Diacritics for Secondary Articulatory Place
Other ways we modify the production of vowels is to vary our secondary articulatory placements. Vowels, like consonants, can be produced with nasalization, with sound resonating in the nasal cavity because the velum is relaxed during production. Vowels are transcribed narrowly using the same diacritic that is used for transcribing nasalized consonants, the tilde,

as in [mæ̃n]. In English, we most frequently nasalize vowels when they precede nasal consonants, a phenomenon that we will explain in Chapter 8. Do you remember our earlier discussion of how we can express *no* using the utterance *uh-uh*? When we produce *uh-uh*, the vowels are nasalized; therefore, a more accurate transcription of *uh-uh* would be [ʔʌ̃.ʔʌ̃].

Two other secondary place modifications involve the lips. One modification affects the four rounded back vowels [u, ʊ, oʊ, ɔ] when they are produced with less than typical lip rounding, as can occur when they are paired with nonrounded consonants, as in the word *hoot*, for example. We can note decreased lip rounding using the left half ring diacritic, [̜], as in [hu̜t]. There are other instances when a nonrounded vowel becomes slightly rounded in the context of a lip-rounded consonant, as in the word *she*, for example. When a nonrounded vowel is produced with lip rounding, we can use the right half ring diacritic placed under the vowel symbol to capture that variation, as in [ʃi̹].

We will teach one final secondary articulator placement and diacritic: rhoticity. When a vowel is produced with [ɹ] coloring, we say it has rhoticity. We place the diacritic for rhoticity on the right-hand side of the vowel phonetic symbol to indicate that the vowel has rhoticity. This diacritic is called a rhotic hook and is symbolized as [˞]. For example, the words *share* and *fear* could be transcribed narrowly as [ʃɛ˞] and [fɪ˞], respectively, with the rhotic hook conveying the influence of [ɹ] on the vowels. In Chapter 3, we taught you phonetic symbols representing rhotic vowels. Technically, either method is correct—using the rhotic phonetic symbols or using the rhotic hook diacritic—but in speech-language pathology, we typically transcribe rhotic vowels using the actual rhotic vowel symbol that represents schwar, [ɚ].

Vowel Diacritics for Articulatory Manner

The duration of vowels also can be marked like consonants. Vowels that are produced with a longer than typical duration are transcribed using the long diacritic, as in [iː], and those produced with a shorter than typical duration are transcribed using the extra short diacritic, called the breve, [˘], as in [ĭ]. English does not phonemically contrast vowels by length; however, we do vary our vowel durations, which you will learn more about in Chapter 7. In addition, some children acquiring closed word shapes also have been found to vary vowel length, seemingly to signal a final consonant prior to being able to produce that final consonant. Be careful that you do not confuse this diacritic with the mark that is often used in dictionaries and grade-school classrooms to indicate a "short vowel," such as the "short e," [ɛ], in the word *bed*.

A chart of the vowel diacritic symbols and their character codes from Unicode are displayed in Table 4–10.

TABLE 4–10. Character Codes and Unicode Names for Diacritical Symbols for Vowels

Name	Diacritic	Character Code	Unicode Name
Breathy voice	x̤	324	Combining diaresis below
Creaky voice	x̰	330	Combining tilde below
Raised	x̝	31d	Combining up tack below
Lowered	x̞	31e	Combining down tack below
Advanced	x̟	31f	Combining plus sign below
Retracted	x̠	320	Combining minus sign below
Nasalized	x̃	303	Combining tilde
More rounded	x̹	339	Combining right half ring below
Less rounded	x̜	31c	Combining left half ring below
Rhoticity	x˞	2de	Modifier letter rhotic hook
Long	xː	2d0	Modifier letter triangular colon
Extra short	x̆	306	Combining breve

?   4–4. Did You Get It?

1. Narrow phonetic transcription differs from broad phonetic transcription because narrow transcription includes the use of _____, marks that indicate articulatory details.

2. Name two states of the glottis.

   _____ _____

3. Match each primary articulatory placement with its corresponding diacritical mark.

   dental _____   a. [◌̪]
   apical _____   b. [◌̺]
   laminal _____   c. [◌̻]

4. Match each secondary articulatory placement with its corresponding diacritical mark.

   labialized _____   a. [◌̃]
   palatalized _____   b. [◌ʷ]
   velarized _____   c. [◌ʲ]
   nasalized _____   d. [◌̴]

5. Narrowly transcribe each of the following words using the appropriate diacritical mark.

   a. *sun* produced by lateralizing [s]

   [_____]

   b. *sick* produced by unreleasing the stop

   [_____]

   c. *bus* produced by prolonging the final consonant   [_____]

   d. *bugle* produced with a syllabic final consonant   [_____]

6. Write the vowel and diacritic described.

   a. advanced production of [u]   [_____]
   b. raised production of [æ]   [_____]
   c. rounded production of [æ]   [_____]
   d. extra short production of [æ]   [_____]

Suprasegmental Diacritical Marks

Diacritical Marks for Stress

You learned about primary and secondary stressed syllables in words in Chapter 1. You then learned how the physical speech systems are used to produce syllable stress in Chapter 2. Now you will learn the diacritical marks used to denote stressed syllables in your phonetic transcriptions.

As you have learned, the strongest stress on syllables in multisyllabic words is called the primary stress. Primary stress is transcribed by placing the superscript vertical line [ˈ] before the strongly stressed syllable (Unicode character code 2c8). For example, the word *building* has two syllables, "buil" + "ding," and the first syllable carries the primary stress. Primary stress is marked in the transcription as [ˈbɪl.dɪŋ]. In the three-syllable word *regretful*, primary stress is on the second syllable, transcribed as [ɹə.ˈgɹɛt.fəl].

Multisyllabic words also may contain a syllable with a degree of stress that is between primary stress and no stress. This degree of stress is called second-ary stress and it is transcribed by placing the sub-script vertical line [ˌ] before the affected syllable (Unicode character code 2cc). Be careful to place this stress mark *before* the syllable, because it could be easily confused with the syllabic consonant diacritical mark. Consider the three-syllable word *animal*. Which syllable carries primary stress? Yes, the first syllable. Which carries secondary stress? Yes, the second syllable. Transcribing the word *animal* to include primary and secondary stress would be [ˈæˌnə.ml̩] (note the stress marks before the syllables and the syllabic consonant mark under the consonant). Next, try to transcribe the four-syllable word *television* including the primary and secondary stress diacritics. With the first syllable carrying the most stress and the third syllable carrying the second-most stress, the phonetic transcription of *television* would be [ˈtɛ.lɪˌvɪ.ʒən]. It can be very difficult to hear the varying degrees of stress, but it is important to learn to hear at least primary stress because there are some disorders of speech for which stress errors are differentially diagnostic. Practice identifying primary stressed syllables as you say multisyllabic words aloud. Check your answers by looking up word pronunciations in a dictionary. You will get better with practice.

? 4–5. Did You Get It?

Include the primary stress diacritic in your phonetic transcription of each of the following words.

above _____

coffee _____

believe _____

giraffe _____

crystal _____

tablet _____

kitchen _____

canal _____

Diacritical Marks for Clinical Populations

We turn now to diacritical marks that were developed to capture production variations in disordered speech, that is, articulatory variations that are not characteristic of a speaker's language or dialect. There are many different diacritics available for clinical use; however, we will narrow our discussion to the ones we use most frequently in our clinical practice. We will explain 11 diacritics that detail atypical variations in the airstream mechanism, primary and secondary places of articulation, and manner of articulation. You can find an overview of these diacritics in Table 4–11. For a comprehensive set of phonetic symbols and diacritical marks for disordered speech, refer to the chart called Extensions of the International Phonetic Alphabet for Disordered Speech (ExtIPA), which is easily found online.

Airstream Mechanism Diacritic for Disordered Speech

The first diacritic listed is related to the airstream mechanism, specifically the direction of the airflow used to produce speech. As you learned in Chap-

ter 2, all the consonants and vowels in English are produced on exhaled air. Because using the correct type of airstream mechanism is implied in a broad transcription, we do not use a diacritical mark to denote exhaled airflow. However, if an individual were to produce, for example, the phonemes /b/ or /i/ on inhaled air, called **ingressive** air, we would note that incorrect production by using the ingressive airflow diacritic, the downwards arrow [↓], as in [b↓] and [i↓]. Try to say the word *hello* using an ingressive airstream—it is difficult, isn't it? In addition to being difficult to produce speech using an ingressive airstream, the sound quality of the production is odd to listen to. Some individuals with disordered speech have been observed to articulate sounds, syllables, and words using inhaled speech, and noting such productions with the ingressive airflow diacritic can pinpoint exactly where the airflow deviations occurred. In Chapter 9, we will discuss how different airstreams are used to produce select phonemes in languages other than English.

Primary Place of Articulation Diacritics for Disordered Speech

We will discuss four production deviations that affect primary place of articulation. The first is when an individual misarticulates a nonlabiodental sound by placing the upper teeth on the lower lip. To review, what are the labiodental sounds when you *would* place your upper teeth on your lower lip? You would use this articulatory position when producing [f] and [v]. Individuals with disordered speech, however, may use this position to produce the bilabial sounds [p, b, m]. Try saying the word *mama* by articulating the two [m] phones with your upper teeth on your lower lip, instead of by bringing both lips together. To note such misarticulations, you would use the subscript bridge diacritic, as in ['m̪a.m̪a]. Hopefully this diacritic has gotten your attention, as you have seen it before. It is the diacritic that marks dentalization in typical speech. When you use this diacritic with bilabial phonemes, remember that it refers to a *labio*dental place of articulation.

The opposite articulatory place to labiodental is placing the lower teeth on the upper lip. This articulatory place, called **dentolabial**, does not describe the production of any phonemes in any language. Nonetheless, individuals with disordered speech

TABLE 4–11. Diacritical Symbols for Disordered Speech

Name	Diacritic	Explanation
Airstream Mechanism		
Ingressive airflow	x↓	Consonant or vowel produced on an inward flowing airstream
Primary Articulatory Placement		
Labiodental	x̪	Consonant, typically a bilabial stop or nasal, produced with upper teeth on lower lip
Dentolabial	x̺	Consonant, typically a bilabial stop or nasal, produced with lower teeth on upper lip
Interdental	x̪̺	Consonant, typically an alveolar, produced with the tongue tip or blade protruding through the upper and lower teeth
Linguolabial	x̼	consonant, typically *l*, produced with the tongue touching the upper lip
Secondary Articulatory Placement		
Labial spreading	x̹	Consonant or vowel produced with the lips spread
Sliding articulation	x̗	Sounds produced with the articulators sliding into one another, resulting in slurred speech
Articulatory Manner		
Nasal emission	x̃	Consonant or vowel produced with airflow through the nostrils
Denasal	x̃	Consonant or vowel produced without nasal resonance
Strong articulation	x̎	Consonant produced forcefully
Weak articulation	x̗	Consonant produced weakly

Note. x represents a consonant or vowel phonetic symbol.

may use this posture to produce bilabial stops and nasals. Try to articulate the word *mama* again, this time by placing your lower teeth on your upper lip when you articulate [m]. The dentolabial diacritic also is the bridge; however, the dentolabial bridge is placed on top of the affected phoneme. For example, your place misarticulations of *mama* would be narrowly transcribed as ['m̺a.m̺a].

Another common misarticulation in disordered speech is an interdental placement of the tongue tip or blade, commonly called an **interdental lisp**, a type of distortion of alveolar consonants. The diacritic to designate an interdental production is a superscript and a subscript bridge placed directly on top of and under the affected consonant. If you can picture the bridge symbol as resembling a tooth, then you can think of the interdental diacritic as the misarticulated sound surrounded by an upper and lower tooth. Practice saying the word *ten* using an interdental articulation for both alveolar consonants, as in [t̪̺ɛn̪̺]. Also, practice saying the word *zoo* with an interdental consonant articulation, as in [z̪̺u].

The final primary place of articulation diacritic we will discuss is **linguolabial**, when the tongue tip touches the upper lip. This place misarticulation most commonly occurs on production of the lateral [l] phoneme in English. The diacritic for this linguolabial place of articulation is called the seagull: [◌̼]. Practice singing *la-la-la* using a linguolabial articulation for [l], as in [l̼a.l̼a.l̼a]. Interestingly, while there are no linguolabial phonemes in English, they do exist in a few other languages.

Secondary Place of Articulation Diacritics for Disordered Speech

The first diacritic we will discuss that involves a second place of articulation is a movement gesture that is the opposite of rounding: **labial spreading**. Labial spreading is when a sound is produced with the lips spread widely, similar to a smile, but without the corners of the lips upturned. The labial spreading diacritical mark is a left-right arrow placed directly under the affected sound: [◌↔]. Individuals with disordered speech may use this secondary place of articulation for a variety of non-lip-spread consonants and vowels. An example would be an individual who pronounces the word *zip* with his or her lips spread for articulation of initial [z̳].

Sliding is a term used to indicate two rapid articulations that result in a consonant diphthong. Remember that vowel diphthongs occur when two vowels are articulated so quickly that only a single vowel sound is produced. Similarly, when two consonants are articulated so rapidly that a single consonant sound is produced, we term the production "sliding," which is how we produce diphthongs. We note that production by drawing a right-pointing arrow under the affected consonants: [◌͢]. In typical speech, we might slide the phones [sθ] in the word *kinesthetic*, producing [kɪ.nə.ˈs͢θɛ.ɹɪk]. The term "slurring," as used in music when two notes are sung together, also can be used to describe this type of misarticulation.

Manner of Articulation Diacritics for Disordered Speech

When sounds are produced with a small amount of air blowing through the nostrils, we call that airflow nasal emission. Nasal emissions are typical in the speech of individuals who have difficulty closing the velopharyngeal port by raising their velum during speech, such as individuals with a history of a cleft of the soft palate. Nasal emissions most frequently occur on sounds requiring high intraoral pressure, such as the voiceless oral stop consonants; however, nasal emissions can occur on any speech sound. To produce a nasal emission, try saying the word *puppy* by sharply blowing small bursts of air through your nose while you produce the /p/ phonemes. It may take you repeated practice, so take your time. It will be beneficial for you to understand how the velopharyngeal mechanism works to produce these misarticulations. A sound that contains a nasal emission is symbolized with the diacritic called homothetic: [◌̃]. This diacritic looks like a tilde with one small dot above the line and another small dot under the line. The nasal emission diacritic is placed above the affected phoneme. For example, if you could produce *puppy* with nasal emissions on the stop phonemes, you would transcribe your production as [ˈp̃ʌ.p̃i].

In Chapter 2, we talked about hypernasality and hyponasality. Hypernasal speech is speech produced with an excess of nasal resonance. Hyponasal speech is speech produced with too little nasal resonance, making the speaker sound as though he or she has a stuffy nose. When individuals with disordered speech produce hyponasal speech sounds, we use the denasal diacritic to note those misarticulations. If you remember, the nasal diacritic is the tilde placed on top of the affected phoneme. The denasal diacritic is the tilde with a line drawn through it, as though to cancel it out: [◌̃̄]. Hypernasal and hyponasal speech also can affect the consonants produced. For example, if you say the word *Bobby* with significant *hyper*nasality, you are likely to produce a word that sounds like [ˈma.mi]. Contrastively, if you say the word *mommy* with significant *hypo*nasality, it is likely to sound like the name *Bobby*, as in [ˈbɑ.bi]. Practice saying these words with varying degrees of hyper- and hyponasality.

Individuals with disordered speech may produce sounds with too much articulatory effort, or not enough. When forceful effort is expended, we call the production a strong articulation and place the diacritic called a double accent (i.e., [◌̋]) below the affected phoneme. When a sound is produced with insubstantial articulatory effort, we call the production a weak articulation and place the diacritic called a left angle (i.e., [◌̖]) below the affected phoneme.

It takes a lot of experience and time to develop an ear for hearing these small articulatory differences in the productions of individuals with speech sound disorders, in part because their consonants and vowels may be misarticulated in obvious and subtle ways. When you are first learning to transcribe disordered speech, it is probably wise to start by creating broad transcriptions. As you gain experience both listening to and transcribing disordered speech, then you may find more success creating narrow transcriptions.

Putting It All Together

In this chapter, we discussed how to transcribe using broad consonant and vowel phonetic symbols, as well as how to transcribe narrowly using diacriti-cal marks that provide detailed information about the articulation of consonants and vowels. There are situations when completing a broad transcription will meet your goals, and other situations that will require you to complete a narrow transcription. The best way to learn the different diacritical marks is to practice narrow transcription, something that you are ready to practice now. It also helps when you learn how to visualize those subtle articulatory changes, a skill that you will learn in our chapter on acoustic phonetics. In addition, learning when the articulation of consonants and vowels varies from the idealized targets you learned in Chapters 2 and 3 also helps increase your understanding of diacritics. Again, you are in luck, because we will cover these patterns in Chapters 7 and 8. So stay with us, there is more learning ahead.

Applied Science: Revisited

Summary
Now that you have read about broad and narrow transcription, and learned some of the ways speech sounds are produced by different speakers and the diacritics we can use to better capture those differences, you hopefully have a height-ened awareness of speech production in its many nuanced forms. It can be very difficult to hear these subtle differences if you do not know the range of articulatory possibilities. However, once you become aware of the range of possibilities, especially for a particular language, you can listen for and transcribe those differences when appropriate, for the goal of your transcription. Next, let us revisit the clinical scenario.

One Step at a Time

1. When the speech-language pathology colleague listened to the audio recordings of the young daughter, she focused her attention on the daughter's articulation of the words with final consonants. The speech-language pathologist heard subtle differences between the vowels in the misarticulated words and the vowels in the correctly articulated words. The difference she heard was that the vowels before the target words that contained final consonants were produced slightly longer. The speech-language pathology colleague transcribed those vowels as [Vː], as in [hæː] for /hæt/, [tʌː] for /tʌb/, [bʊː] for /bʊk/, [mɑː] for /mɑm/, and [buː] for /bʌɪn/.

2. The speech-language pathology colleague then researched the literature on vowel lengthening and final consonant dele-tion. She discovered that some children have been reported to prolong the vowel preceding a final consonant that they omit. This vowel lengthening phenomenon was reported to occur right before some children started to produce word-final consonants, as though they were signaling that they knew there was another sound in the word, but could not produce it. The speech-language pathology colleague believed that the daughter's vowel lengthening was an indicator that she was on the cusp of being able to produce final consonants.

Answer
In this scenario, we know from research that young children omit final consonants from at least some of their words as they acquire speech.

However, we also know from research compiled after acute observation and narrow transcription that many children "signal" that they realize there is a consonant sound at the end of a word by going through a stage when they lengthen the vowel that precedes a final consonant. In children who produce this type of vowel lengthening, soon after the emergence of lengthened vowels they begin to produce word-final consonants. Because the daughter already produced sounds that were developmentally appropriate for her age and showed signs of realizing the existence of final consonants, the speech-language pathology colleague could predict that the daughter's articulatory ability soon would "catch up" to her understanding of final consonants.

If you, as the speech-language pathologist who screened the daughter, had paid closer attention to the daughter's articulation of the words with final consonants and used the lengthening diacritic (i.e., [ː]) to note that phonetic detail on the affected vowels, then you could have searched for research regarding your observation. Luckily, your speech-language pathology colleague had learned how to transcribe narrowly, preventing you from unnecessarily enrolling the daughter in speech intervention. Instead, you could carefully monitor her speech for several months to ensure that final consonants developed in her speech as predicted by her usage of vowel lengthening.

Science Applied

Applying phonetics to this problem was the solution to understanding how to more effectively capture speech production, and by doing so, developing a deeper understanding of speech acquisition and usage. Ultimately, if we do not know what to listen for in speech production and how to capture what we hear, then we will miss the beauty of what phonetics can offer in increasing our understanding of language. It also was made clear that knowing the primary and diacritic symbols is not enough. We also need to understand how words typically are acquired and produced by speakers of a language, which encompasses understanding the phonology of a language. We will discuss this aspect of phonetics in Chapters 7 and 8.

Interest Piqued?

Recommended materials to further your understanding of topics covered in this chapter.

Print Resources

Bleile, K. M. (2003). *Manual of articulation and phonological disorders* (2nd ed.). San Diego, CA: Singular.

International Phonetic Association. (2013). *Handbook of the International Phonetic Association: A guide to the use of the International Phonetic Alphabet*. Cambridge, UK: Cambridge University Press.

McLeod, S., & Singh, S. (2009). *Seeing speech: A quick guide to speech sounds*. San Diego, CA: Plural.

Online Resources

http://www.internationalphoneticalphabet.org/ipa-charts/diacritics/
Diacritics for typical speech.

http://ipa.typeit.org
To access an online broad phonetic symbols keyboard.

http://ipa.typeit.org/full
To access an online narrow phonetic symbols keyboard.

http://teaching.ncl.ac.uk/ipa/consonants-extra.html
Diacritics for disordered speech.

https://teaching.ncl.ac.uk/ipa/practical-exercises.html
For practice listening to consonants and vowels and transcribing them.

ANSWER KEY

4–1.

1. A speech-language pathologist interested in capturing a client's tongue placement and precise movements during articulation of words containing [s] would employ a <u>speaker</u>-oriented approach to transcribing.

2. A speech-language pathologist who wants to determine how many of a client's spoken words he or she can understand would employ a <u>listener</u>-oriented approach to transcribing.

Circle the correct word in the following sentences.

3. When transcribing a speech sample in a language you do not speak or understand, your transcription will be <u>impressionistic</u> in nature.

4. When transcribing the target words included on a test of articulation, your transcription will be <u>systematic</u> in nature.

Circle the type of phonetic representation system you would use for each of the following scenarios.

5. A teacher reports a student in his class with a monotone voice. You need to note intonation when you transcribe the student's speech. You would use a <u>suprasegmental</u> representation system.

6. You want to transcribe how a child articulated each consonant phoneme in a list of words. You would use a <u>segmental</u> representation system.

4–2.

1. The words seize-key-believe-meat all contain which vowel? <u>/i/</u>

2. Orthographically, write one word that has more alphabet letters than phonemes.
   <u>Answers will vary; examples could include</u> <u>*cough*, *special*, *match*, etc.</u>

3. List one situation or routine that you take advantage of to practice transcribing every day.
   <u>Answers will vary; could include taking</u> <u>notes in class, writing a to-do list, sending a</u> <u>text.</u>

4. The four consonants in the English alphabet that are not also phonetic symbols in English include "<u>c, q, x, y.</u>"

5. The words tries-dog's-buns all end with the morpheme "s." How do you know that the morpheme "s" is produced as [z] in these words?
   Because the phonemes immediately preceding the morpheme "s" are voiced.

6. Is the final sound in these words typically produced as [s] or [z]?

   taxis <u>[z]</u>   taxes <u>[z]</u>   Texas <u>[s]</u>
   axis <u>[s]</u>   axes <u>[z]</u>   access <u>[s]</u>

7. Next to each of the following words, write whether the word contains a consonant digraph or a cluster.

   Example, echo <u>consonant digraph</u>
   a. shut   <u>consonant digraph</u>
   b. skip   <u>consonant cluster</u>
   c. cheese   <u>consonant digraph</u>
   d. sound   <u>consonant cluster</u>

8. Next to each of the following words, write whether the word contains a vowel digraph or a diphthong.

Example, soil   <u>vowel diphthong</u>

a. beat   <u>vowel digraph</u>
b. caught   <u>vowel diagraph</u>
c. height   <u>vowel diphthong</u>
d. sound   <u>vowel diphthong</u>

4–3.

Write "yes" or "no" next to each word to designate if the medial consonant can be replaced with a tap.

high-tops   <u>no</u>
butter   <u>yes</u>
filter   <u>no</u>

little   <u>yes</u>
letter   <u>yes</u>
listen   <u>no</u>
attach   <u>no</u>
city   <u>yes</u>

4–4.

1. Narrow phonetic transcription differs from broad phonetic transcription because narrow transcription includes the use of <u>diacritics</u>, marks that indicate articulatory details.

2. Name two states of the glottis. <u>Any two from: voiceless, breathy voice, modal voice, strained voice.</u>

3. Match each primary articulatory placement with its corresponding diacritical mark.

dental   <u>b</u>   a. [̪]
apical   <u>c</u>   b. [̺]
laminal   <u>a</u>   c. [̻]

4. Match each secondary articulatory placement with its corresponding diacritical mark.

labialized   <u>b</u>   a. [̃]
palatalized   <u>c</u>   b. [ʷ]

velarized   <u>d</u>   c. [ʲ]
nasalized   <u>a</u>   d. [~]

5. Narrowly transcribe each of the following words using the appropriate diacritical mark.

a. *sun* produced by lateralizing [s]   [sˡʌn]
b. *sick* produced by unreleasing the stop   [sɪk ̚]
c. *bus* produced by prolonging the final consonant   [bʌsː]
d. *bottle* produced with a syllabic final consonant   ['ba.tl̩]

6. Write the vowel and diacritic described.

a. advanced production of [u]   [u̟]
b. raised production of [æ]   [æ̝]
c. extra rounded production of [æ]   [æ̹]
d. extra short production of [æ]   [æ̆]

4–5.

Include the primary stress diacritic in your phonetic transcription of each of the following words.

above   [ə.'bʌv]
coffee   ['kɔ.fi] / ['ka.fi]
believe   [bə.'liv]

giraffe   [d͡ʒɚ.'æf]
crystal   ['kɹɪs.tl̩]
tablet   ['tæ.blət]
kitchen   ['kɪ.t͡ʃn̩]
canal   [kə.'næl]

5

SUPRASEGMENTAL FEATURES OF SPEECH

Learning Objectives

By reading this chapter, you will learn:

1. the definition and examples of the various suprasegmental features
2. the phonetic use of suprasegmental features in American English
3. how we produce and use stress in spoken language
4. how we produce and use intonation in spoken language
5. ways to describe the steady and changing pitch in intonational contours
6. the components and study of prosody

Applied Science

Read the following utterances. What do you think the speaker of each utterance is trying to convey to his or her listener? Can you think of an alternate message the speaker could be trying to convey? Write the meaning(s) of each utterance.

1. Yes _____

2. No way _____

3. I'd like to be your friend _____

4. Sure, I'll go _____

5. I'll see you later _____

6. Don't even _____

7. Who are you _____

8. Whatever _____

Verbal Communication

Have you ever overheard or had a phone conversation that went something like this?

Alex: *Hello.*

Mia: Hi, Alex!

Alex: *What's up?*

Mia: Hey, it's Mia!

Alex: *Hi, Mia. I knew it was you. I saw your name on my screen.*

Mia: Alex, you don't sound happy to hear from me.

Alex: *Happy?*

Mia: You don't sound it.

Alex: *What? Mia, all I've said so far is hello.*

Mia: But I can tell, Alex. What's the matter? Are you upset with me about something?

Alex: *No. Why would you say that?*

Mia: Because. I can just tell.

Alex: *Well, nothing's wrong and I'm not upset with you.*

Mia: Yes, you are, Alex.

Alex: *Okay, whatever. I don't want to argue.*

Mia: I'm not arguing! Now, you're just trying to pick a fight.

Alex: *Look Mia, call me back when you're less upset, okay?*

Click.

What do you think happened in this conversation, to have it end so badly?

Let us assume that the person who answered the phone, Alex, *was* happy to hear from Mia. Alex said hello and began to engage in a conversation with Mia, but Mia became upset almost immediately. If we look at the words they exchanged, Alex never said anything negative. If what Alex said was not negative, then why did it provoke a negative response from Mia? If you are hypothesizing that maybe it was not *what* Alex said, but possibly *how* Alex may have said it, then you are thinking about a feature of speech production that is as important to a verbal message as the speech sounds themselves. We call those features of speech production suprasegmentals. As introduced in Chapter 2, suprasegmentals are features overlaid on phonemes that add additional meaning to utterances.

In addition to containing the consonant, vowel, and diacritical phonetic symbols you already have learned, the IPA also contains a set of marks we can use when transcribing. As you have learned, the segmental system consists of the consonants, vowels, and word shapes in a language. The *suprasegmental* system is an additional aspect of spoken language. The adage, "It's not what you say, but how you say it" captures the gist and importance of suprasegmentals. Suprasegmentals add meaning to words beyond the meaning of the words themselves, the result of changes to speech intensity, frequency, and timing. Suprasegmentals are not aspects of production that are specific to one person, such as someone's voice secondary to physical characteristics of height, weight, biological sex, or age, or education, or geographic background, but rather, the deliberate use of speech intensity, frequency, and timing to imbue meaning when talking. Generally speaking, there are four suprasegmental features. Two of the four suprasegmental features we will discuss in this chapter: stress and intonation. The two other suprasegmental features, tone and length, are not phonemic in American English, so we will discuss them in Chapter 9 when we talk about the phonetics of languages other than English. We will begin our discussion of suprasegmentals by revisiting stress, one feature that you were introduced to in the first chapter.

Stress

In Chapter 1, we introduced you to the concept of stress, including different types of stress (i.e., contrastive, lexical, and grammatical), different degrees of stress (i.e., primary, secondary, and tertiary), and production of stress (i.e., articulatory, respiratory, and phonatory). To briefly review, contrastive stress is the degree of emphasis a speaker places on a sound, syllable, or word depending on what the speaker wants to convey as most important in an utterance (e.g., with stress indicated by the uppercase letters, as in, *I'd like YOU to go* versus *I'd like you to GO*). Lexical stress is the inherent stress pattern of a word—it is part of how we pronounce a word (e.g., *poTAto*, not *POtato*). One specific type of lexical stress is grammatical stress, when a change in a word's stress pattern results in a word that means

something different (e.g., *The CONtents of the box spilled everywhere* versus *The baby was conTENT to sleep all day*). We produce stress that ranges from weak to strong as we actively engage one or more of the speech production systems (e.g., there are three different degrees of stress in the trisyllabic word *buttercup*, [ˈbʌ.ɾɚ.ˌkəp]).

Let us further explore the different types of stress. You know that individual words have an inherent pattern of stress that we realize in citation speech. For example, consider three words: *provide*, *one*, and *example*. The word *provide* has two syllables and its lexical stress pattern is weak-STRONG; the word *one* has one syllable, so that one syllable is stressed; the word *example* has three syllables and its lexical stress pattern is weak-STRONG-weak. Now that we have established the lexical stress patterns for each word, we want to find out if those stress patterns remain the same regardless of the speaking context, or if they change as speaking context changes, and if they do change, how and why they do so. To investigate, form a sentence with the three words. In class, your phonetics instructor might ask you to *Provide one example*. Did each word maintain its inherent stress pattern, even when strung together in a sentence? Repeat the sentence aloud a few times. Did the lexical stress stay the same for any or all the words when you pronounced them in a sentence? The lexical stress patterns in *provide*, *one*, and *example* likely changed when articulated in the sentence.

Lexical stress typically is not maintained when words are spoken in sentences, for a variety of reasons. One reason is that speakers of American English tend to space out stress, because, if overdone, stress placed on every word can make speech sound artificial, whereas stress omitted from every word can make speech sound monotone. We call a pattern of stress the **rhythm** of an utterance. Rhythm is how we group words together in an utterance, and in English the rhythm of a sentence is not fixed but determined by the speaker. Have you ever watched a Charlie Brown movie? If so, you heard the muffled trombone sounds used to characterize the voices of the adults in the movies. The adults' voices were made to sound like they were droning on with little expression. No one likes to listen to speech for long periods of time when it sounds monotone or robotic, but we also can become fatigued listening to overly stressed speech. We tend to prefer to listen to utterances produced with a balance of stressed and unstressed units of speech. For example, if we articulated an utterance containing five one-syllable words, such as *Please hand me that glass*, we would not vocally stress every word, even though each individual word has a strong monosyllabic lexical stress pattern. Stressing every word would be like capitalizing every letter in a text or email—something we largely avoid doing when writing. We call the vocal patterns of emphasis in connected speech **sentential stress**. Word stress in sentences usually differs from lexical stress.

Another reason that lexical stress changes in sentence contexts is because a speaker must decide what he or she thinks is the most important information to convey and then emphasize that information, which results in stress patterns that can change from production to production, as well as from speaker to speaker. As a speaker's intention varies, so do the degrees of stress placed on the words spoken. Try to imagine saying the sentence *I am hungry* in response to three different scenarios in which you would stress a different word in the sentence each time, as in **I** am hungry, I **AM** hungry, and I am **HUNGRY**. In the first scenario, you want your listener to know that it is you who is hungry. In the second scenario, you want your listener to know that indeed, you are hungry. And in the third scenario, you want your listener to know that you really want to eat soon.

We mark stress in one of several ways, or in a combination of ways. To mark stress in American English, speakers increase loudness, pitch, duration, and/or articulatory effort of the stressed speech unit (syllable or word) relative to the rest of the sounds in the utterance. Fundamentally, speakers exert more muscular effort on the speech units they stress, which results foremost in a slight increase in loudness of those speech units. Many people mistakenly believe that stress is indicated primarily by loudness. However, an increase in loudness alone is not sufficient to indicate stress. Why would loudness alone be insufficient to indicate stress? To answer that question, you want to think back to Chapter 1 when you learned about the sonority of speech sounds. The wider your mouth is open when you articulate a sound, the more sonorant that sound will be. This production phenomenon results in sounds with inherently different degrees of loudness, or sonor-

ity. Therefore, because some sounds naturally are louder than other sounds, only a *slight* increase in loudness alone is unlikely to be perceived by a listener as indicating stress.

The most efficacious way for a speaker to indicate stress is to increase the pitch of the stressed speech unit. You have learned that pitch is produced by varying the tension of the vocal folds; the tenser the vocal folds, the higher the pitch we perceive. In the case of increased pitch in stressed speech, the increase in pitch may be secondary to increased laryngeal tension, or it also may be secondary to increased expiratory effort. Increasing expiratory muscular effort will result not only in an increase in loudness, but also in pitch; therefore, the two events can occur simultaneously, resulting in stressed speech units that are both slightly louder and higher pitched.

Pitch variants can be sudden jumps or gradual increases. For demonstration purposes, we will diagram pitch in sentences using horizontal lines of varying heights. In the case of diagramming pitch, the higher the line, the higher the pitch. (You also could use the same procedure to diagram loudness.) Practice with the sentence *Provide one example*. In a situation where you want to stress the word *one*, as in you want someone to give a single example, you would articulate the sentence to emphasize the number *one*. Figure 5–1 shows pitch diagrammed. In this example, you see a sudden jump in pitch on the word *one*. Notice also in this example that the stress in the other two words remained the same, as it would have been if the words were spoken in isolation. Nonetheless, stress on the word *one* was greater than the stress marked on any other syllable or word, as indicated by increased pitch. It is this increase in pitch that provides the most salient auditory cue for stress.

Consider another example. Pretend for a moment that you are talking with a close friend who has an upcoming birthday. You want your friend to tell you something that he or she would like as a gift, so you say, *Tell me one thing you'd like*. Imagine that you are exasperated because your friend will not give you any suggestions. You show that exasperation in your voice as you gradually increase your pitch on the word *one*. Note that while doing so, you also increase the duration of the production and the clarity of your articulation, and, perhaps you even increase loudness. Such an example shows the effect of multiple changes in production that indicate to listeners what you, the speaker, most want them to focus on in your spoken language. Practice saying the sentence *Tell me one thing you'd like* by gradually increasing your pitch as indicated in Figure 5–2, as well as increasing the duration and articulation of the word *one*. Try to say the word *one* so that your production reveals frustration in your voice.

Next, consider that your friend still is not complying with your request. In this situation, you might stress that you really want to know what your friend

would like. How might you do so? There are many ways to emphasize this point. One way would be to produce either a sudden jump or a gradual increase in pitch on one or more of the words. Figure 5–3, below, is an illustration of a gradual increase in pitch on the words *thing* and *you'd*.

In addition to increasing loudness and pitch, we also can indicate stress by increasing the duration of the stressed speech units. These changes often are subtle increases of only a few milliseconds; nonetheless, the cues are salient to listeners. These increased durations are secondary to speaking with increased

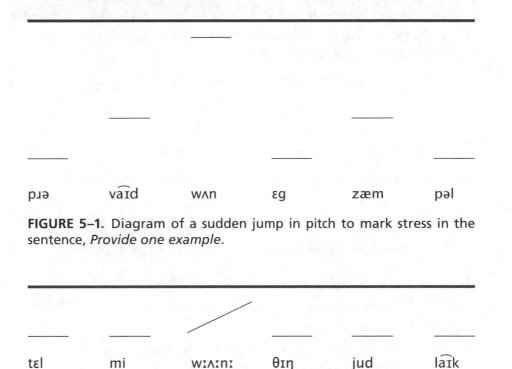

pɹə   va͡ɪd   wʌn   ɛg   zæm   pəl

FIGURE 5–1. Diagram of a sudden jump in pitch to mark stress in the sentence, *Provide one example*.

tɛl   mi   wːʌːnː   θɪŋ   jud   la͡ɪk

FIGURE 5–2. Diagram of pitch, loudness, and lengthening increases to mark stress in the sentence, *Tell me one thing you'd like*.

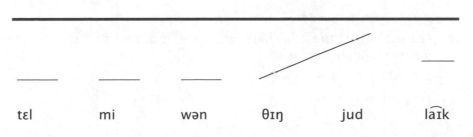

tɛl   mi   wən   θɪŋ   jud   la͡ɪk

FIGURE 5–3. Diagram of a gradual pitch increase to mark stress in the sentence, *Tell me one thing you'd like*.

muscular effort; however, we also can deliberately slow our speech rate, which serves to increase the duration of the speech unit. Imagine a situation in which your friend gave you a long list of gifts he or she wanted, and you wanted to clarify the word *one*. You could stress that word by stretching out one or more segments, as in [wːʌːnːː].

The phonetics of stress are complex, and include secondary articulatory effects that occur on stressed speech units. Consonants and vowels in stressed contexts tend to be articulated precisely. The reverse also is true: consonants and vowels in unstressed contexts tend to be articulated with less precision. For example, in unstressed contexts, voiceless stops are not fully aspirated, voiced consonants are devoiced, and consonants such as [h] may be omitted. In unstressed contexts, peripheral vowels tend to be neutralized as schwa and back vowels lose their lip rounding. In summary, stressed speech units tend to be relatively louder, higher pitched, longer in duration, and more precisely articulated than sounds and syllables in the rest of the utterance.

? 5–1. Did You Get It?

1. Write the typical lexical stress patterns of the following words. The first word has been done for you.

   benefit   <u>STRONG-weak-weak</u>   beneficial   _____

   pole   _____   polemic   _____

   method   _____   methodical   _____

   complain   _____   complainant   _____

2. Match the type of stress clarified by each example pair of words.

   _____ lexical   a. obJECT and OBject

   _____ grammatical   b. YOU go and you GO

   _____ contrastive/sentential   c. ZEbra and girAFFE

3. In American English, we produce stress on syllables and words by increasing _____, _____, _____, and/or _____.

4. Draw a lexical stress contour for the following words, marking each syllable. The first one has been done for you.

   ‾‾‾‾
   ___
   TA   ble   restaurant   hotel   schoolhouse

5. Practice saying the following sentences so that they fit the following pitch pattern.

   I should leave now.

   Do your work now.

   _____

   _____

   _____   _____

Intonation

Intonation can be described as the melody of speech. Technically, it is the pattern of pitch that extends over a phrase unit. A phrase unit can be a complete utterance or part of an utterance that is bounded by a pause on each side and (typically) contains one stress unit. A phrase unit often is related to syntactic units, such as clauses. For example, the utterance, *The little boy went to his friend's house before he walked to the store to buy himself a candy bar,* could be articulated as a single phrase unit, as in a single sentence without pauses. The actual word that carries the intonation peak will depend on which word the speaker wants to emphasize. However, because of the grammatical structure of the utterance, it is most likely that a speaker would produce that utterance in three phrase units that correspond to the clause structure, as in, *The little boy went to his friend's house, before he walked to the store, to buy himself a candy bar.* Each phrase unit would have its own pitch pattern overlaid on the syllables and words. Used linguistically, intonation tells about the grammatical aspects of an utterance.

Punctuation can help us parse utterances into syntactical phrase units. Consider a few examples. Say the following utterance aloud: *A woman without her man is nothing.* What phrase units did you produce? Say the utterance again, this time using different phrase units. Pause right now to think about a different way you could parse the words into phrases. Can you produce the utterance two different ways? If you can, then you know that the meaning of the utterance changes significantly. If you produced the utterance with two syntactical phrase units, you likely would have said, *A woman without her man, is nothing.* Spoken with three syntactical phrases, you would have said, *A woman: without her, man is nothing.* Quite a difference in meaning!

While some phrases are based on syntactical units, others are based on informational units, depending largely on how a speaker wants to convey a message. There is no way to predict exactly how someone is going to articulate an utterance, but its meaning will be influenced by the intonation pattern produced. Consider the utterance, *She said she'd like to see me again.* If the speaker is happy about this information, he or she may use a pleasant singsong intonation pattern to say it, as shown in the fluctuating intonation diagram in Figure 5–4. If the speaker is unhappy, he or she may use a flat intonation pattern, as shown in Figure 5–5. Or perhaps the speaker shows that he or she doubts the information by articulating the utterance as a question

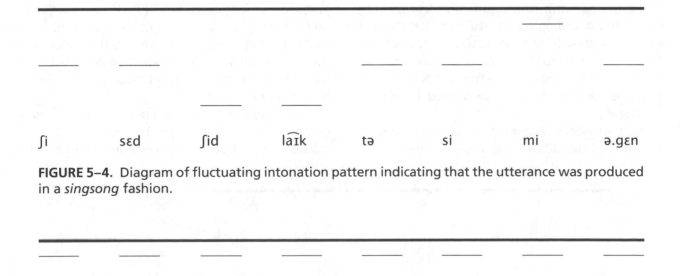

FIGURE 5–4. Diagram of fluctuating intonation pattern indicating that the utterance was produced in a *singsong* fashion.

FIGURE 5–5. Diagram of flat intonation pattern indicating that the utterance was produced in monotone fashion.

rather than a statement, by raising pitch at the end of the utterance, as shown in Figure 5–6. Notice also in Figure 5–6 that the speaker stressed the word *me* in the utterance, as if doubting exactly who the person wanted to see again. When analyzing intonation, the stressed word is said to carry the **pitch accent**.

As you saw in the intonation diagrams above, pitch can be steady, rising, or falling. There is an easier way to indicate pitch than drawing a diagram, and that is to use diacritics in your phonetic transcriptions. The diacritic for rising pitch is an upward arrow (i.e., [↑]), falling pitch is a downward arrow (i.e., [↓]), a global rise is a northeast arrow (i.e., [↗]), and a global fall is a southeast arrow (i.e., [↘]). For example, the question, *She said she'd like to see ME again?*, with the word *me* stressed and lengthened, could be transcribed phonetically as [ʃi sɛd ʃid laɪk tə si 'miː↑ ə.'gɛn↑]. This latter example demonstrates that even though intonation most often is described as pitch related, like stress, intonation is more complex than that. While intonation is the pattern of pitch that is overlaid on a phrase, it also involves establishing the phrase; deciding on the pitch contour; and deciding which speech unit will be stressed, and how. Because intonation affects meaning, it is vital for speakers to understand how it is used and how to produce it correctly. In speech-language pathology, you will work with clients who have difficulty understanding and/or producing intonation. Sometimes the difficulty is secondary to a known neurological or structural deficit, such as a motor speech or voice disorder, respectively. Other times, atypical intonation signals that English is a second language for a speaker. And in some cases, the specific cause of disordered intonation is unknown.

Most sentences in American English are produced with falling intonation, in that pitch lowers at the end, including questions that begin with the wh-words *who*, *what*, *where*, *when*, and *why*. Figure 5–7 displays falling-intonation diagrams for a declarative sentence and a wh-question. A falling intonation pattern is called **declination**. Listeners perceive declination as a signal that the speaker has finished saying a sentence. Alternatively, using rising intonation when saying a list of words, for example, indicates that a speaker has not finished naming items, so listeners, please keep paying attention. When a speaker gets to the final item, intonation falls, signaling the end of the list. Take a moment to try to hear rising intonation and declination as you say a list of items. Imagine that your friend offers to pick up a few things for you at the drugstore. You are trying to remember the three things you want your friend to get for you: shampoo, toothpaste, and gum. You say *shampoo* using rising intonation, because you know you need to pause to think of the other items and you do not want your friend to leave. You then remember *toothpaste*, and again you use rising intonation as you try to remember the third item. You finally say *gum* using a falling pitch, indicating that your list is complete.

Two expected exceptions to declination include yes/no (and other non–wh-word forced-choice) questions and mid-utterance pauses. Examine yes/no questions first. Say the following three yes/no questions aloud, trying to discern the intonation pattern you use: (1) *Are you hungry?* (2) *Do you want to go?* and (3) *Will you read it?* Hopefully, you could hear that your pitch rose as you spoke each question, with the highest pitch on the final syllable or word. An intonation diagram of the question, *Are you hungry?* is shown in Figure 5–8.

In addition to yes/no questions, we also produce questions by raising our pitch when we are asking a listener to select an answer from a closed set of

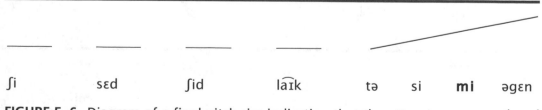

ʃi   sɛd   ʃid   laɪk   tə   si   **mi**   əgɛn

FIGURE 5–6. Diagram of a final pitch rise indicating that the utterance was produced as a question, with the word *me* stressed (shown in bold).

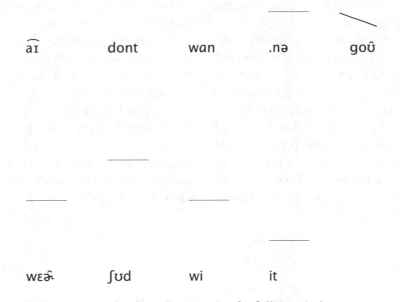

aɪ̂ dont wan .nə goʊ̂

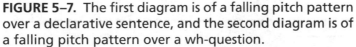

wɛ̂ɚ ʃʊd wi it

FIGURE 5–7. The first diagram is of a falling pitch pattern over a declarative sentence, and the second diagram is of a falling pitch pattern over a wh-question.

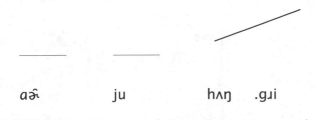

aɚ̂ ju hʌŋ .gɹi

FIGURE 5–8. Diagram of rising intonation at the end of the yes/no question, *Are you hungry?*

possibilities, such as *Me or you?*, *Ranch or vinaigrette?*, or *Pencil, pen, or marker?* Similarly, pitch rises when we pause midway through an utterance, for example, when we need to pause to think of what we want to say next. The pitch rise signifies that we are not yet ready to yield the floor to another speaker. For example, we might say, *She said she was going⬆* (pause) *to see a movie⬇*. This utterance, with two intonation phrases, is diagrammed in Figure 5–9.

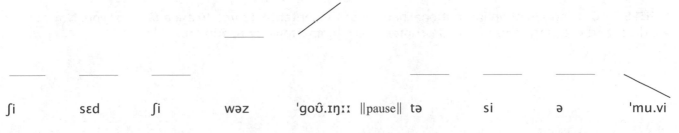

ʃi sɛd ʃi wəz ˈgoʊ̂.ɪŋːː ‖pause‖ tə si ə ˈmu.vi

FIGURE 5–9. A declarative statement with a pause mid-utterance, produced with two intonational phrases.

By raising our pitch at the end of the first phrase, we held on to our turn; by lowering our pitch at the end of the second phrase, we signaled we were finished speaking. This phenomenon is similar to our use of rising and falling intonation when we name items in a list, as discussed previously.

Describing the different ways that pitch changes in intonation of words and sentences is a skill that you will use clinically. One easy set of descriptors you can learn was developed by speech-language pathology professors Harold Edwards and Kathy Strattman (1996; see also Edwards, 2003). They used the descriptor "walk" to describe speech produced at a speaker's habitual pitch, which is a person's average pitch. When pitch increased to mark a stressed syllable, they described it using the term "jump."

After we articulate the stressed syllable, we incrementally lower our pitch, which they called "step down." The lowest pitch that occurs at the end of an utterance is what they called "fall." Refer to Figure 5–10 to see how we can use these terms to describe the intonation of the utterance, *I came to ask a favor of you.*

Again, be aware that the intonational pattern for an isolated word often changes when it is articulated in a sentence. Figure 5–11 displays two intonational patterns for the word *autobiographical.* In the first diagram, *autobiographical* is articulated as an isolated word, and the intonation pattern for the seven syllables is walk-walk-walk-walk-jump-step down-fall. In the 10-syllable utterance, *The book is autobiographical,* the pattern could change to walk-jump-step down-step down-step down-walk-walk-walk-walk-fall.

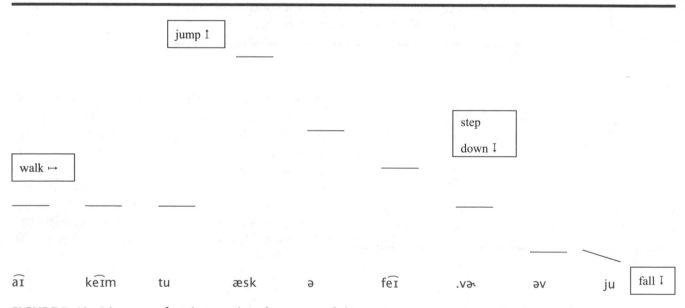

FIGURE 5–10. Diagram of an intonational pattern of the sentence, *I came to ask a favor of you.* Notice how we described the pattern using the descriptors walk, jump, step down, and fall.

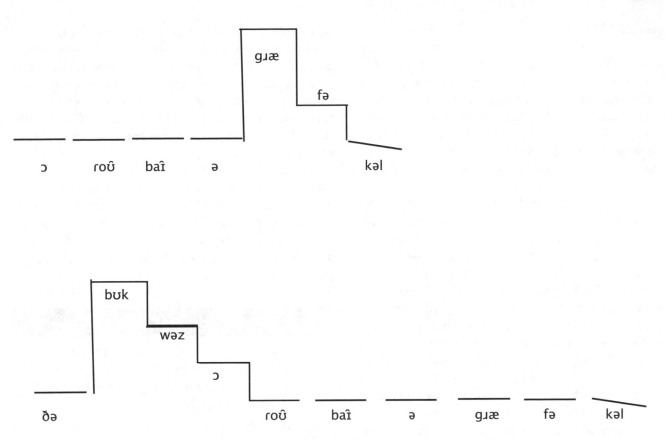

FIGURE 5–11. Diagrams of the intonation contour of the word *autobiographical* as spoken as a single word versus in a sentence. Notice how the contour changed across the two contexts.

? **5–2. Did You Get It?**

1. Saying the utterance, _She went to school, after she ate breakfast_ in two phrases, as underlined, is an example of producing intonation based on syntactical or informational units? _____

2. Saying the utterance, _She went to school_ in two phrases, as underlined, is an example of producing intonation based on syntactical or informational units? _____

3. Say the following utterance aloud using two different intonational phrase patterns, each signifying a different meaning. Underline the phrases and give the meaning of each production.

   Let's eat grandma. Meaning: _____

   Let's eat grandma. Meaning: _____

4. Write if the pitch typically falls or rises on each of the following utterances.

   Is she funny?   _____

   What's your name?   _____

Prosody

Although we tried to discuss the suprasegmentals of stress and intonation as autonomous features, the different production features interact, so stress and intonation involve pitch, loudness, hyper- and hypoarticulation, pausing, etc. And while the term suprasegmental technically means features overlaid on the segment, as you just learned, consonant and vowel articulation also changes in different stress and intonation contexts. For accuracy, we often refer to the combination of these features as prosody. We study the production and perception of prosodic features in speakers and listeners to better understand these phenomena. One example of studying prosody is infant-directed speech (IDS). Think about how we speak to babies and young children for a moment. Can you hear in your head how you would say to an infant, for example, *Ohhhhh, you're such a sweet baby*? Your speech would be slower, your volume lower, your pitch higher, and your intonation fluctuating. Each of these characteristics has been studied singly and in combination to help scientists better understand IDS. Another example of studying prosody is the investigation of how emotion is conveyed by speakers and perceived by listeners. We do not need to hear the exact words that a speaker is saying to know how the speaker feels about what he or she is saying. You play with prosodic features when you play games such as *Mad Gab*, a game in which you vary your articulation, stress, and intonation to figure out the common expression in a nonsensical phrase. For example, the game phrase "day fib let Herman" is the name of former talk show host David Letterman. The phrase, "Juno watt I'm mean" is the question, *Do you know what I mean*? These are fun explorations of the phonetics of prosody and suprasegmental features.

As clinical speech-language pathologists and audiologists, we work with individuals with a variety of diagnoses that affect their production and perception of prosody. Individuals who are deaf or hearing impaired often have difficulty correctly producing prosodic features because they cannot hear them or cannot hear them well. Individuals who are learning a second language oftentimes exhibit more difficulty mastering prosodic features than mastering the actual speech sounds of the language. Children and adults with motor speech disorders also can exhibit difficulty with the production of stress, pitch, and intonation, as well as with the understanding of others' use of prosodics. Individuals with autism spectrum disorder also frequently have trouble producing and understanding prosodic features. With practice, you will increase in your ability to understand these features that enhance verbal communication.

In the next chapter, you will learn the technical aspects of visualizing speech using acoustics and acoustic instrumentation. What may be difficult for you to hear will become easy for you to see. Applying acoustic phonetics to these articulatory and perceptual features will help your practice of phonetic science.

? 5–3. Did You Get It?

1. Say each phrase aloud several times while varying your articulation, stress, and intonation to change the meaning of each production.

   You want to go out for pizza?

   I could hardly believe that I ran into her.

Putting It All Together

In this chapter, you learned two of the four suprasegmental features, stress and intonation, that we vary to convey meaning beyond the meaning of the words we speak. When we communicate verbally, we decide how we want to divide our words into phrases, which word we want to stress in each phrase, and how we want to fluctuate our pitch throughout each phrase. It is a very complicated undertaking, yet we do this in millisecond speed simultaneously while articulating the consonants and vowels. Given the complexity of speech production, we should not be surprised that some individuals have difficulty producing not only speech sounds, but suprasegmental features as well. Your understanding of prosody is foundational for accurately diagnosing and treating individuals with related disorders.

In Chapter 9, the final chapter in this book, we will discuss two other suprasegmental features—tone and length. Tone refers to how pitch is used phonemically in languages such as Mandarin Chinese and Vietnamese to convey lexical and grammatical information. Length refers to phonemic changes in how long consonants and vowels are articulated to convey lexical and grammatical information in languages such as Italian. While we have discussed pitch changes and articulatory durations in this chapter when describing stress and intonation, in English these features are allophonic.

References

Edwards, H. T. (2003). *Applied phonetics: The sounds of American English* (3rd ed.). Clifton Park, NY: Delmar Learning.

Edwards, H. T., & Strattman, K. H. (1996). *Accent modification manual: Materials and activities.* San Diego, CA: Singular.

White, T. (2008). *Mad gab.* Game produced by Mattel.

Interest Piqued?

Recommended materials to further your understanding of topics covered in this chapter.

Print Resources

de Boer, B. (2011). *Infant-directed speech and language evolution.* In K. R. Gibson & M. Tallerman (Eds.), *The Oxford handbook of language evolution.* Oxford, UK: Oxford University Press.

Gray, J. (1992). *Men are from Mars, women are from Venus: A practical guide for improving communication and getting what you want in relationships.* New York, NY: HarperCollins.

In a book written for the general population, Gray discusses the role of suprasegmentals in verbal communication notably in *Chapter 9: How to Avoid Arguments*, focusing on the differences between how many men and women use and interpret suprasegmentals.

Truss, L. (2003). *Eats, shoots and leaves: The zero tolerance approach to punctuation.* London, UK: Profile Books.

Online Resources

http://www.dailymotion.com/video/x15wh1v_phonetic-description-of-annoying-sounds-teenagers-make-low-240p_fun

Here is a video and phonetic description of "the annoying sounds made by teenagers."

http://www2.leeward.hawaii.edu/hurley/ling102web/mod3_speaking/3mod3.7_suprasegmentals.htm

An instructor's fun examples of suprasegmental use (and misuse).

https://www.youtube.com/watch?v=b61R50gj5p4

A video clip of prosody.

https://www.youtube.com/watch?v=eIho2S0ZahI&t=346s

A video clip of prosody.

https://www.youtube.com/watch?v=65AgbiwQ6ko

A video clip showing stress.

http://www.youtube.com/watch?v=zIavvxoqxvs

Here is a short video clip of sarcasm.

Applied Science: Revisited

Summary

Now that you have read the suprasegmental chapter, do you want to make any changes to your list of meanings of the eight utterances? If so, go ahead and make those changes.

Let's see how we might answer.

One Step at a Time

1. When you first read the eight utterances, you may have provided literal meanings, similar to the ones that follow.

Yes	An affirmative response.
No way	A negative response.
I'd like to be your friend	Someone requesting a positive action.
Sure I'll go	A positive response indicating that the person will go somewhere.
I'll see you later	Indicating goodbye until the people meet again.
Don't even	A negative command.
Who are you	Someone asking someone else his or her name.
Whatever	Someone expressing neutrality.

2. In addition, you may have provided alternate meanings, based on how each utterance was articulated. Use your new knowledge about stress and intonation to provide different interpretations of the eight utterances. A variety of possible interpretations are possible, a few of which follow.

Yes	If said with rising intonation, it could signal a question, not a response.
No way	If said with rising intonation, it could signal a question like, "Really?"
I'd like to be your friend	If said with sarcasm, it could mean that the person does not want to be friends.
Sure, I'll go	If said with sarcasm, it could mean that the person will not go.
I'll see you later	If said with excessive stress on "you," it could mean that the person is in trouble.
Don't even	If said with fluctuating intonation, the speaker could be kidding.
Who are you	If said with increased length and fluctuating intonation, it could indicate that the speaker was surprised or upset by the person.
Whatever	Someone responding with stress and intonation that basically means *I don't care.*

3. Hopefully, you could think of several nonliteral meanings for each of the eight utterances, depending on the suprasegmental features added during articulation.

Answer
Your responses are correct if you provided a variety of ways that those utterances could have been spoken. Without information regarding the suprasegmentals used during production, there is no way to know what those eight utterances mean just by reading them.

Science Applied
Applying the phonetics of suprasegmentals to these utterances increases the range of correct responses. Being aware of how meaning is imbued in the speech we produce is vital to understanding verbal communication, and being able to capture that in your phonetic transcriptions will help you to identify individuals with deficits in understanding and/or using suprasegmental features in conversational speech.

? Did You Get It?

ANSWER KEY

5–1.

1. Write the typical lexical stress patterns of the following words. The first word has been done for you.

benefit	STRONG-weak-weak	beneficial	weak-weak-STRONG-weak
pole	STRONG	polemic	weak-STRONG-weak
method	STRONG-weak	methodical	weak-STRONG-weak-weak
complain	weak-STRONG	complainant	weak-STRONG-weak

2. Match the type of stress clarified by each example pair of words.

  <u>c</u> lexical   a. obJECT and OBject

  <u>a</u> grammatical   b. YOU go and you GO

  <u>b</u> contrastive/sentential   c. ZEbra and girAFFE

3. In American English, we produce stress on syllables and words by increasing <u>loudness</u>, <u>pitch</u>, <u>duration</u>, and/or <u>articulatory effort</u>.

4. Draw a lexical stress contour for the following words, marking each syllable. The first one has been done for you.

```
 ___            _____         _____        _____
   ___
TA  ble         RE             stau          rant


_____         _____                        _____
ho              TEL            SCHOOL         house
```

5. Practice saying the following sentences so that they fit the following pitch pattern.
   <u>These are verbal practice sentences. The pitch should drop incrementally on each word.</u>

5–2.

1. Saying the utterance, *She went to school, after she ate breakfast* in two phrases, as underlined, is an example of producing intonation based on syntactical or informational units?   <u>syntactical</u> units

2. Saying the utterance, *She went to school* in two phrases, as underlined, is an example of producing intonation based on syntactical or informational units?   <u>informational units</u>

3. Say the following utterance aloud using two different intonational phrase patterns, each signifying a different meaning. Underline the phrase units and give the meaning of each production.

<u>Let's eat grandma.</u>   Meaning: <u>We are hungry and want grandma to feed or eat with us.</u>

<u>Let's eat grandma.</u>   Meaning: <u>We are going to eat grandma!</u>

4. Write if the pitch typically falls or rises on each of the following utterances.

Is she funny?   <u>rises</u>

What's your name?   <u>falls</u>

5–3.

1. Say each phrase aloud several times while varying your articulation, stress, and intonation to change the meaning of each production.

You want to go out for pizza?

I could hardly believe that I ran into her.

<u>These are verbal practice sentences. Productions will vary.</u>

6

ACOUSTIC PHONETICS

Learning Objectives

By reading this chapter, you will learn:

1. basic physical properties of the acoustic signal
2. how sound travels
3. what acoustic phonetics adds to our understanding of speech
4. how acoustic phonetics can be applied in the clinical sciences
5. the difference between transverse, longitudinal, and surface waves
6. the difference between sine, complex periodic, complex aperiodic, and complex periodic and aperiodic waves
7. subjective and objective ways we measure sound
8. what a waveform tells us
9. what a spectrum tells us
10. about Fourier analysis and the source-filter theory
11. about formants, fundamental frequency, and harmonics
12. what a spectrogram is and how to read vowels, consonants, and pitch on them
13. the difference between wide- and narrowband spectrograms

Applied Science

To explore the use of acoustic phonetics in the clinical sciences, we examine how acoustics can be used to understand speech development. In the early 1990s, a linguist described a young girl's mispronunciations of several words as she was developing speech and language (Macken, 1992). Her mispronunciations at four ages are displayed in Table 6–1. Note the four target words: *pretty, tree, drink, cradle*. What similarity across the four target words do you see? (Hint: Look at how each word begins.) Yes, all four words begin with a stop + /ɹ/ consonant cluster: /pɹ, tɹ, dɹ, kɹ/.

The data show how the child produced each target word during the first time period (T1) when she was between 1 year, 6 months and 1 year, 10 months of age. What speech error pattern do you see? The child omitted the /ɹ/ from each cluster, producing [p] for /pɹ/, [t] for /tɹ/, [d] for /dɹ/, and [k] for /kɹ/. In addition, she strongly aspirated most of the stop consonants.

Before determining the error patterns, we need to review background information. Speech-language pathologists and researchers ask a series of questions in their attempt to understand how children acquire speech. For this particular child we first ask, "What is her specific error?" followed by, "Do other children make the same error?" and finally, "Why did she make that error?" We have already answered the first question: the error this child made was to delete /ɹ/ in the target clusters. There is extensive research evidence showing children reduce consonant clusters to singleton consonants during speech development. In addition, children typically delete the consonant in a cluster that is later to be mastered. With regard to stop + /ɹ/ clusters, the liquid /ɹ/ is mastered later than the stop phonemes; therefore, we would expect a young child to delete /ɹ/ and retain the stop consonant.

Why might this child, and most children, exhibit this specific error pattern? Generally speaking, singleton consonants are mastered earlier than consonant clusters. We can hypothesize that to reduce the articulatory difficulty of producing two sequential consonants in a cluster, the child retained the early-mastered stop consonant and deleted the later-mastered consonant, /ɹ/. It seems likely that the child simplified her production of the clusters because of the difficulty involved in articulating sequential consonants. This indeed was Macken's suggested explanation when she contemplated the data from T1.

Now we turn to the other three time periods. At T2, the child's productions of two of the words were the same as at T1, but the child produced two words differently: [fi] for /tɹi/ and [fɪŋkʰ] for /dɹɪŋk/. By T3, the child substituted [f] for all four of the clusters, a pattern that continued into T4

TABLE 6–1. Misarticulations of Four Target Words Across Four Time Periods by a Child Developing Speech*

Time Period	Age (years; months)	Target Words and Productions			
		/pɹɪ.ɾi/	/tɹi/	/dɹɪŋk/	/kɹeɪ.dəl/
T1	1;6–1;10	[pʰɹ.tʰi]	[tʰi]	[tɪŋkʰ]	[kʰeɪ.dəl]
T2	1;11	[pʰɹ.tʰi]	[fi]	[fɪŋkʰ]	[kʰeɪ.dəl]
T3	1;11–2;1	[fɹ.tʰi]	[fi]	[fɪŋkʰ]	[feɪ.dəl]
T4	2;2	[pʰɹ.tʰi]	[fi]	[fɪŋkʰ]	[feɪ.dəl]

*For clarity, the transcription of the vowel phonemes in *drink* and *cradle* have been changed from the original manuscript to match the transcription conventions used in this textbook.

for three of the clusters. Across the latter three time periods, the child changed from deleting /ɹ/ in each stop + /ɹ/ cluster to substituting [f] for each stop + /ɹ/ cluster. Macken searched to find an explanation for why the child may have made the [f] substitution for the target stop + /ɹ/ clusters. Given that the cluster reductions at T1 were argued to be articulatory based, we may speculate that there is a production-based reason why the child may have substituted [f] for each of the four stop + /ɹ/ clusters. Before we present Macken's explanations, what explanations can you hypothesize?

Macken asserted that production-, or phonetics-based, explanations (albeit not necessarily strong ones) could be made for the substitution of [f] for three of the four clusters: /pɹ, tɹ, dɹ/. Macken suggested that the [f] for /pɹ/ substitution might be explained phonetically because /f/, like /ɹ/ in the target cluster, has a labial component to its production. She thought that the [f] substitution for /pɹ/ was best explained phonetically, given that the production of a /tɹ/ cluster is strongly aspi-

rated and has a labial component in the /ɹ/ segment, with the [f] substitution being a labiodental fricative. By extension, Macken proposed that the child's representation of /tɹ/ and /dɹ/ could be categorized as coronal + /ɹ/ clusters; therefore, the same substitution pattern would be expected.

However, according to Macken, the [f] substitution for /kɹ/ could not be explained by production-based—or by any phonetic-based—reason. She presumed that the child's phonological system, as opposed to her phonetic system, was the reason for the [f] for /kɹ/ substitution pattern. She concluded that the child had a phonological rule that substituted stop + /ɹ/ clusters with the labiodental fricative phoneme /f/.

Do you agree with Macken that these errors can only be explained phonologically? Is there a phonetic-based reason that could account for this error? Could there be a reason based on acoustic properties? Or does this specific error provide otherwise unexplainable evidence of a child's phonology at work? Ponder these questions as you read this chapter on acoustic phonetics.

Acoustic Phonetics and Clinical Scientists

In previous chapters, we have focused on what the speaker is doing to produce speech that clearly communicates her message to the listener. We have covered the anatomy and physiology of the speech system and how the respiratory, phonatory, oronasal, and articulatory systems interact to produce the phonemes of English. But what about what the listener hears—does this matter? Actually, it matters less how the speaker moves her mouth to make sound than what sounds reach the listener's ear, regardless of how the sounds were produced. During speech development, caregivers typically emphasize what words sound like rather than how to produce speech sounds. In fact, computer-generated speech, made without any articulation, is completely intelligible to the listener. What makes computerized speech clear is that the audio signal has captured the acoustic characteristics of the speech signal. As clinical scientists, we must have a thorough knowl-

edge of the process of speech production, as well as the acoustic properties of speech sounds that allow a listener to comprehend speech.

In this chapter, we explore how sound energy travels and how the speech system is manipulated to contrast phonemes, words, and phrases in speech. Acoustic phonetics provides the tools for analyzing the acoustic signal. This analysis is useful in describing how similar *sounds* are acoustically, and thus why those sounds might be confused. For instance, /f/ and /θ/ have similar acoustic structures, are lower energy, and are often confused by non-English speakers and young children. Acoustic phonetics also allows us to specify why some sounds differ when their differences cannot be easily described by articulation, such as vowels. The acoustic structure of sound determines what we hear; if sounds are too similar or too different from adult speech targets, the speaker will sound confusing to the listener and may not be understood. In contrast, since speech sounds, such as the English /ɹ/, can be produced different ways, acoustic phonetics helps us understand what properties in the acoustic signal are required for a listener to correctly identify them as /ɪ/. Remember, adults did not tell us how to produce speech and no one ever stood over us and said, "Move your articulators this way to make [ɪ] and [i] sound different from each other." What we did learn is whether our listener understood what we said or whether we needed to produce speech sounds differently in our mouth to aid our listener's understanding.

Acoustic phonetics is the branch of phonetics that studies the acoustic characteristics of speech at multiple levels, exploring the physical properties of sound, including frequency, intensity, and duration of speech. In acoustic phonetics, we gain an understanding of how speech is conveyed to the listener, how articulatory differences affect speech sounds, and what the listener hears.

We can visualize sound properties using instrumentation. These visualizations of the acoustic signal display acoustic differences in speech sounds and reveal individual speaker differences. They can also help explain how languages form sound patterns and why we are often able to differentiate speech sounds even when listening to disordered speech.

Acoustics

We begin our study of acoustic phonetics with a review of basic acoustic principles. Acoustics is a branch of physics that explains the properties of sound. At its most basic level, sound results from repeated vibration of an entity, or **sound source**. Our ears hear this repetitive vibratory motion because the vibration travels from the sound source to our ears through a medium, such as air. For example, if we are in the kitchen, we may be able to hear a noise generated by the fan in the bathroom. Our ears are not directly hearing the sound generated by the fan; we are hearing vibratory waves made by molecules in the air as a result of the fan blades moving. The vibratory sound waves, but not the molecules themselves, travel from the fan to our ear via air.

A guitar string is another sound source. When not vibrating, a guitar string is at rest and makes no sound. If the string is plucked, it moves from its resting position as far as it is pulled. When the string is

released, it travels opposite the direction in which it was pulled, passing and not stopping at its original resting position. When the string is released, it returns to its resting position but does not stop there. Instead, the string travels beyond its original position in the opposite direction. Because it is elastic, the string will go back and forth across the resting position, decreasing its **displacement** (distance from its original position) with each back and forth cycle, until the string finally settles back to its original resting position. The string's **elasticity** is why it moves back and forth repetitively as it crosses the original resting place. And as the string moves back and forth, it vibrates.

A plucked string will be displaced the furthest when it is first plucked, although it will keep moving back and forth, diminishing in displacement and decreasing in vibration until it eventually returns to the original position. If the string continues to be plucked, it will continue to vibrate. How far the string is pulled, or displaced, affects how long the string vibrates, as well as the **intensity** of the sound it makes. The intensity of a sound is how loud it is.

Why does guitar string movement result in sounds that we hear across the room? Adjacent to the string are air molecules, each of which obeys basic physical properties. These molecules are motionless in their resting position and are spaced equidistant from each other. These molecules remain evenly spaced until a sound source—a string, an engine, a tuning fork, the vocal folds—is moved. The movement of the sound source displaces adjacent air molecules, pushing these molecules in the direction of the movement closer together and leaving the molecules behind the sound source farther apart. As the object moves back and forth, it continues to displace air molecules. While these vibrating molecules do not reach our ear, the plucking movement propagates a sound wave, with the adjacent molecules pushed away from their resting position, which in turn push against molecules in the air adjacent to them. The pushing of molecules continues until those molecules adjacent to the listener's ear are pushed against the ear drum. Figure 6–1 demonstrates this molecular movement over time. The first line shows molecules A through E at rest (the connecting springs have been added to highlight the molecules' elasticity). The second line shows how a

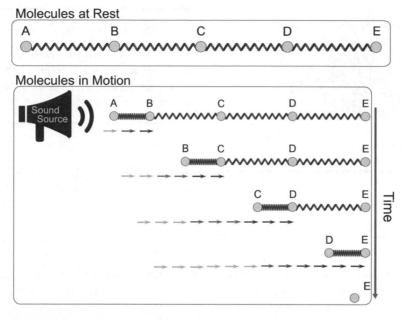

FIGURE 6–1. Diagram of sound source moving molecule A and resulting in the wave of movement of molecules B through E.

sound source pushes molecule A closer to molecule B, which then pushes molecule B closer to C (in line 3), through line 6, where molecule D, which has been pushed by molecule C, pushes molecule E.

Wave Motion

Sound that reaches our ear results from a disturbance of an object from its resting position. Some vibratory motions do not last long, pushing molecules toward the ear only for a short period of time. For example, dropping a book results in an abrupt, time-limited sound. However, there are many sounds that last for an extended period of time as the sound source continues to vibrate. Examples include a tuning fork, the strings of string instruments, drums, as well as prolonged vibration of the vocal folds as a vowel is produced. The movement of these sound sources consists of a repetitive vibratory movement, with the particles' simple wave of movement shown in Figure 6–1 repeated multiple times.

Movement of a sound source results in waves that can travel through many media, as long as the **medium** has molecules to carry the sound wave. Media that can propagate waves of sound include solids, liquids, and gases. Examples of these media include rock, bone, water, and air. We most frequently hear speech traveling through air. Like particles in rock, water, and bone, air molecules are spaced evenly apart. Air is also an elastic medium, allowing individual molecules to move independently from each other. The elasticity of air results in the back and forth movement of the particles and in their eventual return to a resting state once the perturbation (such as pulling on the guitar string) has ended. Sound cannot travel through a vacuum because there are no molecules in a vacuum to displace.

Sound Wave Propagation

Molecules are displaced by movement of the sound source. As was shown in Figure 6–1, these displaced molecules push against neighboring molecules in a wavelike movement that is propagated through the medium. Particles can be moved by three types of waves: **transverse, longitudinal,** and **surface**. A Slinky toy, shown in Figure 6–2, can be used to demonstrate transverse and longitudinal waves.

Pretend you have a Slinky and that you have spread it horizontally on a table. If you raise and

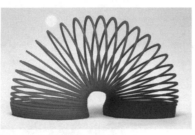

FIGURE 6–2. Picture of a Slinky.

Direction of Particles **Direction of Energy**

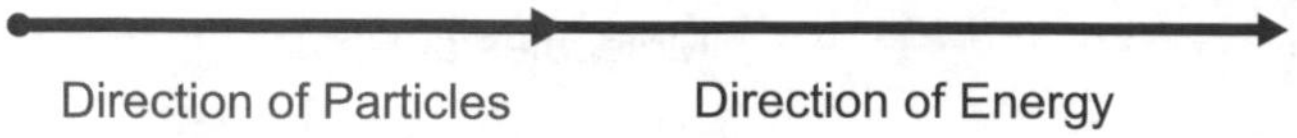

FIGURE 6–4. Longitudinal wave movement. Longitudinal waves result from parallel movement, where particles push other particles and the energy movement is from side to side in the same direction.

lower one end of the Slinky for several seconds, your continuous movement creates a wave that travels from one end of the Slinky to the other. This movement is shown in Figure 6–3. Notice that the wave is being initiated by an *up-and-down* movement, while the wave is traveling through the Slinky *side-to-side*. These opposing or perpendicular directions of movement are characteristic of a transverse wave. The particles of a wave (where you are holding on to the Slinky) are moving in the opposite direction from the energy traveling down the Slinky. Another way to visualize a transverse wave is to think of "the human wave," people standing up and sitting down in succession at a concert or sports event, creating a traveling wave. Note that people are standing up and sitting down (like particles of a wave), while the direction of the wave (energy transfer) is side-to-side.

Back to the Slinky on the table. This time, bump one end of the Slinky forcefully toward the other end. This quick bump creates a pulse that travels down the Slinky. In this scenario, the direction of the particles moving (initial bump on one end) is the same as the energy transfer (wave traveling down the Slinky). This parallel movement is characteristic of a longitudinal wave, and illustrates the way in which sound waves travel. Sound waves force molecules to collide into one another in the direction of travel, similar to how the initial bump of the Slinky sent the energy in the same direction. A longitudinal wave is shown in Figure 6–4.

A third type of wave is a surface wave, a wave on the surface of two different media. Surface waves can be seen in the disturbance of water. Imagine the ripples on a pond after you throw a pebble into the water. The pebble displaces water at the point of contact. Because of the displacement, we see ripples in the water. The water molecules move back and forth around the same spot, but the ripples or waves they generate travel in all directions. What we do not see, but what we do hear, is the sound made by the movement of molecules in the air, above the water. Thus the vibratory wave travels through the water below the pebble and through the air above the water. Eventually, the water and air settle back to their resting position.

How are sound waves processed by the human brain? Sound waves reach the ear as a transmission of variations in air pressure. The auditory system converts the physical energy resulting from air pressure disturbances into neurological information. Thus, physical aspects of sound reach the ear and travel to the brain, where they are converted into psychological aspects of sound. The conversion of sound waves into neurological energy is not an aspect of acoustic phonetics, so it will be left for hearing science courses.

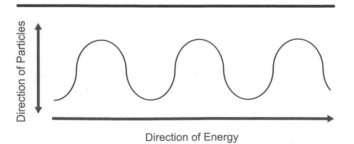

Direction of Particles

Direction of Energy

FIGURE 6–3. Transverse wave movement. Transverse waves are initiated by up and down movement of particles resulting in energy movement from side to side.

Sound Waves

So how do sound waves travel through air? Prior to the movement of the sound source, there is silence: molecules in the air are evenly spaced and at rest. Then the sound source is disturbed and molecules adjacent to the sound source are forced from their resting state. This disturbance could be a guitar string being plucked, a tuning fork being hit, or vocal folds vibrating as air particles are pushed out of the lungs. As a result of the sound source movement, the molecules are pushed away from the disturbance and closer to the molecules in front of them, an event called **compression**. The compressed molecules in front of the disturbance result in the molecules behind the wave of compression being farther apart, referred to as **rarefaction**. This compression and rarefaction of molecules is repeated as the vibration travels through the air, creating a longitudinal wave of vibration.

Figure 6–5 is a demonstration of the process of compression and rarefaction, showing how the movement of the tuning fork results in many air particles being pushed (compression) and that behind the pushed particles there are fewer air particles (rarefaction). Because of the original tuning fork movement, the pushed particles push other particles, creating a wave of compression and rarefaction in both directions. If the sound source is no longer perturbed, the molecules will eventually return to their resting state where they are equidistantly spaced. Longitudinal sound moves in all directions, or spherically, although it is easiest to visualize sound as simple two-dimensional waves.

Sound does not move linearly but spherically; that is, sound leaves its source and travels in all directions. Figure 6–6 provides a simplistic image of the spherical sound wave leaving the sound source. This spherical wave propagation eventually arrives at the human ear.

Compression and rarefaction are periods of high pressure and low pressure, respectively. Figure 6–7

shows the tuning fork and the periods of compression and rarefaction resulting from the tuning fork movement. These periods of compression and rarefaction can be transferred to a **waveform**, a graph of pressure changes fundamental to acoustic phonetics. On a waveform, the *x*-axis represents time, while the *y*-axis represents pressure or amplitude, shown at the bottom of Figure 6–7. The dotted horizontal line represents atmospheric pressure at zero (0). On a waveform, increased pressure resulting from compression of molecules is shown when the line is above 0 on the graph, while decreased pressure resulting from rarefaction is seen when the line is below the 0 mark.

Describing Sound Waves

We measure repeating sound waves by measuring their pressure variations. The measurements are determined by measuring the time from resting through maximal compression and rarefaction dispersion. This period of time is referred to as one **cycle**. The time it takes to complete one full cycle is called a **period**. We measure the **frequency** of these cycles or periods by counting the number of times this compression-rarefaction cycle occurs in a second. For sound, the measurement unit for cycles per second is the **hertz**, abbreviated **Hz**. The human ear can hear a vast range of cycles per second or fre-

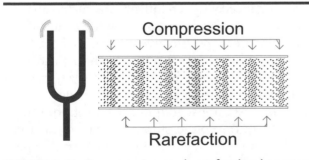

FIGURE 6–5. Compression and rarefaction in a sound-wave resulting from a tuning fork movement.

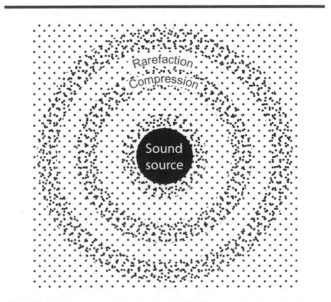

FIGURE 6–6. Sound waves traveling spherically from the sound source.

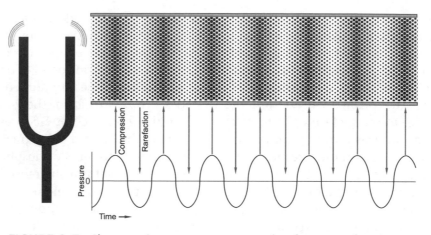

FIGURE 6–7. Changes in pressure as a result of waves of compression and rarefaction. The *x*-axis represents time and the *y*-axis represents pressure.

quency differences. We can hear sounds with very few cycles per second, that is, with a very low frequency, as low as 20 Hz, and we can hear sounds with a very high frequency, as high as 20,000 Hz. This frequency range represents the number of vibrations of sound that happen per second. Low and high frequency sounds are perceived as low and high pitch, respectively. We perceive a 20 Hz sound as being very low pitched, and a 20,000 Hz sound as being very high pitched.

The speech signal is composed of sounds at many frequencies. The most meaningful components of speech sounds in languages range from 250 to 8000 Hz. The fundamental frequency (F0) is the objective measurement of pitch: how high or low a person's voice is. F0 is the number of cycles of a sound wave occurring per second. Fundamental frequency is dependent on how often the vocal folds vibrate as well as the length of the vibratory portion of the vocal folds. If the vocal folds vibrate 200 times per second (200 cps), the person's F0 is 200 Hz. While there is not a 1:1 correspondence, sounds of high frequency are perceived as being high-pitched and low frequency sounds are perceived as low-pitched. Larger vocal tracts tend to have larger and longer vocal folds which vibrate at a lower rate. A biologically male voice has an F0 between 80 and 200 Hz, biologically female voices have an F0 range up to 400 Hz, and the average F0 for children ranges between 250 and 400 Hz, but can be as high as 800 Hz.

Intensity is a measure of how high or low the pressure changes in the sound wave are. Intensity is also referred to as the **amplitude** of air pressure variations. Intensity is measured in **decibels**, written dB. Sounds with greater air pressure changes are heard as louder. A bigger original disturbance of the sound source will cause air molecules to be displaced farther from rest, causing a greater rise and fall in air pressure. Loudness is the subjective measurement of intensity, which also is measured in dB.

The human ear detects sound with a loudness range of 0 to 140 dB, although most phonemes are approximately 60 dB when they reach our ear. Differences in amplitude for speech sounds are related to the shape of the vocal tract during the sound's production. In speech, sonorants have the greatest amplitude and obstruents have the smallest amplitude. Sonorants are speech sounds produced with a relatively unobstructed airway; obstruents are sounds produced with a relatively obstructed airway. Sonorants are vowels, nasals, liquids, and glides. Obstruents are stops, fricatives, and affricates. Vowels have slightly more amplitude than nasals, liquids, and glides. Sibilant fricatives (/s, z, ʃ, ʒ/), are slightly less intense than sonorants. In descending order, the least intense sounds are nonsibilant fricatives /f, v, θ, ð/, voiced stops, and voiceless stops. Actual sound intensity of a phoneme also is dependent on additional factors, including the position of a word in a sentence, whether the word or syllable is stressed or unstressed, and individual speaker characteristics.

Sound waves can differ in amplitude and frequency. Figure 6–8 shows sound waves that share amplitude but differ in frequency. Figure 6–9 shows sound waves that have the same frequency but differ in amplitude.

Frequency and amplitude are concrete, physical dimensions of sound. They can be measured accurately and reliably with instruments that measure frequency in hertz and amplitude in decibels. Alternatively, pitch and loudness refer to perceptual or psychological dimensions that are measured subjectively (without instrumentation). Amplitude and frequency are independent of one another; that is, sounds with high amplitude can be low frequency. Take a moment to apply this concept to speech. Say [u], prolonging its production for several seconds. Now say [u] with a higher than typical pitch and vary loudness from quiet to loud. Next, produce a quiet, low-pitched [u], and then say it loudly, keeping pitch the same. Your ability to do these tasks exemplifies the independent nature of pitch and loudness.

Frequency and amplitude are important to our understanding of phonetic differences in acoustic phonetics. There are frequency differences that tell us the difference between /i/ and /u/ and loudness differences that cue us into whether a sound is a vowel or a consonant. As you will see, though, frequency and amplitude are not sufficient measurements to understand how we distinguish sounds. We will also need information on **quality** and **duration** of sounds.

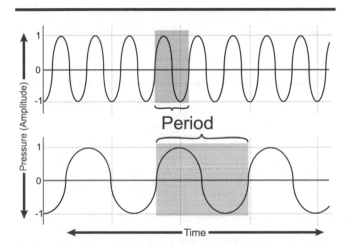

FIGURE 6–8. Two sound waves of the same amplitude but different frequencies.

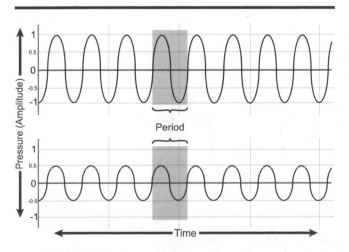

FIGURE 6–9. Two sound waves that share the same frequency but different amplitudes.

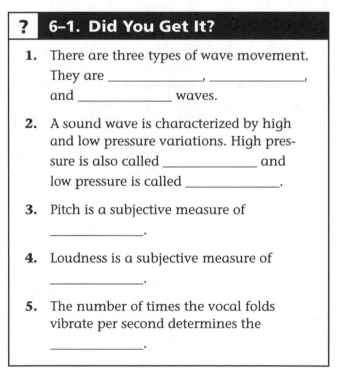

? 6–1. Did You Get It?

1. There are three types of wave movement. They are _____, _____, and _____ waves.

2. A sound wave is characterized by high and low pressure variations. High pressure is also called _____ and low pressure is called _____.

3. Pitch is a subjective measure of

_____.

4. Loudness is a subjective measure of

_____.

5. The number of times the vocal folds vibrate per second determines the

_____.

Sound Waves and Vocal Fold Vibration

As we have seen, sound can be generated from a sound source such as a guitar string or a tuning fork. One sound source for speech is the open-and-close cycle of the vocal folds during vocal fold vibration. At rest the vocal folds are abducted, or apart, and air flows out of the lungs inaudibly. To produce voiced sounds, we adduct the vocal folds. As the vocal folds are brought together, we force air out of our lungs, resulting in a pressure buildup below the vocal folds. As air continues to leave the lungs, the pressure below the vocal folds builds up to such an extent that the elastic vocal folds are forced apart. Air particles then flow rapidly through the approximated vocal folds. However, because the vocal folds are close together and air is traveling very rapidly between them, the air pressure decreases and the elastic vocal folds come back together. This cycle of pressure buildup and release results in high and low pressure periods that are repeated between 80 and 400 times per second, with lower frequency repetitions heard as lower pitch.

Waveforms

A variety of sound waves can be shown on a waveform. The simplest sound wave is a **sine wave** (or **sinusoid**), a smooth, repeating sound wave. Simple sine waves are rare and do not occur in speech. Sine waves are produced by a tuning fork or created with computer technology in a lab. Figure 6–10 is a waveform of a sine wave. In this wave, we have marked one period, indicating where one vibratory

cycle starts and where it ends. Note that the same cycle repeats multiple times in this sine wave, not changing in amplitude or frequency.

As Figure 6–10 shows, waveforms capture air pressure variations over time. The y-axis represents amplitude, or pressure. At the midpoint on the y-axis is 0.0, indicating 0 pressure and the resting state of a molecule. Look carefully at the sine wave in Figure 6–11, noting how much time has passed on the x-axis. There you can see that the sine wave starts at 0.0 amplitude and travels to 1.0 in approximately 0.125 seconds. Time is shown on the x-axis. The sine wave in Figure 6–11 travels from its resting point (at 0 amplitude), reaches maximum **dispersion** and returns to its resting point at the x-axis after 0.25 seconds. The wave continues beyond its resting point to its maximal negative pressure at

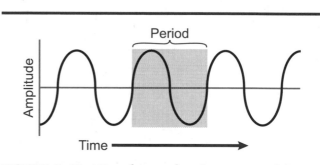

FIGURE 6–10. Waveform of a sine wave with one cycle of pressure variation marked.

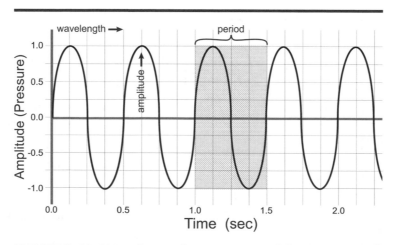

FIGURE 6–11. Waveform of a sine wave with a wavelength of 2 Hz.

0.375 seconds. This sine wave completes a full cycle every 0.5 seconds and then repeats itself. There are two cycles of the sound wave in a second, meaning that this sine wave travels at a frequency of 2 cycles per second, which equals 2 Hz.

The waveforms in Figures 6–10 and 6–11 are of **sine waves**. Sine waves are simple, recurring sound waves. Their cycles and amplitudes do not change and are sinusoidal. In contrast, speech is made up of **complex sound waves**. Complex waves are made up of energy from the sound source traveling at many different frequencies. In other words, complex waves are made up of sets of simple waves added together. The combination of these different frequencies creates a unique sound pattern. A complex wave can still demonstrate periodic cycles, or **periodicity.** However, due to the wave's complexity, a complex wave has a richer sound quality than a sine wave. Figure 6–12 compares a sine wave to a complex speech wave. Note that both waves have the same amplitude and the same time period; however, the pressure variation differs. The sound in Waveform B does not have the sinusoidal quality of Waveform A. Also note that Waveform B does not have a repeating cycle.

Complex sound waves can be periodic or aperiodic. **Periodic waves** have a rhythmic, repeating pattern, in which each cycle is a repetition of the preceding and following cycle. In speech, vowels are periodic waves. Voiced continuant consonants also

have a complex periodic component. Figure 6–13 is the complex periodic wave of an English vowel. The start and end of one cycle has been marked. Look carefully at this waveform to see how this cycle is repeated.

Aperiodic waves are characterized by unpredictable and chaotic properties. There is no repeating pattern of vibration. Aperiodic sounds are perceived as noisy and hiss-like. An example of an aperiodic sound is white noise. In speech, voiceless phones are aperiodic. Examples of aperiodic waves in speech are those for voiceless stops, like the phonemes [t] and [p], and fricatives, such as [s] and [ʃ]. Figure 6–14 is a waveform of the voiceless fricative [ʃ], which does not have the repeating pattern that the vowel has in Figure 6–13.

Some speech sounds are both periodic and aperiodic. That is, they have a repeating pattern as a result of vocal fold vibration, as well as non-repeating patterns resulting from turbulent noise created by obstruction in the vocal tract. Can you think of any sounds that are both periodic and aperiodic? Voiced fricatives are an example. Figure 6–15 is a waveform of [ʒ], showing a repeating cycle of pressure variation and a chaotic aperiodic wave superimposed on the periodic pattern. The periodic sound source for /ʒ/ is vocal fold vibration. The aperiodic sound source is the partial obstruction in the oral cavity as the blade of the tongue nears the hard palate, creating turbulence (friction).

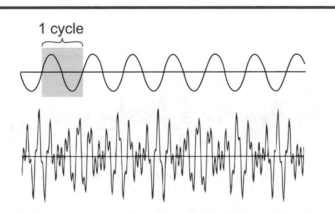

1 cycle

FIGURE 6–12. Waveforms demonstrating the same cycle length and the same amplitude but differing in the type of sound wave. Waveform A demonstrates a sine wave while Waveform B represents a complex wave.

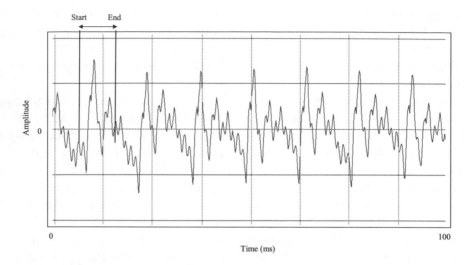

FIGURE 6–13. A complex periodic wave of an English vowel, with the beginning and end points of one cycle marked.

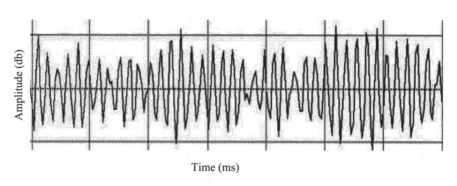

FIGURE 6–14. A complex aperiodic wave of the voiceless fricative [ʃ].

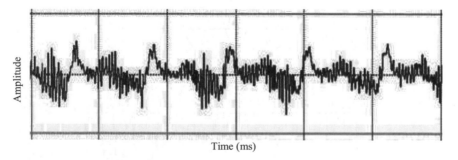

FIGURE 6–15. Waveform of the voiced fricative [ʒ], demonstrating a complex periodic and aperiodic wave.

? 6–2. Did You Get It?

Below are three waveforms, labeled A, B, and C. Use these waveforms to answer the questions below.

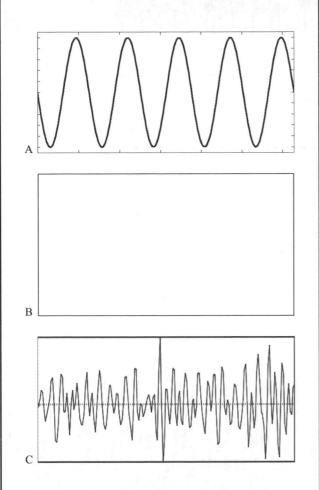

1. Which sound wave(s) is/are periodic? Aperiodic? Simple? Complex?

2. Which sound wave(s) represent/s a pure tone? Which sound wave(s) represent/s speech sounds?

3. How are the axes labeled for a waveform? What information does a waveform provide?

4. Which elements of speech are represented in periodic waveforms? Which are represented in aperiodic waveforms?

Determining Fundamental Frequency on a Waveform

We have covered the types of sound waves that occur in speech, as well as how speech sounds appear on a waveform. We can use a waveform to determine the fundamental frequency, F0, of a sound. F0 is calculated by counting the number of cycles in a period of time and dividing that number by the amount of time passed in seconds. The formula is:

$$F0 = \text{\# cycles / time in seconds.}$$

We measure F0 by counting the number of cycles of pressure variation that occur in a second on a few waveforms. Before we do so, remember that there are hundreds of pressure variations in a second. Figure 6–16 is a waveform of 7.25 seconds of the vowel /i/ (time is noted in the lower right corner of the waveform). You cannot tell anything about frequency in this waveform—too many vibratory cycles have occurred. Figure 6–17 is another waveform of the vowel /i/, but only 0.073 seconds. This waveform represents a tiny slice of the vowel /i/, but it allows us to count the number of cycles per second to determine F0. To do so, find the repeating pattern in Figure 6–17 and count the number of times it occurs. The repeating cycle occurs 19 times in the 0.073 seconds shown in this waveform. Using the formula above, we know that the number of cycles divided by the amount of time passed will tell us the fundamental frequency. In this case, our formula is 19 divided by .073. The fundamental frequency equals 260 Hz.

Figure 6–18 is a waveform of a vowel [ɛ]. What is the F0 for this waveform? You should have counted 19 cycles that occur over 0.10 seconds. Using our formula, we know that this [ɛ] was produced at 190 Hz.

Practice calculating F0 for the vowel [o͡ʊ] produced at high and low pitches for 0.08 seconds, as shown in Figure 6–19. For the [o͡ʊ] on top, you should have calculated 32 cycles produced over 0.08 seconds, which equals an F0 of 400 Hz. The [o͡ʊ] on the bottom shows 6 cycles in 0.08 seconds, which equals an F0 of 75 Hz. Since there are more cycles per second in the upper [o͡ʊ], it will be perceived as higher pitch than the [o͡ʊ] produced at 75 Hz.

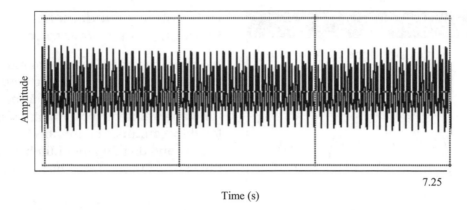

FIGURE 6–16. Waveform of the vowel [i] produced for 7.25 seconds.

FIGURE 6–17. Waveform of the vowel [i] produced for 0.073 seconds.

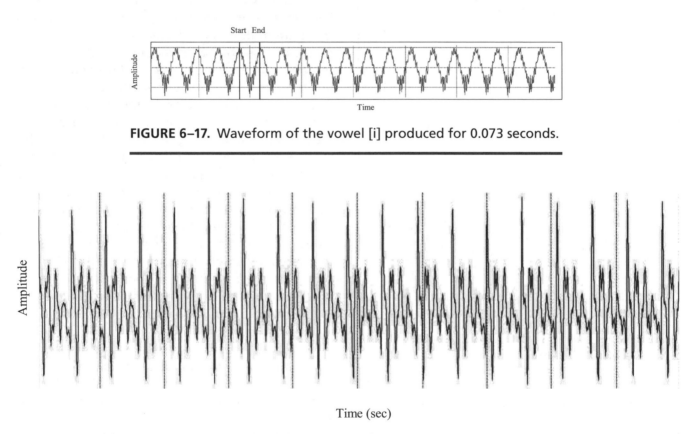

FIGURE 6–18. Waveform of the vowel [ɛ] produced for 0.10 seconds.

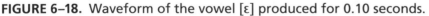

Fourier Analysis

The complex waves of speech are **non-sinusoidal waves**. Non-sinusoidal waves are made up of many sine waves. Not only do complex waves travel at different frequencies, they also have different ampli-

tudes and phasing. **Phasing** refers to the timing of the cycles of the complex sound wave, since not all waves start, nor will they cross the *x*-axis, at the same point in time.

Fourier analysis is a method of separating a complex non-sinusoidal wave into its constituent

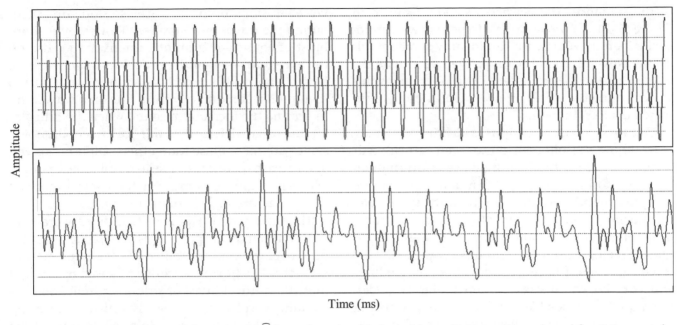

FIGURE 6–19. Waveforms of the vowel [oʊ] produced at high and low pitch, each produced for 0.8 seconds.

sine waves of different frequencies, amplitudes, and phases. If you conduct Fourier analysis on a complex wave, you will divide that wave into a series of sine waves, allowing you to determine each sine wave's frequency and phase. With Fourier analysis, scientists can build complex waves by combining sine waves into a single wave. They can also deconstruct complex waves into their sinusoidal component waves. All complex waves can be broken down into sets of sine waves. We will not examine Fourier analysis in any detail; however, it is important to be aware of the fact that we can deconstruct complex waves to analyze the sine waves they comprise. Figure 6–20 shows three sine waves with different frequencies, amplitudes, and phases, combined in the complex sound wave at the bottom of Figure 6–20.

Identifying Types of Sounds on a Waveform

In summary, we have learned that phones can comprise periodic, aperiodic, and combinations of periodic and aperiodic waves. We have analyzed waveforms of single speech sounds, examining them over short periods of time. However, a waveform of running speech looks quite different. A waveform

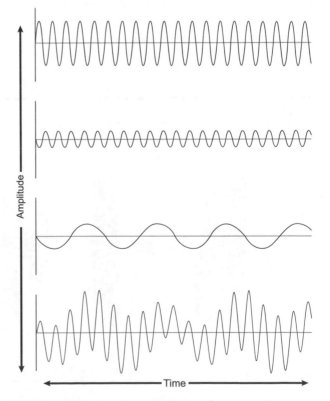

FIGURE 6–20. Fourier analysis of a complex wave, deconstructing the complex wave into sine waves. Note the differing frequencies and amplitudes of the sine waves.

of the sentence, *The teacher is smart,* is shown in Figure 6–21. In waveforms of speech, we cannot easily identify F0, but we can identify some sounds on the waveform, and perhaps even determine the words that the speaker uttered. It is near impossible to determine the words on a waveform if not given forced choices, though.

Can we segment waveforms to identify phonemes, if we know the phonemes that were articulated? While it is difficult to identify place of articulation on a waveform, we can identify manner. To start, we compare sounds that differ in intensity, specifically comparing sonorants and obstruents. Sonorants are high-amplitude sounds such as vowels, nasals, glides and liquids. Of the sonorants, vowels will tend to be the highest in amplitude, although loudness will vary based on stress patterns. Nasals, glides, and liquids will look like vowels on a waveform, but with a little less energy. Obstruents (stops, fricatives, and affricates) tend to have decreased intensity compared with sonorants. Obstruents will be slightly louder if they are voiced or sibilant fricatives. Stops can be identified by a sharp burst in intensity, resulting from the pressure change when the articulators come apart. You can also differentiate voiced from voiceless stops because voiceless stops are silent during the articulator closure, followed by a sharp burst of sound—a dramatic intensity increase on the waveform—when the articulators are released. Voiced stops will have a little sound energy during their production and a vertical line on a waveform, indicating the increase in sound when the articulators are released. Fricatives will have aperiodic noise, some with more noise than others. Diphthongs will often have a gradual change in amplitude. Changes between sonorant sounds, such as vowel to nasal consonant, are slightly more abrupt.

The waveform in Figure 6–22 is of the word *ship.* Can you identify the phonemes in *ship?* Follow along the waveform and try to identify the phonemes in the word *ship,* [ʃɪpʰ]: a fricative followed by a vowel (note the vertical lines, or striations, indicating the vibrating vocal folds), followed by silence for the [p]. You can tell that [pʰ] was aspirated because of the small burst of sound after the silence.

Figure 6–23 shows waveforms of two words: *muddy* and *exit.* The phonemes on the waveforms have been marked [mʌ.ɾi] and [ɛg.zɪt]. Note that in *muddy* there was a very short decrease in intensity for the tap, and then a long vowel at the end. How can

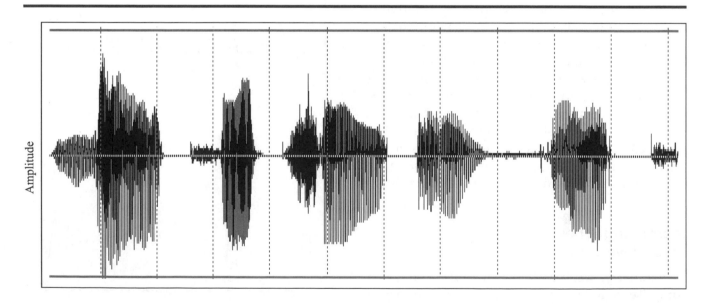

Time (ms)

FIGURE 6–21. Waveform of the sentence *The teacher is smart.*

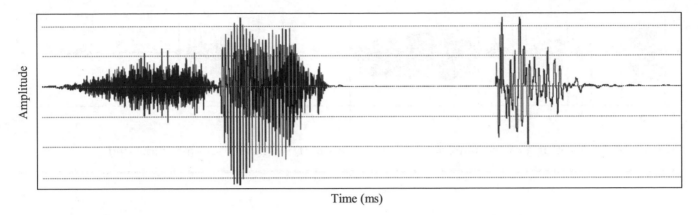

FIGURE 6–22. Waveform of the word *ship* [ʃɪp].

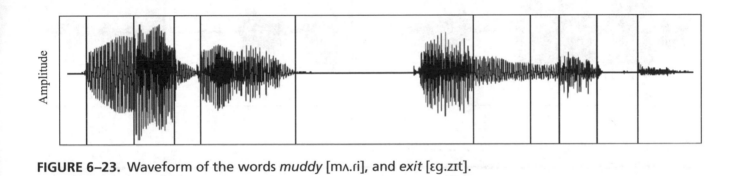

FIGURE 6–23. Waveform of the words *muddy* [mʌ.ɾi], and *exit* [ɛg.zɪt].

you tell that the word *exit* was said [ɛg.zɪt] and not [ɛk.sɪt]? Yes, you could tell that *exit* was articulated with voiced medial consonants because of the continuous voicing until the closure for [t].

Now that we have segmented words, we can segment the sentence in the waveform back in Figure 6–21. The first step to segmenting a waveform is to transcribe. So we start by transcribing the sentence: [ðə ˈti.t͡ʃɚ ɪz ˈsmɑɚt]. The sentence has five vowels, so we need to look for five intensity peaks on the waveform. At first glance, the waveform has six peaks, not five. However, note that the third peak does not have the vertical striations of the others, suggesting that this peak is not a vowel. Continuing with this hypothesis, label the vowels on the five peaks with striations. Now that you have identified the vowels, start figuring out the adjacent consonants. The first word has a long-ish [ð] followed by [ə]. Then there is silence, followed by a [tʰ] (there is

quite a bit of aspiration), and then [i]. Then there is [t͡ʃ], shown as a period of silence and the noise of the sibilant, followed by [ɚ]. The word *teacher* is followed by silence between words and another vowel, [ɪ], which is followed by the sibilant fricative [z]. It appears this [z] was voiceless, and really was combined with the [s] in *smart*. We then see an increase in amplitude. This peak represents two sonorant sounds: the nasal [m] and the vowel [ɑɚ]. The last phoneme is [t], again characterized by silence followed by aspiration. Figure 6–24 is the same sentence, *The teacher is smart*, but this time we have segmented it for you.

The waveform in Figure 6–25 is of the phrase *Vitamin C prevents the flu*. It is your turn to segment this waveform. Try to find the vowels first, and remember that silence can be a phoneme. If you get stuck, you might try working from the end of the phrase backward.

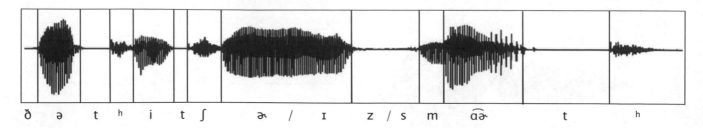

| ð | ə | tʰ | i | t | ʃ | ɚ | / | ɪ | z | / | s | m | a͡ɚ | t | ʰ |

FIGURE 6–24. Waveform of the sentence *The teacher is smart,* with the phonemes indicated.

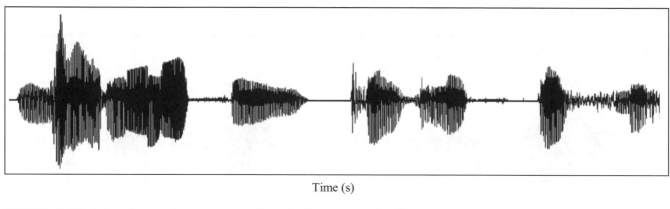

Time (s)

FIGURE 6–25. Waveform of the phrase *Vitamin C prevents the flu.*

Figure 6–26 is the same waveform, this time with the phonemes segmented. The first thing we did to segment the waveform into phonemes was to transcribe the phrase as ['vaɪ.ɾɪ.mɪn 'si pʰɹə.vɛnˈs ðə flu]. Compare your segmented waveform with ours. How did you do?

In addition to determining fundamental frequency and segmenting phonemes, we can use a waveform to compare the lengths of sounds. Figure 6–27 allows us to compare the three words *chop, choppy,* and *choppiest* in a waveform . These three words all contain one identical syllable, but the words increase in length. Can you see that the repetition of amplitude changes at the beginning of each word? You should see a burst of energy at the beginning of each, representing the latter portion of the affricate [t͡ʃ]. Each of these affricates is followed by the low vowel [a], which tapers off in amplitude before the closure of the articulators and complete silence of the [p]. Notice that there is a burst in amplitude, represent-ing the aspiration following the voiceless stop [pʰ]. Can you see how each syllable [t͡ʃa] gets shorter as the words get longer?

Spectrum of a Sound Wave

Thus far we have seen how vibratory sound can be represented on a waveform. Waveforms show time on the *x*-axis, and intensity or amplitude on the *y*-axis. They are helpful for measuring fundamental frequency and intensity and for seeing the repetition of vibratory cycles of sound. A waveform can show us number of cycles per second for sine waves as well as complex waves. However, because waveforms provide only amplitude and time measurements, we cannot use waveforms to define unique sound qualities of specific phonemes.

A **spectrum** is another visual representation of sound that graphs a single moment in time. The

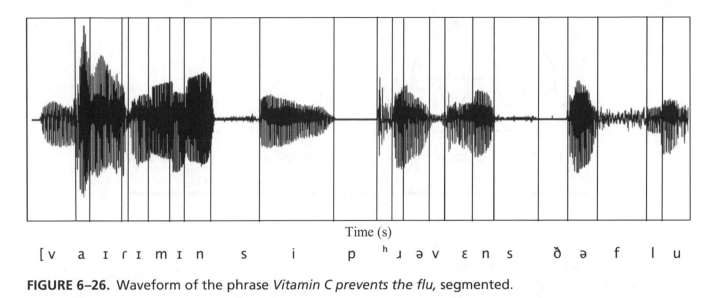

[v a ɪ ɾ ɪ m ɪ n   s   i   p ʰ ɹ ə v ɛ n s   ð ə   f l u

FIGURE 6–26. Waveform of the phrase *Vitamin C prevents the flu*, segmented.

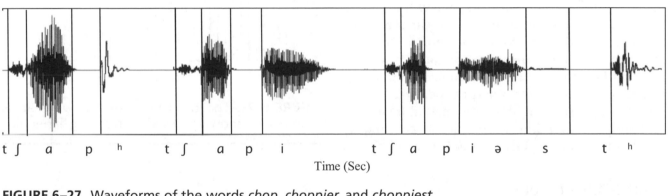

t ʃ   a   p ʰ   t ʃ   a   p   i   t ʃ   a   p   i   ə   s   t ʰ

FIGURE 6–27. Waveforms of the words *chop*, *choppier*, and *choppiest*.

spectrum shows amplitude on the *y*-axis and frequency (not time) on the *x*-axis. The spectrum is useful for understanding the various frequencies of vibrations inherent in complex sound waves. Acoustic spectra do not provide any time information; they are in fact a slice in time. We can compare information about sine waves on a spectrum and a waveform.

Figure 6–28 shows the pressure variations over time of a sine wave on a waveform on the left, representing the pressure variations over time. Remember that a sine wave has a sound source vibrating at only one frequency. On the right of Figure 6–28 you see the same sine wave on a spectrum. The spectrum

is a single moment in time and shows frequency, not time, on the *x*-axis, and amplitude, or intensity, on the *y*-axis. Given that a sine wave has pressure variations at one frequency only, the spectrum of the sine wave is a single vertical line.

As Fourier analysis shows, complex waves are made up of a number of sine waves traveling at different frequencies. The sound spectrum can be used to display the different frequencies that comprise the sound. These different frequencies are dependent on the sound source and on the shape of the vocal tract, which causes certain frequencies to be emphasized and other frequencies to be deemphasized or dampened.

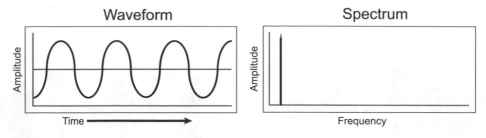

FIGURE 6–28. Sine wave information on a waveform and on a frequency spectrum.

As we learned, periodic sounds have a fundamental frequency, determined by the frequency of vocal fold vibration. In a complex sound, F0 has additional sound energy called **harmonics**. Harmonics are whole number multiples of the fundamental frequency. Thus, if the F0 is 100 Hz, the first harmonic is the fundamental frequency, the second harmonic is two times F0 or 200 Hz, the third harmonic is 300 Hz, and so on. Harmonics decrease in amplitude as they increase in frequency, with F0 (the first harmonic) having the highest amplitude. Figure 6–29 is a spectrum of a periodic wave at its sound source, showing the fundamental frequency and the corresponding harmonics, decreasing in amplitude as they increase in frequency.

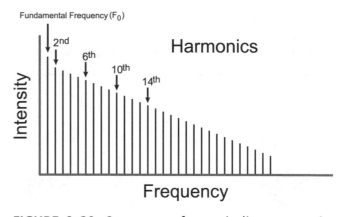

FIGURE 6–29. Spectrum of a periodic wave at its sound source showing F0 and the resulting harmonics.

Source-Filter Theory

To produce the characteristic resonant properties of speech sounds, we need a sound source coupled with a unique vocal tract shape. The **source-filter theory** describes speech sounds using a two-step process. Sound must originate at a source that provides a spectral shape. That sound is filtered by the vocal tract, which gives the source a speech sound's characteristic resonant qualities.

All sounds originate at a sound source. For vowels and voiced consonants, the source is the airstream from the lungs and phonation resulting from vocal fold vibration. For voiceless sounds, the source is turbulent noise. Following the sound being originated at its source, sounds travel through the vocal tract where they are altered, or filtered. The shape of the vocal tract determines the specific frequencies of the sound it will transmit, giving the sound its unique pho-

netic properties. For any speech sound, certain frequencies of sounds will be filtered by lips, tongue position, velum placement, and other articulatory movements during the sound's production. The perception of different vowels is dependent on the filter, with changes in the vocal tract shape due to different tongue, lip, and other articular placement, emphasizing sounds at certain frequencies. Figure 6–30 demonstrates how the sound source, filtered through a particular vocal tract shape, has a unique output spectrum that reflects the sound source and the filter.

Figure 6–31 shows how sounds with differing source properties are affected by the filter. Sound source A, with an F0 of 100 Hz, will have twice as many harmonics as a source with an F0 of 200 Hz. This results in sound A having more sound energy in the output spectrum.

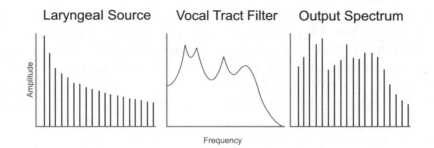

FIGURE 6–30. Source-filter model of speech production.

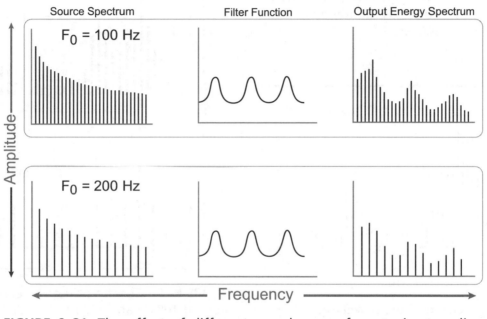

FIGURE 6–31. The effect of different sound source frequencies traveling through the same filter on the output spectrum.

The sound source, with its characteristic fundamental frequency and resulting harmonics, will be affected by the filter of the vocal tract shape. Changes in vocal tract shape in turn, will, emphasize certain frequencies of sound and deemphasize others. The fundamental frequency and harmonics coupled with the filter properties results in a particular phoneme's emphasized sound frequencies. The emphasized harmonics are called **formants**, also called overtones. Formants are a group of harmonics that form a band of acoustic energy that corresponds to a resonating frequency of the air in the vocal tract. These formants are the sound characteristics of a particular vowel (or voiced consonant). We number formants in ascending order, with the lowest formant, formant 1, abbreviated F1, representing the lowest frequency band of energy, F2 the second lowest band of energy, and so on. Thus production differences in phonemes such as [i] and [u] are not a result of a change in fundamental frequency. Rather, the differences between [i] and [u] are the unique characteristics of the emphasized harmonics in the complex sound wave as a result of the filter.

Figure 6–32 is the output spectrum for the vowel [ɑ]. We can see F0 at 100 Hz. We also see emphasized harmonics at 500 and 600 Hz, comprising the first formant. The second formant can be seen at the next emphasized harmonics at 800 and 900 Hz. The third formant, F3, is at approximately 3000 Hz.

A periodic wave, resulting from vocal fold vibration and a unique vocal tract shape, repeats itself at regular intervals. Aperiodic waves can have sound at all frequencies. Figure 6–33 shows waveforms and sound spectra of aperiodic sounds. The first sound has acoustic energy at all frequencies, while the second aperiodic sound wave has slightly more sound frequency at about 2,500 Hz.

Sound spectra can show differing amounts of acoustic energy at different frequencies. Figure 6–34 shows two sound spectra for the low central vowel /ʌ/. The first is a spectrum with an F0 at 100 Hz and the second is a spectrum vibrating at 200 Hz. Note that the harmonics in each spectrum increase

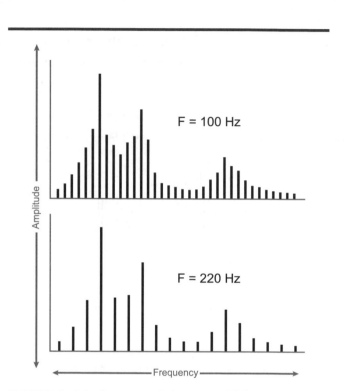

FIGURE 6–34. Spectra of the vowel [ʌ] spoken with an F0 at 100 Hz and 200 Hz.

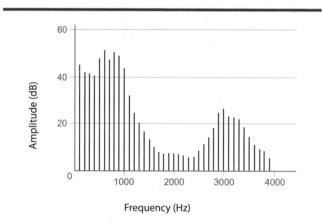

FIGURE 6–32. Spectrum of the vowel [ɑ].

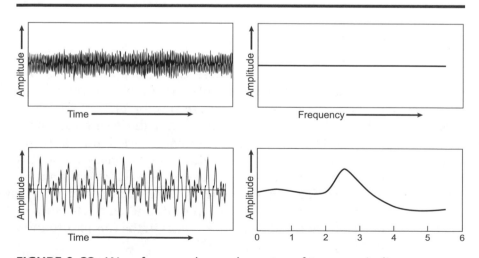

FIGURE 6–33. Waveform and sound spectra of two aperiodic waves.

and decrease in amplitude in a similar manner. This harmonic pattern reflects the filter shape. Note also that the spectrum of the sound at 100 Hz has twice as many harmonics as the sound at 200 Hz. Why is that? Harmonics are multiples of the fundamental frequency. The higher the F0, the larger the frequency difference between harmonics, and the fewer harmonics there will be in a complex sound wave.

Vowel Differences

The source-filter theory describes how the shape of the vocal tract results in a phoneme's characteristic sounds. The effect of the filter, or vocal tract shape, on sound quality is particularly evident with vowels. Vowels can have the same fundamental frequency and same intensity level, but the emphasized harmonics, or formants, will differ and are determined by the shape of the oral cavity during production. As we have learned, the change in shape of the oral cavity acts as an acoustic filter for passing sound. This changing shape lets resonant frequencies pass through most easily, giving a specific vowel its characteristic formants. For example, the tongue is low and back during the production of /a/, and mid and central for /ʌ/, and these differences in tongue position contribute to different vocal tract shapes for these two vowels. Compare the frequency peaks for /a/ in Figure 6–32 to the frequency peaks for /ʌ/ in Figure 6–34. These peaks represent formants or the emphasized harmonics for each vowel. These characteristic formants, or overtones, are produced by the molecules vibrating the oral, nasal, and pharyngeal structures and causing unique resonances.

Spectrograms

We have represented speech on two-dimensional diagrams: waveforms showing amplitude differences over time, and spectra showing the characteristics of sound at different frequencies at a single point in time. A **spectrogram** provides a more comprehensive picture of speech sounds, showing all of the emphasized frequencies of complex sound waves over time. On a spectrogram, time is represented on the x-axis, frequency on the y-axis. The intensity of sound at different frequencies is represented through gradations of darkness on the spectrogram,

with greatest intensity sounds the darkest. Because sounds with greater amplitude are darker, all else being equal, vowels will be the darkest on a spectrogram, followed by nasals, liquids, and glides, and then sibilant fricatives and other obstruent sounds.

A spectrogram shows intensity of various aspects of the acoustic signal for individual sounds. It is much easier to identify phones on a spectrogram than on a waveform or a spectrum. In the next section, you will learn how to identify phones on a spectrogram.

? 6–3. Did You Get It?

1. How are the axes labeled for a spectrogram? What is the purpose of the darkness of the spectrogram? What sound information does a spectrogram provide?

2. The images below are labeled A, B, and C. Which of the images is a waveform, spectrum, and spectrogram? How do you know which is which?

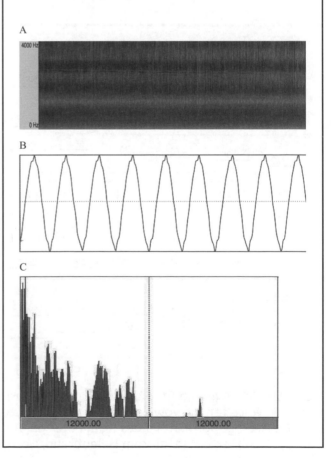

Vowel Identity

Vowels are perceived differently because of their unique formant structure, determined by the particular overtones of the vowel. Vowels differ from each other in vowel quality because of specific harmonics that are emphasized in relation to vocal tract shape. Some harmonics will increase in energy due to vocal tract resonance, with emphasized harmonics equaling formants or overtones. These overtones result from air vibrating in the oral, nasal, and pharyngeal structures plus tongue gestures changing the shape of these cavities. This changed shape results in different resonance characteristics.

Vowel identity is fairly straightforward. We hear a particular vowel based on the frequency of the first and second formants as well as the distance between F1 and F2. You can alter your voice to focus on each formant. The first formant, or F1, can be heard if you say a series of vowels in a creaky voice. By speaking in a creaky voice you lessen the sound effects of the higher formants. Try saying the vowels [i, ɪ, ɛ, æ] with a creaky voice. As you say these vowels, you should hear a rising tone. The rising tone you are hearing is an increase in frequency of the first formant. Now say the vowels [ɑ, ɔ, ʊ, u] with a creaky voice; you should hear the first formant decreasing. We can also isolate the second formant. To do so, say the following vowels in a whisper. Whisper the vowels [i, ɪ, ɛ, æ, ɑ, ɔ, ʊ, u]. By whispering them, you should hear a descending pitch: from highest frequency in [i] to lowest for [u]. What you are hearing is F2 decreasing.

Thus the first formant is an inverse of vowel height, with high vowels having a low F1, and low vowels having a high F1. The second formant is directly related to tongue advancement: the farther forward in the mouth the vowel is produced, the higher F2 is; the farther back in the mouth, the lower the F2. Vowel identity is primarily dependent on F1 and F2, with the distance between F1 and F2 also aiding the listener in vowel identification. It's important to become familiar with the 1st and 2nd formant frequency for vowels. Figures 6–35 and 6–36 show average formant frequencies for the 1st,

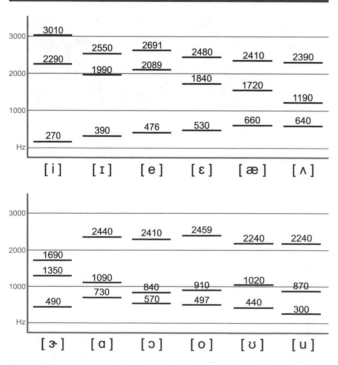

FIGURE 6–35. Average F1, F2, and F3 of an American male voice for the vowels [i, ɪ, e, ɛ, æ, ʌ, ɝ, ɑ, ɔ, o, ʊ, u]. Average formant values from Peterson and Barney (1952), except [e, o] from Hillenbrand, Getty, Clark, and Wheeler (1995).

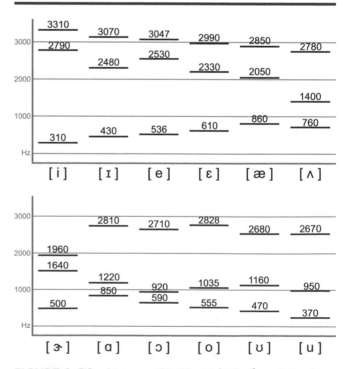

FIGURE 6–36. Average F1, F2, and F3 of an American female voice for the vowels [i, ɪ, e, ɛ, æ, ʌ, ɝ, ɑ, ɔ, o, ʊ, u]. Average formant values from Peterson and Barney (1952), except [e, o] from Hillenbrand, Getty, Clark, and Wheeler (1995).

2nd, and 3rd formants for the monophthong vowels [i, ɪ, e, ɛ, æ, ʌ, ɝ, a, ɔ, o, ʊ, u] in American English (Hillenbrand, Getty, Clark, & Wheeler, 1995; Peterson & Barney, 1952). Figure 6–35 shows the averages for biologically male voices and 6–36 shows the averages for biologically female voices. Examine Figures 6–35 and 6–36 to confirm the increase in F1 for low vowels and the decrease in F2 as vowels are made further back in the mouth. Note that for the purposes of simplicity, we are not covering the effects of lip rounding, which has an effect on F3 and is most noticeable in /ɝ/ in these vowels.

Vowel formants are identified on a spectrogram by their darkness. Now that you more or less know what frequency each formant should be for each vowel, see if you can identify them in Figures 6–37, 6–38, and 6–39. Figure 6–37 shows spectrograms of the vowels [i, ɪ, e, ɛ], Figure 6–38 is a spectrogram of

the vowels [æ, ʌ, ɝ, u], and Figure 6–39 is a spectrogram of the vowels [ʊ, o, ɔ, a]. Note that frequency up to 4400 Hz is shown and that there are many dark bands of energy averaging about 500 Hz in width. If you observe bands that are much wider, it can be two formants close together, as F2 and F3 are in [i] and F1 and F2 are in [a].

Figures 6–40, 6–41, and 6–42 are of the same vowels shown above, this time with the formants indicated. Were your measurements accurate?

Monophthongs tend to be steady state vowels, although you can see a diphthong-like quality at the end of the mid and back vowels in the vowel spectrograms. Figure 6–43 is a spectrogram of the three phonemic diphthongs, [aɪ], [aʊ], and [ɔɪ]. Note the gliding quality of the vowels and how the low central [a] transitions to a high front vowel in [aɪ], and a low back position in [aʊ].

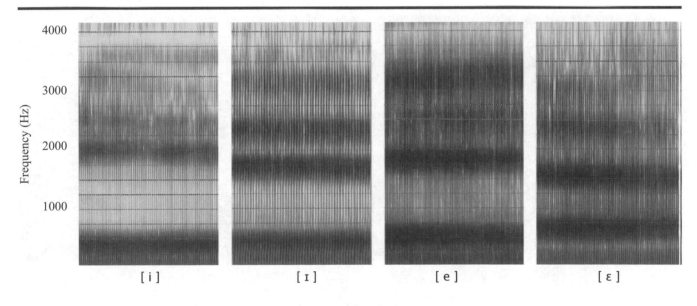

FIGURE 6–37. Spectrograms of the English vowels [i, ɪ, e, ɛ].

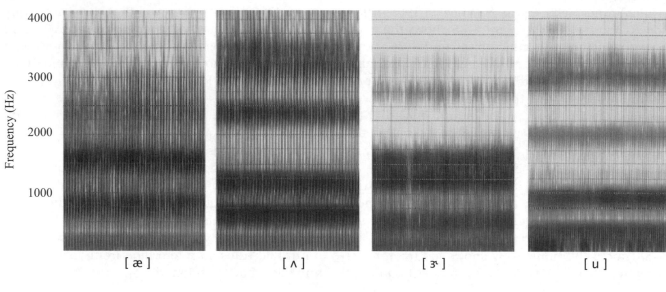

Time (sec)

FIGURE 6–38. Spectrograms of the English vowels [æ, ʌ, ɝ, u].

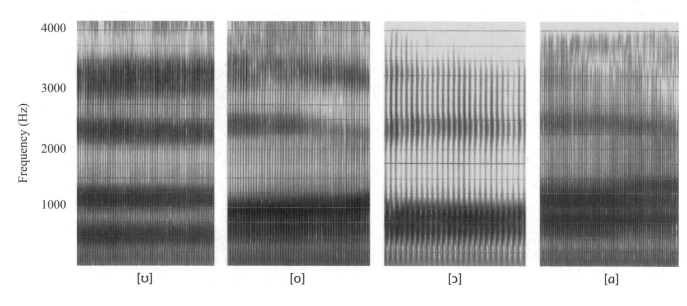

Time (sec)

FIGURE 6–39. Spectrograms of the English vowels [ʊ, o, ɔ, ɑ].

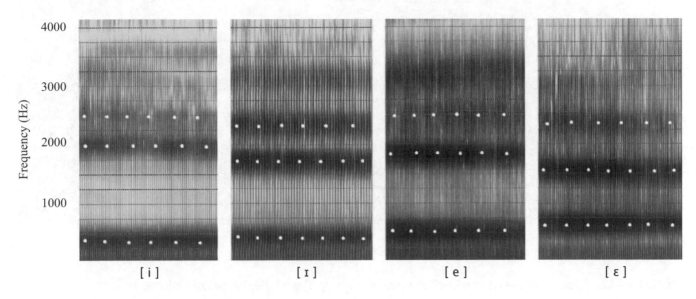

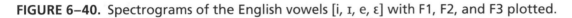

FIGURE 6–40. Spectrograms of the English vowels [i, ɪ, e, ɛ] with F1, F2, and F3 plotted.

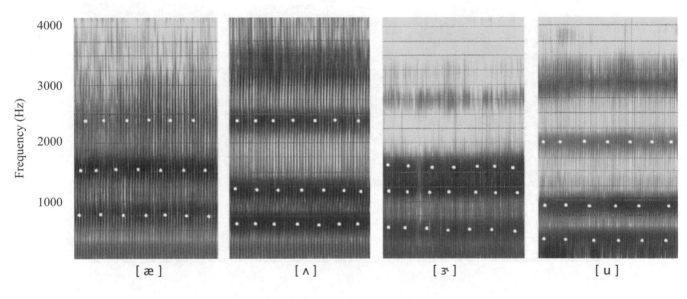

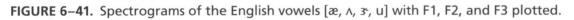

FIGURE 6–41. Spectrograms of the English vowels [æ, ʌ, ɝ, u] with F1, F2, and F3 plotted.

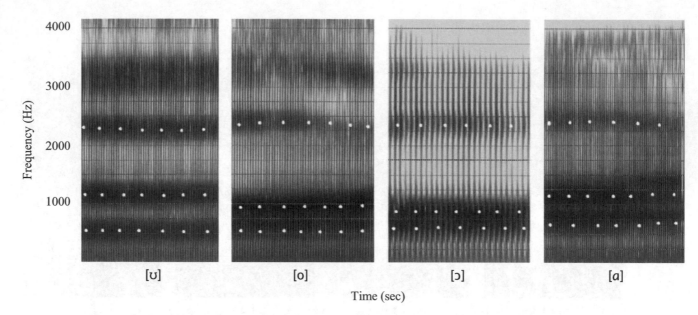

[ʊ] [o] [ɔ] [a]

Time (sec)

FIGURE 6–42. Spectrograms of the English vowels [ʊ, o, ɔ, a] with F1, F2, and F3 plotted.

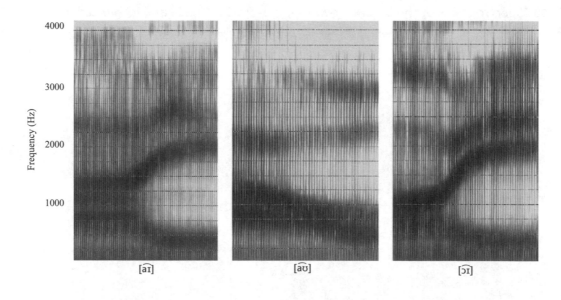

[aɪ] [aʊ] [ɔɪ]

FIGURE 6–43. Spectrogram of the phonemic diphthongs, [aɪ], [aʊ], and [ɔɪ].

The Vowel Quadrilateral Revisited

The relationship between F1 and F2 for vowels is best shown on the vowel quadrilateral. You learned the vowel quadrilateral in Chapter 3 as a way to visualize articulatory properties of vowels. As you saw, though, articulatory properties of vowels are difficult to confirm because of their subtle changes. The vowel quadrilateral also represents acoustic qualities of vowels better than articulatory properties. The average F1 and F2 of biological males is shown in Figure 6–44. Figure 6–45 shows average F1 and F2 for biological females (see Figures 6–35 and 6–36 for the specific frequency values). F1 values are shown on the y-axis and F2 values on the x-axis. Figure 6–46 overlays the male and female F1 and F2 values to compare the acoustic space for each group. Notice how both

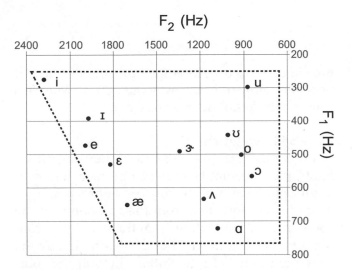

FIGURE 6–44. Vowel quadrilateral of the monophthong vowels of English produced by biologically male speakers. F1 is on the *x*-axis and F2 on the *y*-axis.

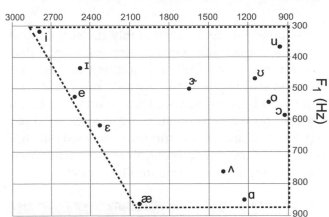

FIGURE 6–45. Vowel quadrilateral of the monophthong vowels of English produced by biologically female speakers. F1 is on the *x*-axis and F2 on the *y*-axis.

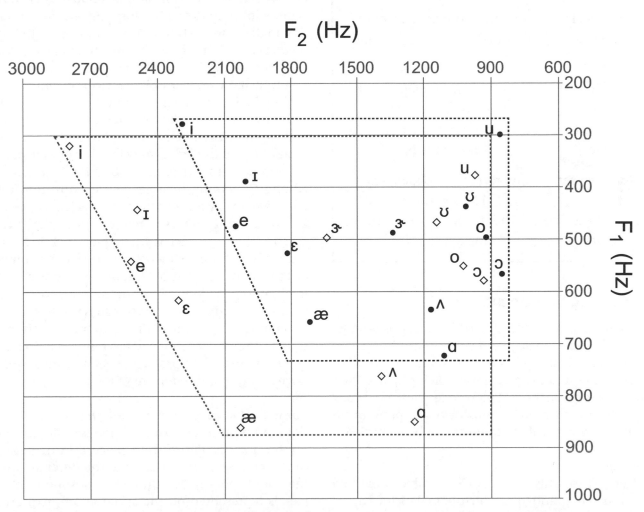

FIGURE 6–46. Comparison of biologically male and female F1 and F2 formant frequencies and respective vowel quadrilaterals. Female vowels are indicated with a diamond and male vowels are indicated with a circle. F1 is on the *x*-axis and F2 on the *y*-axis.

vowel quadrilaterals have roughly the same shape, although the acoustic space for females is larger than that for males. In addition, placement on the vowel quadrilateral explains the acoustic similarities and differences between vowels. Thus /i/ and /ɪ/ are close together on the vowel quadrilateral, indicating perceptual and production similarity, whereas /u/ and /æ/ are far apart, suggesting that these two vowels are articulatorily and perceptually distinct.

? 6–4. Did You Get It?

1. Emphasized harmonics are called _____. The frequency of these _____ are dependent on the size and shape of the vocal tract.

2. Vowel identity is primarily dependent on which two formants? _____ and _____.

3. A vowel's first formant varies dependent on _____. This relationship is direct/inverse. That is, the higher F1 is, the _____ the tongue is.

4. A vowel's second formant is dependent on _____. This relationship is direct/inverse. That is, the higher F2 is, the _____ the tongue is.

Identifying Consonants

Consonant production differs from vowel production with respect to degree of vocal tract constriction. As we have learned, consonants can be classified along three main dimensions: voicing, place, and manner of productions. Below we explore how voicing, place, and manner appear on a spectrogram and how individual consonants can be identified.

Voicing
Voiced consonants, like vowels, involve vocal fold vibration chopping up the airstream. Voicing can be seen in vertical striations on the spectrogram, representing vocal fold vibration. Voiced consonants also are characterized by a **voice bar**, a dark band of periodic energy at or below about 200 Hz. Voiceless consonants do not have a voice bar.

Place of Articulation
While we can see place of articulation for consonants, place cannot be observed in the actual consonant production. Instead, place of articulation is heard in the transition from the consonant to the vowel in a CV context, or from the vowel to a consonant in a VC context. That is, we can identify the consonant place of articulation through the coarticulation of the vowel and consonant.

What do we hear that indicates place of articulation in these transitions? Bilabial consonants tend to have more energy at all frequencies than do alveolar or velar consonants. Bilabials also have slightly lower 2nd and 3rd formants as they transition to the vowel. Alveolar consonants tend to have greater sound energy at higher frequencies, typically between 2000 and 4000 Hz for an adult male. The transition from an alveolar consonant will be slightly higher at the 2nd formant, as well as at the 3rd formant where the alveolar consonant transitions to the vowel. Velar place of articulation is the easiest to identify because velars have their greatest sound energy at around 2000 Hz. You can see F2 and F3 coming together as we transition from the vowel to a velar consonant. This joining of the 2nd and 3rd formants is referred to as the "velar pinch." These characteristic frequency changes for place of articulation are determined by the volume of the cavity in front of the place of constriction. Bilabial sounds do not have an anterior cavity and their lower frequency characteristics result from the resonant quality of the entire vocal tract. In alveolar sounds, smaller anterior cavities result in higher frequencies than when producing velar sounds, which have a larger cavity in front of them.

Consonant Manner of Articulation
Consonant manner of articulation is easier to identify on a spectrogram than place of articulation. In the next section, we explore the different ways the sound energy for different consonant manners is represented on the spectrogram, exploring their interaction with voicing and place resonant characteristics.

Stops. As we have seen, the six oral stops in English are voiceless and voiced bilabial /p/ and /b/, alveolar /t/ and /d/, and velar /k/ and /g/. Stop consonants are produced with the vocal tract completely obstructed. If obstructed, the air from the lungs is trapped behind the constriction, building up air pressure behind the articulators. When the articulators are released, there will be a decrease in pressure that creates a brief turbulent airflow. Thus stops create a brief noise when the articulators are released. The duration of stop consonants is extremely short, typically 5 to 20 milliseconds. This noise burst is dependent on how long the articulators are held together. In English, we make the distinction between voiced and voiceless stops greater due to extended occlusion of the articulators for voiceless stops. In addition, while the transient noise occurs for both voiced and voiceless stops, remember that voiced stops will also have a voice bar.

Stop consonant formant transitions are of very short duration, since the articulators change rapidly from a stop consonant to a vowel position. The place of articulation for stops is observed in these formant transitions. For all voiced stop consonant-vowel combinations, the F1 transition from the stop to the vowel is always rising; there is no F1 transition for voiceless stops. The direction and extent of the F2 transition varies depending upon the following vowel. The F2 transition for bilabial [b, p]-vowel combinations is always rising. The F2 transition for [k, g]-vowel combinations is always falling. The F2 transition for alveolar stops differs depending on the vowel, with [t, d]-front vowel combinations generally rising and the F2 transition from [t, d] to back vowel combinations generally falling.

In the last paragraph, we've explored how place of articulation will differ for stops. The contrast between voiced and voiceless stops is easier to identify. As you have learned, voiceless stops in initial word position in English can be aspirated. **Aspiration** is turbulent noise after the release of the articulators and before the voicing for the vowel. Aspiration results from a delay of voicing for the subsequent vowel. **Voice onset time (VOT)** refers to the length of time after release of the stop consonant before the start of vocal fold vibration for the following vowel. Aspirated voiceless stops have a VOT delay in a consonant-vowel syllable. The time interval in milli-

seconds between articulator release and vocal fold vibration is the VOT delay. For voiced initial stops, VOT is typically 0 milliseconds because the vocal folds start vibrating for voiced consonants at the same time as the release; i.e., there is no voicing delay.

In initial voiceless stops that are aspirated, VOT delay must be enough so that the listener can hear the difference between the voiced-voiceless consonant pairs. The difference in VOT varies between stop consonant pairs. The bilabials [p] and [b] have a difference in VOT, with [p] having a VOT delay of approximately 25 milliseconds and 0 VOT delay for [b]; alveolar [t] versus [d] differ in VOT by around 40 milliseconds, and velar [k] differs from [g] by 45 to 55 milliseconds.

Figure 6–47 is a spectrogram of voiced and voiceless bilabial stops in the words *bye* and *pie,* [ba͡ɪ] and [pʰa͡ɪ]. Note the turbulence or aspiration in the voiceless stop and the onset of voicing without aspiration in the voiced stop. How long is the aspiration that differentiates the voiced and voiceless stops? As an aside, you can see the diphthong quality of [a͡ɪ] in each word, with F1 decreasing as tongue height increases and F2 increasing as the tongue moves back.

Now let's compare spectrograms to see how stop place of articulation is indicated. Figure 6–48 is a spectrogram of the three voiced stop consonants in VCV environments. Can you see the characteristic formant transitions for each place of articulation from and to the vowels? In all three voiced stops, F1 rises in the transition from the consonant to the vowel. You should see the diffuse sound energy in the bilabial, the decrease in F2 in the transition from the alveolar to the low vowel, and the velar pinch of F2 and F3 in the transition to the vowels. The most significant distinctions between voiced and voiceless stops are the noise energy up to about 200 Hz during the voiced stops and the lack of aspiration in their production. Figure 6–49 shows the three voiceless stop consonants in the same VCV environments. In Figure 6–49, note the lack of sound during the articulator obstruction as well as the aspiration, indicating VOT delay.

Fricatives. During fricative production, the vocal tract is markedly constricted and air can only travel through a small opening between the articulators. When particles are forced through a narrow

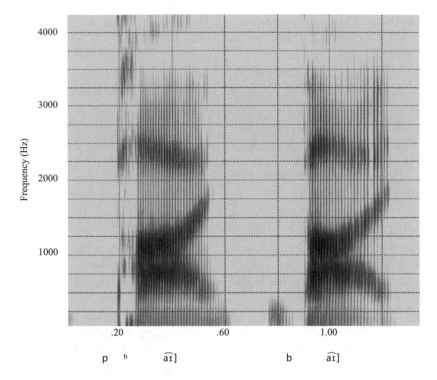

FIGURE 6–47. Spectrogram comparing voiced and voiceless stops in the words [pʰaɪ͡] and [baɪ͡].

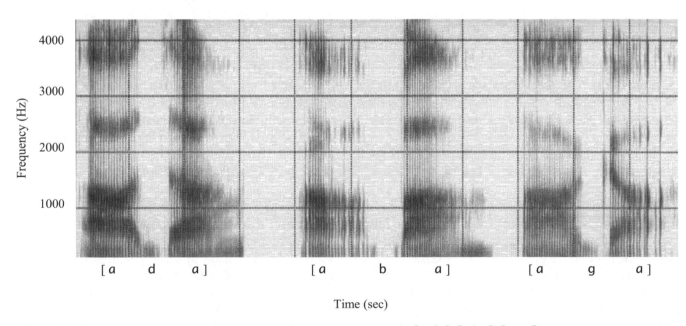

Time (sec)

FIGURE 6–48. Spectrogram comparing voiced stop consonants in [a.da], [a.ba], [a.ga].

opening, the particle movement becomes chaotic, irregular, and turbulent. As we have seen, turbulent airflow produces an aperiodic acoustic output which is a characteristic of all fricatives. Voiced fricatives will have the additional periodic sound source of vocal fold vibration. Fricatives are long in duration

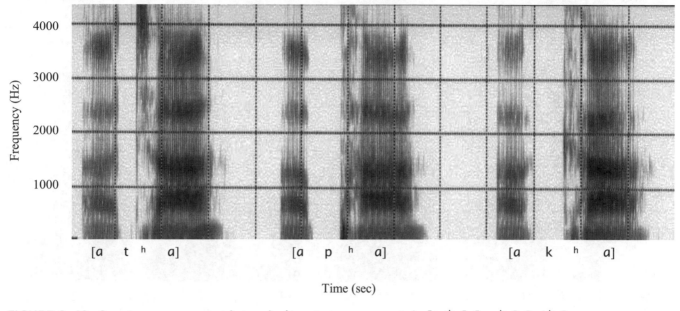

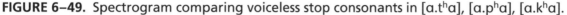

[a   t ʰ   a]   [a   p ʰ   a]   [a   k ʰ   a]

Time (sec)

FIGURE 6–49. Spectrogram comparing voiceless stop consonants in [a.tʰa], [a.pʰa], [a.kʰa].

in comparison to the short duration of stops. Voiceless fricatives, like voiceless stops, have larger amplitudes of the sound source than their voiced cognates.

Different fricatives are made with different-shaped articulations of the vocal tract. The shape of the opening at the constriction is another sound source consideration. These differently shaped openings result in more sound energy—noise—for sibilant fricatives [s, z, ʃ, ʒ], and less noise for nonsibilant fricatives [f, v, θ, ð].

Fricatives sound different from each other because of the spectral properties of the noise in their production. The alveolar and post-alveolar fricatives can be easily differentiated because the primary acoustic energy is higher for alveolar than post-alveolar fricatives. Thus [ʃ] and [ʒ] have acoustic energy that is between 2000 and 6000 Hz, lower in frequency than [s] and [z], which have sound energy between 4000 and 8000 Hz because of the shorter oral cavity in front of their production. Additionally, voicing will differentiate the cognates [s, z] and [ʃ, ʒ] from each other. Figure 6–48 is a spectrogram of all four sibilant fricatives in a vowel-fricative-vowel framework. Unlike previous spectrograms, Figure 6–50 shows frequencies up to 8000 Hz so you can see the acoustic differences between the places of articulation. Note the higher frequency energy in the alveolar fricatives [s, z] compared with the post-alveolar

fricatives [ʃ, ʒ]. Also note the voicing differences as indicated by the voice bar in [z] and [ʒ].

The spectral characteristics of [f, θ] and [v, ð] are similar to each other, since there is little difference in the place of constriction for the labiodental and interdental fricatives, just a difference in lower surface articulator. These four nonsibilant fricatives are low in intensity and have a broad frequency noise. Differences between the labiodental and interdental fricatives are heard based on formant transitions, especially F2, to the vowel. As you see in a spectrogram of the four nonsibilant fricatives in Figure 6–51, the differences in acoustic qualities of the fricatives is slight, with voicing easier to identify than place of articulation.

Affricates. As you know, English has two affricate phonemes: voiceless /t͡ʃ/ and voiced /d͡ʒ/. Affricates are produced by briefly obstructing the vocal tract, immediately followed by partial obstruction, the latter of which creates a turbulent air flow perceived as sustained turbulent noise. Therefore, affricates are produced as a combination of the sound sources for stops and fricatives. On a spectrogram, affricates are seen as a short stop with a longer fricative component. The stop and fricative components of an affricate are shorter in duration than they would be in separate sounds. The major vocal tract constriction

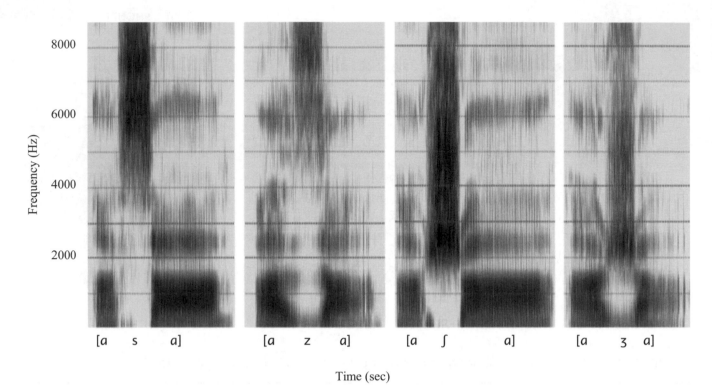

[a   s   a]   [a   z   a]   [a   ʃ   a]   [a   ʒ   a]

Time (sec)

FIGURE 6–50. Spectrogram comparing the sibilant fricatives in the words [ɑ.sɑ], [ɑ.zɑ], [ɑ.ʃɑ], [ɑ.ʒɑ].

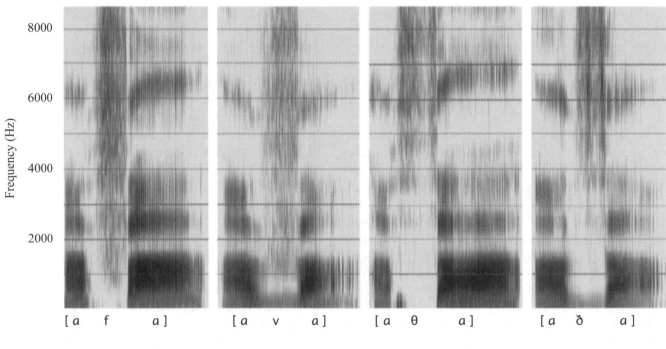

[a   f   a]   [a   v   a]   [a   θ   a]   [a   ð   a]

Time (sec)

FIGURE 6–51. Spectrogram of the nonsibilant fricatives in the utterances [ɑ.fɑ], [ɑ.vɑ], [ɑ.θɑ], [ɑ.ðɑ].

for affricates is behind the alveolar ridge and is classified as alveopalatal. The voiceless affricate [t͡ʃ] is produced as a combination of the voiceless alveolar stop [t] and the voiceless post-alveolar fricative [ʃ], while the voiced [d͡ʒ] is a combination of the voiced alveolar stop [d] and the voiced post-alveolar fricative [ʒ]. Figure 6–52 is a spectrogram of the two English affricates in VCV contexts. Note the complete closure followed by sound energy beginning at about 1800 Hz for the [t͡ʃ], similar to a post-alveolar fricative. The [d͡ʒ] has a voice bar present throughout the stop closure and fricative constriction but has the same turbulent property observed in [t͡ʃ].

Nasals. All nasals are voiced continuants. Nasal consonants have a formant structure like vowels, but fainter. Nasals are produced by lowering the velum so the oral cavity is closed off while the nasal cavity is open, resulting in characteristic resonances and **antiresonances**, the latter of which decrease resonance at certain frequencies. In general, the nasal resonant characteristics result in a relatively low F1, called the **nasal bar**, because the nasal cavity is so large. The nasal bar is typically at or below 250 Hz. Antiresonances result in nasal frequencies at varying

frequencies. The main way to distinguish the place of articulation for nasals is sound energy between 750 and 1250 Hz for [m], 1500 to 2000 Hz for [n], and above 3000 Hz for [ŋ]. See if you can identify the nasals and their resonant frequencies in VCV productions in Figure 6–53, as well as the nasal bar.

Approximants. Our final two manner categories are liquids and glides, both approximants. As you have learned, the approximants in English are /ɹ/, a liquid that can be produced at the alveolar, palatal, or retroflex place of articulation; /l/, an alveolar lateral liquid; /j/, a palatal glide; and /w/, a bilabial glide with secondary articulation at the velum. Approximants share a short steady state period followed by a relatively long gliding formant transition to the formant frequencies of the vowels that follow them. F1 transitions are not consistent, as they are dependent on varying properties of the following vowel. F2 transition frequencies in approximants are dependent on the tongue's height and front/back location for the vowel. F3 transition frequency values vary depending on the degree of lip rounding. Acoustic properties of approximants also differ dependent on whether they are liquids, glides, or rhotacized.

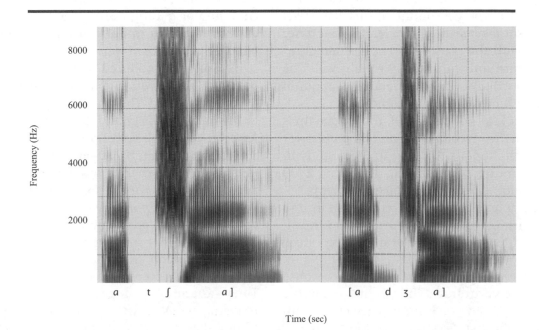

FIGURE 6–52. Spectrogram comparing the affricates in the utterances [a.t͡ʃa], [a.d͡ʒa].

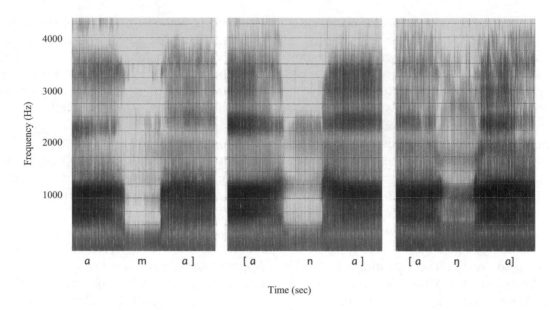

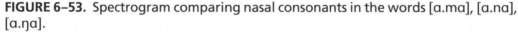

FIGURE 6–53. Spectrogram comparing nasal consonants in the words [ɑ.mɑ], [ɑ.nɑ], [ɑ.ŋɑ].

Liquids. [ɹ] and [l] have similar formant structures to vowels, although their formant structure is fainter. The rhotic liquid [ɹ] and the rhotic vowel [ɝ] are produced with some degree of lip rounding. The distinguishing characteristic of [ɹ] and [ɝ] is the lower F3 and F4. The consonant [ɹ] and the vowel [ɝ] have the same acoustic characteristics but differ in duration, with the consonant shorter and characterized by formant transitions to the vowel. The unstressed [ɚ] will also share these transition qualities, although they are less pronounced.

/l/ is a lateral sound. During [l], the tongue tip is in contact with the alveolar ridge and air passes over both sides of the tongue. For the [l], there are typically faint formants at about 250, 1200, and 2400 Hz, with the higher formants reduced in energy.

The primary acoustic difference between [l] and [ɹ] is the transition to the third formant. F3 transition is related to lip rounding and [ɹ] is produced with some degree of lip rounding, while [l] is not. Lip rounding lowers vocal tract resonances because it lengthens the vocal tract. Thus in the case of the lip rounded [ɹ], the lower resonances associated with lip rounding will be reflected in the low frequency starting point for the F3 transition.

Glides. Glides have a formant structure similar to vowels and have more formant energy than liquids and nasals. The phonemes [j] and [w] are similar articulatorily and acoustically to the vowels [i] and [u]. However, the formant structure is usually changing or gliding during the production of the glides, while the formant structure is steady-state for a longer period for vowels.

[j], like [i], is produced with a high front tongue position; that is, with the body of the tongue raised toward the palate. The starting point for the tongue in the glide [w] is similar to that for the high back rounded vowel [u], with lip rounding in both cases. Speed of articulatory movement is the most important factor in glide versus vowel production. [j] is produced by moving rapidly from the high front vowel position to the preparatory position for the following vowel. During [w] production, the high back position is shorter and not sustained as long as it is for the vowel [u]. Instead, the articulators are rapidly moving to the position required for the following vowel. Thus a fast rate of change in articulator position will result in a [w]+V or [j]+V syllable, such as [wɑ] or [jɛ], while a slower movement of the articulators will yield a two-syllable vowel sequence, such as [u.ɑ] or [i.ɛ].

The steady-state durations for [w] and [j] are shorter than for [ɹ] and [l]. The primary acoustic difference between [w] and [j] lies in the onset frequency and direction of the F2 transition. The starting F2 transition frequency for [w] is usually below approximately 600 Hz, while the F2 transition frequency for [j] is in the range of 2200 to 3600 Hz. The direction and extent of the formant transitions are dependent to some extent upon the following vowel.

Figure 6–54 is a spectrogram of the English approximants in VCV environments. Apply the information on approximants to identify the glide and liquid differences, as well as the transition distinctions that differentiate each approximant. While you may not remember all of the transition information, you should be able to tell that the sounds are liquids and glides because of their clear formants (not fading as they do for nasals), the similarity of [w] and [j] to the vowels [u] and [i], and the very low F3 and F4 in the [ɹ]. Can you identify any other helpful properties?

Identifying Words and Phrases

You have now learned the identifying characteristics of all vowels and consonants of English. It is a lot of information, but you do not always need all of the information to identify words on a spectrogram. Below are a few phrases to practice your newfound skills.

Figure 6–55 is a spectrogram of the words *baby*, *juice*, and *key*. You should be able to identify the stops, distinguishing voiced from voiceless ones. Also note the affricate and the fricative. There are mid and high front vowels and a high vowel. Can you segment these words and identify the key properties?

Types of Spectrographic Analysis

We have been looking at sound properties on **wideband spectrograms**. Wideband spectrograms are very clear on the time dimension but not as clear on the frequency dimension. By averaging broader

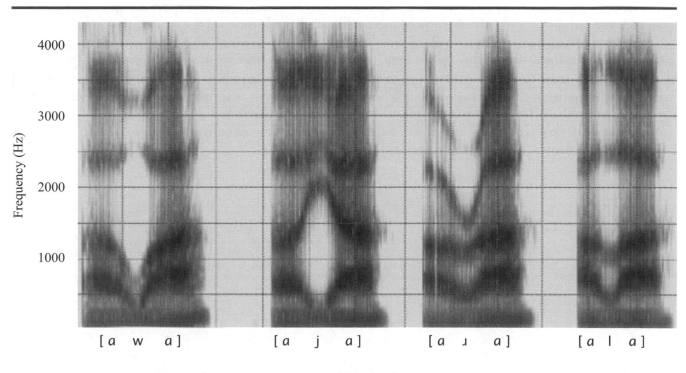

[a   w   a]   [a   j   a]   [a   ɹ   a]   [a   l   a]

Time (sec)

FIGURE 6–54. Spectrogram comparing English approximants in the words [a.wa], [a.ja], [a.ɹa], [a.la].

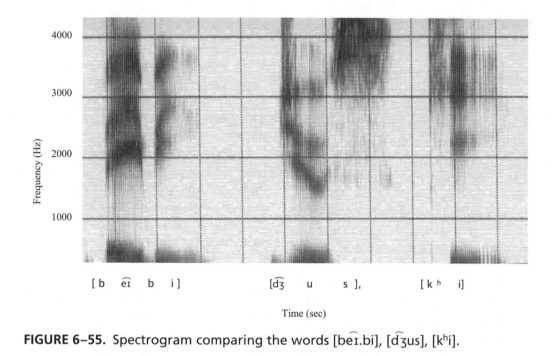

[b e͡ɪ b i]   [d͡ʒ u s],   [k ʰ i]

Time (sec)

FIGURE 6–55. Spectrogram comparing the words [be͡ɪ.bi], [d͡ʒus], [kʰi].

bands of energy, wideband spectrograms make it easier to interpret changes over time. Vertical striations are vocal fold vibrations—the fundamental frequency—and we can see sound bursts as straight lines. Because wideband spectrograms average broad bands of energy, it is more difficult to interpret frequency information. Figure 6–56 is a wideband spectrogram of the sentence *Today is our party.*

Narrowband spectrograms average smaller bands of sound energy. They are more accurate in the frequency dimension at the expense of time details. In narrowband spectrograms, it is easier to see the fundamental frequency and harmonics. Narrowband spectrograms also show how F0 changes as pitch changes. Note how in the narrowband spectrogram in Figure 6–57, also of the words *beat* and *bet,* you can see harmonics, but the bursts of sound for stop consonant release are blurred, unlike the wideband spectrogram in Figure 6–56.

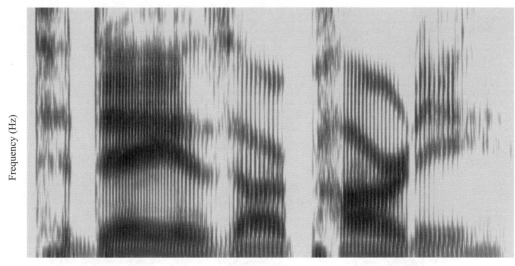

FIGURE 6–56. Wideband spectrogram of the sentence *Today is our party.*

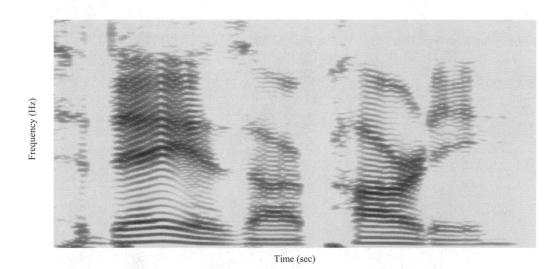

FIGURE 6–57. Narrowband spectrogram of the sentence *Today is our party.*

1. Below are spectrograms of six one-syllable words. These words are labeled A, B, C, D, E, and F.

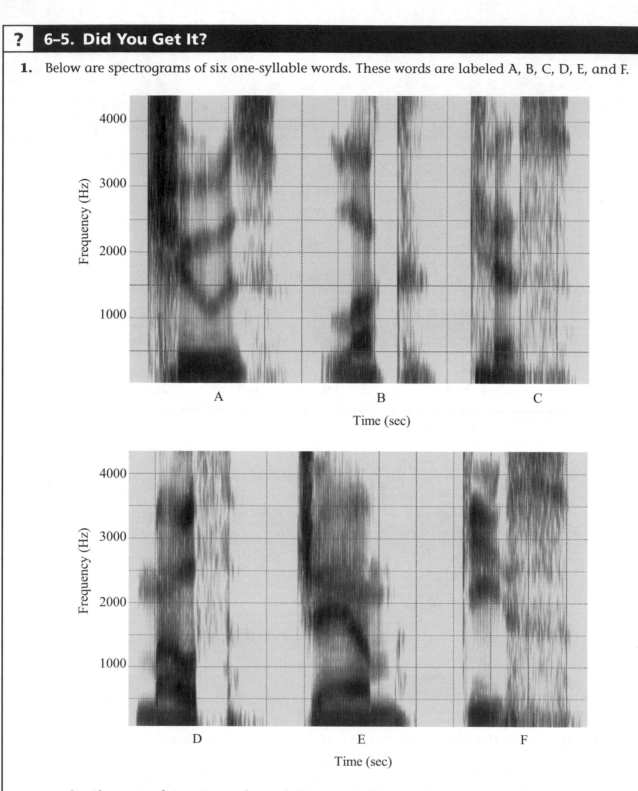

a. See if you can determine each word. First, mark distinguishing acoustic characteristics. Do you see turbulence, formants, silence, bursts, nasality, voicing? Mark them. Then begin segmenting possible phonemes, being careful to note different phoneme possibilities. Do you see a segment that could be an aspirated stop? Or could it be an affricate? List both possibilities. Then mark vowel formants, noting possible vowels based on your F1 and F2 measurements. For consonants, see if you can determine the *manner* and *voicing* categories. Once you have noted possibilities, look at the formant transitions between consonants and vowels to guess place of articulation. Now put all of these together: manner, place, voicing, vowel, consonant information, and guess the word for each spectrogram.

In the answer key, check your answer against the list of possible words for A, B, C, D, E, and F. Is your word one of the options? If so, congratulations! We actually expect that almost no one will get the words right. It is very difficult if not impossible to identify words on a spectrogram without clues.

b. If your word is not on the list, review the list of words provided in the answer key. Which word fits each spectrogram best? Review the phonetic information in the spectrograms again and pick the best word from the list of choices.

2. Spectrograms A and B below are of the same sentence, spoken at a high and a low pitch. Examine these two spectrograms. What is the difference between the spectrograms, and what causes this difference?

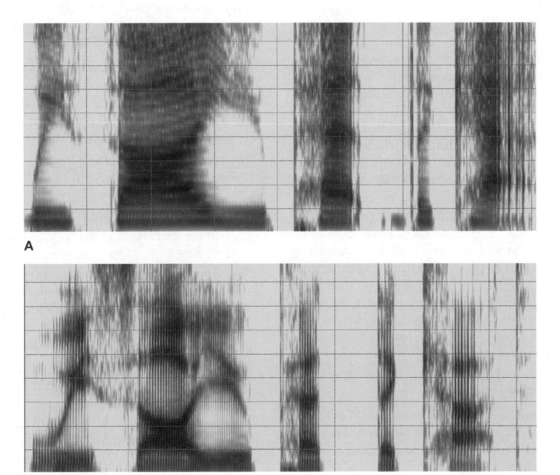

A

B

Spectrograms of the sentence *We saw you pet the cat,* spoken with a high F0 (**A**) and a low F0 (**B**).

Putting It All Together

This chapter introduced the acoustics of speech. As clinical scientists, you now see how different articulations translate into acoustic properties. You are now able to measure speech in a variety of ways to better understand typical speech. While we have not explored disordered speech, you have the tools to distinguish differences in typical and atypical speech. This chapter is an overview; we encourage you to explore the multitude of resources available to further the depth of your knowledge of speech. We also suggest you download software for making spectrograms and waveforms. There are several resources listed at the end of this chapter to do so.

You can use acoustic analysis in speech research and in tracking progress clinically. With acoustic phonetics, we can use instrumentation to record acoustic phonetic information, objectively comparing acoustic differences between sounds or improvements in the production of speech over time. It is easier to objectively measure acoustic phonetics than it is articulatory phonetics because we can represent acoustic information visually, keeping track of change over time. We will apply your acoustic phonetics knowledge as we further explore phonetics in later chapters.

Applied Science: Revisited

Summary

Macken (1992) presented what she regarded as evidence for an autonomous phonological component of a young child's developing speech system. The particular stage in the child's speech development considered to provide critical evidence was a stage from ages 1;11 to 2;1. The child substituted [f] for certain initial stop + /ɹ/ clusters. The child's mispronunciations included: [fɹ.tʰi] for /pɹɪ.ɾi/, [fi] for /tɹi/, [fɪŋkʰ] for /dɹɪŋk/, [feɪ.dəl] for /kɹeɪ.dəl/. Macken argued that while the first three exemplars of [f] possibly could be explained on the basis of phonetic similarity, the mispronunciation of /kɹeɪ.dəl/ as [feɪ.dəl] could not. Consequently, [feɪ.dəl] for /kɹeɪ.dəl/ was considered as evidence of a phonological rule component. We asked you to think about Macken's assertions and to see if you could come up with an alternative phonetic-based explanation as you read this chapter on acoustics. Below we share what we found.

One Step at a Time

1. At one year of age, the young child did not yet have the articulatory skill to be able to produce sequential consonants (i.e., consonant clusters).

2. To simplify the consonant cluster production, she deleted the later-mastered /ɹ/, and produced only the initial stop phoneme, which she articulated with strong aspiration.

3. We note that when a strongly aspirated stop precedes a vowel, the formant transition into that vowel will be flat.

4. After learning the acoustic properties of consonant productions, we take note of the following characteristics of the target words:

   a. The liquid /ɹ/ in all four target words is followed by high vowels.

   b. [ɹ] has a characteristic low F3.

   c. All three of the post-cluster vowels have a high F2.

   d. The low F3 of [ɹ] will rise significantly in the transition period into the high vowel.

   e. The beginning of the voiced portion of the target words would be a sloping rise in the formant frequency, and that sloping rise provides the most prominent spectral information regarding place of articulation.

   f. [f] has a low F2, similar to the low F3 for [ɹ].

5. We then hypothesize that substituting [f] for the /ɹ/ clusters would facilitate simulation of the greater formant increases in the target words, unlike the substitution of aspirated stops that result in a flat formant transition into a vowel. To test our hypothesis, we made spectrograms comparing target words to their expected simplifications to single-

tons, and to this child's mispronunciations. That is, for each we have shown the target word, the word as it would be expected to be produced without the /ɹ/, and the word produced as the child said it. These spectrograms are shown below. Figure 6–58 is a spectrogram of the productions of [pɹɪ.ɾi], [pʰɪ.ɾi], and [fɪ.ɾi]. Figure 6–59 is of [tɹi], [ti], and [fi]. Figure 6–60 is of [dɹɪŋk], [dɪŋkʰ], and [fɪŋkʰ]. Last, Figure 6–61 is a spectro-gram comparing productions of [kɹeɪ.dəl/, [keɪ.dəl], and [feɪ.dəl].

Answer

What do you see in the spectrogram comparisons? The spectrograms revealed that the substitution of [f] for the clusters in all four words did indeed simulate the steeply rising formant transitions found in correct articulations of the r-clusters.

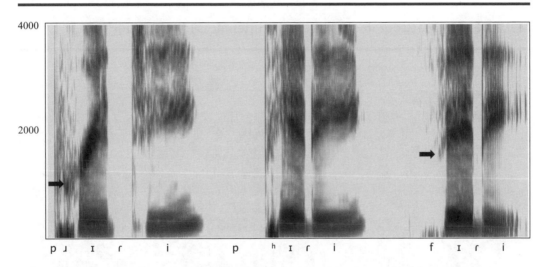

FIGURE 6–58. Spectrograms comparing the utterances [pɹɪ.ɾi], [pʰɪ.ɾi] and [fɪ.ɾi].

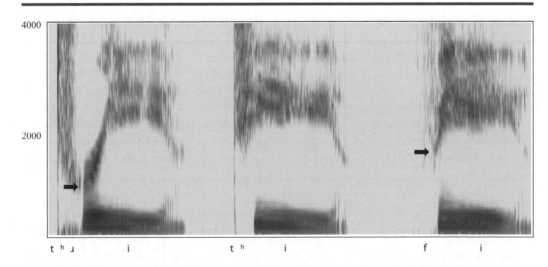

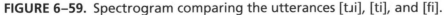

FIGURE 6–59. Spectrogram comparing the utterances [tɹi], [ti], and [fi].

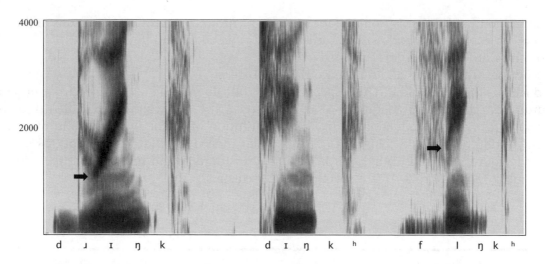

FIGURE 6–60. Spectrogram comparing the utterances [dɹɪŋk], [dɪŋkʰ], [fiŋkʰ].

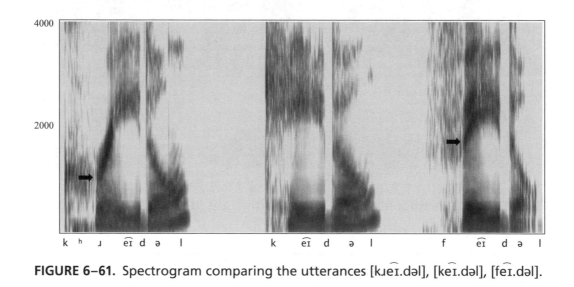

FIGURE 6–61. Spectrogram comparing the utterances [kɹeɪ.dəl], [keɪ.dəl], [feɪ.dəl].

Science Applied

Acoustic analysis of the misarticulated words indicates that the substitution pattern of [f] for the four /ɹ/-clusters may be characterized by a phonetic perspective. Phonetically based behaviors, rather than phonological rules may be a more appropriate characterization of the four exemplars. Applying acoustic phonetics to this problem provided a compelling alternative explanation for understanding this child's misarticulations.

References

Hillenbrand, J., Getty, L. A., Clark, M. J., & Wheeler, K. (1995). Acoustic characteristics of American English vowels. *Journal of the Acoustical Society of America (97)*, 3099–3111.

Jakielski, K. J., MacNeilage, P. F., & Davis, B. L. (1996, November). */fedəl/ for /kɹedəl/: Innate phonological rules ver-*

sus phonetic explanations for child mispronunciations. Poster session presented at the Annual Convention of the American Speech-Language-Hearing Association, Seattle, WA.

Macken, M. A. (1992). Where's phonology? In C. A. Ferguson, L. Menn, & C. Stoel-Gammon (Eds.), *Phonological development: Models, research, implications* (pp. 249–269). Parkton, MD: York Press.

Peterson, G. E., & Barney, H. L. (1952). Control methods used in the study of vowels. *Journal of the Acoustical Society of America, (24)*, 175–184.

Zsiga, E. C. (2013). *The sounds of language: An introduction to phonetics and phonology.* West Sussex, UK: John Wiley & Sons.

Interest Piqued?

Recommended materials to further your understanding of topics covered in this chapter.

Print Resources

Kent, R., & Read, C. (2001). *Acoustic analysis of speech* (2nd ed.). Boston, MA: Cengage Learning.

Ladefoged, P. (2005). *Vowels and consonants: An introduction to the sounds of languages* (2nd ed.). Malden, MA: Blackwell.

Zsiga, E. C. (2013). *The sounds of language: An introduction to phonetics and phonology.* West Sussex, UK: John Wiley & Sons.

Online Resources

https://americanenglish.state.gov/resources/colorvowelchart

Useful for learning the vowel chart and identifying phonemes

http://www.audiostretch.com/

AudioStretch is a free app to record a word or sentence and share the audio file. Once you open the app, it will create a waveform. You can scroll over the waveform to hear each part and see what it looks like. Try recording one of the sentences in this book to compare the book's waveform with the ones they made.

http://www.fon.hum.uva.nl/praat/

PRAAT is a free open source software that allows you to record and see phonetic patterns.

http://home.cc.umanitoba.ca/~robh/howto.html

How to read spectrograms and what features look like on spectrograms

https://itunes.apple.com/us/app/spectrumview/id472662922?mt=8

https://play.google.com/store/apps/details?id=net.galmiza.android.spectrumview&hl=en

SpectrumView is a free app that records your voice and shows a spectrogram.

http://www.linguistics.ucla.edu/people/hayes/103/SpectrogramReading/ShortComparisons/

Great for spectrogram transcription practice

http://www.phon.ucl.ac.uk/home/mark/vowels/

Demonstrates the effect of altering source and filter

http://scienceprimer.com/types-of-waves

A visual moving example of different wave types

http://www.sens.com/products/vowel-demonstrator/?utm_source=Template+for+Vowel+Demonstrator+Email&utm_campaign=FREEWhistIOSConsumerEmail11212014&utm_medium=email

Sensimetrics is a vowel demonstrator which is described as an interactive introduction to vowel acoustics and the production of vowels. Great for understanding source-filter theory, the interaction between the vowel quadrilateral with acoustic properties and vocal tract shape. Costs $10.

https://www.speechandhearing.net/

A wealth of acoustic resources

http://userpages.chorus.net/cspeech/

TF32 (time-frequency 32 bit) analysis software program. There is a free downloadable version which shows spectrograms and frequency, intensity, and duration information.

https://wavesurfer-js.org/

Free software that allows you to record and see phonetic patterns. Real-time recording. Good for seeing VOT and formant structure.

ANSWER KEY

6–1.

1. There are three types of wave movement. They are <u>transverse,</u> <u>longitudinal</u>, and <u>surface</u> waves.

2. A sound wave is characterized by high and low pressure variations. High pressure is also called <u>compression</u> and low pressure is called <u>rarefaction</u>.

3. Pitch is a subjective measure of <u>frequency</u>.

4. Loudness is a subjective measure of <u>intensity or amplitude</u>.

5. The number of times the vocal folds vibrate per second determines the <u>fundamental frequency</u>.

6–2.

1. Waveform A is a simple, periodic waveform due to its clear repetitions. Waveform B is complex and periodic. Waveform C is complex and aperiodic, not displaying a clear pattern or repetitions as the first waveform does.

2. Waveform A is representative of a pure tone because of its periodic, sinusoidal characteristics. Waveforms B and C represent speech sounds. Waveform B is periodic and C is aperiodic.

3. A waveform's *x*-axis is labeled *time*, and the *y*-axis is labeled *amplitude*. These two labels give us information about a waveform's energy or displacement (*amplitude*) over the course of a period of time.

4. In terms of speech, vowels are represented with periodic waveforms due to their vocal fold vibration. Consonant waveforms contain aperiodic waves due to the effects of their more complete obstruction on the sound waves.

6–3.

1. The *x*-axis of a spectrogram is time (in seconds) and the *y*-axis is frequency (in hertz, Hz). Darkness denotes amplitude (in decibels, dB), such that the darker the input, the greater the amplitude. A spectrogram tells us the amplitude of the frequency components of a sound source over time.

2. A is a spectrogram; the *x*-axis is time, the *y*-axis is frequency, and the gray scale indicates amplitude. B is a waveform; the *x*-axis is time and the *y*-axis is amplitude. C is a spectrum; the *x*-axis is frequency and the *y*-axis is amplitude.

6–4.

1. Emphasized harmonics are called <u>formants</u>. The frequency of these <u>formants</u> are dependent on the size and shape of the vocal tract.

2. Vowel identity is primarily dependent on which two formants? <u>F1</u> and <u>F2</u>.

3. A vowel's first formant varies depending on <u>tongue height.</u> This relationship is <u>inverse</u>.

That is, the higher F1 is, the <u>lower</u> the tongue is.

4. A vowel's second formant is dependent on <u>tongue advancement</u>. This relationship is <u>direct</u>. That is, the higher F2 is, the <u>farther forward</u> the tongue is.

6–5.

1. a. The correct answer for each spectrogram is provided, along with five other possibilities.

Spectrogram A:

book	shout	mouth	read	fast	niece

Spectrogram B:

chain	jam	shock	call	jeans	ring

Spectrogram C:

geese	sky	kings	bruise	cause	teach

Spectrogram D:

mist	steers	crop	choose	flute	cheat

Spectrogram E:

juice	squish	wreck	geese	kiss	type

Spectrogram F:

make	quail	luck	lost	blog	rap

b. The words on the spectrograms and their phonetic transcription are found below.

Spectrogram A: mouth /maʊθ/

Spectrogram B: jam /d͡ʒæm/

Spectrogram C: geese /gis/

Spectrogram D: choose /t͡ʃuz/

Spectrogram E: luck /lʌk/

Spectrogram F: kiss /kɪs/

2. Spectrogram A was produced at a higher pitch than Spectrogram B. Thus the F0 in A was higher than the F0 in B. A higher F0 results in harmonics that are further apart, since harmonics are whole integer multiples of the fundamental frequency. Fewer harmonics means there is less sound energy. For these reasons, the formants on A are harder to read than B—there are fewer emphasized harmonics at the sound energy peaks of formants. In addition, the vertical striations in A are harder to distinguish than they are in B, also indicating that the vocal fold vibrations are less frequent.

7

LINGUISTIC PHONETICS AND PHONOLOGY OF CONSONANTS

Learning Objectives

By reading this chapter, you will learn:

1. the relationship between phonetics and phonology

2. explanations and examples of anticipatory and carryover coarticulation

3. how to identify phonemes using minimal pairs

4. the definitions of contrastive, free variation, and complementary sound distributions

5. the study of syllables as the unit of speech planning

6. the syllable components of onset, rime, nucleus, and coda

7. allophonic patterns affecting American English consonants in typical speech

8. clinical uses of phonological patterns affecting American English consonants in atypical speech

Applied Science

A second-grade child, Luis, was referred to his school diagnostic team by his classroom teacher due to speech concerns. Luis's teacher worried that these errors could affect his development of spelling and reading. Puerto Rican Spanish is Luis's home language, although he attends a monolingual English education program. The monolingual English-speaking speech-language pathologist collected a speech sample and noted the following [s] productions in the middle of eight words, four that Luis articulated correctly and four that he misarticulated. The speech-language pathologist also noted that Luis misarticulated [s] in the one word that ended in [s], while correctly articulating the medial [s] in the same word.

['daɪ.nə.sɔɚ]   for *dinosaur*

['pɛn.səl]   for *pencil*

['mʌ.səl]   for *muscle*

['ɹi.sɛh]   for *recess*

['mʌh.tæʃ]   for *moustache*

['beɪh.bɔl]   for *baseball*

[mɪh.'teɪk]   for *mistake*

['kɹɔh.wɔk]   for *crosswalk*

Based on these findings, the speech-language pathologist determined that Luis's articulation of [s] in words is inconsistent. The clinician needs to decide whether a formal speech evaluation is warranted. Are Luis's misarticulations inconsistent? How should the speech-language pathologist proceed?

Phonetics and Phonology

Up to now, you have studied articulatory phonetics, how we produce speech sounds; acoustic phonetics, how we analyze the auditory signals that result from producing speech sounds; and broad and narrow phonetic transcription, how we use phonetic symbols to represent speech in print. You have learned that speech sounds as articulatory units are called phones, and variations of a single phone are called allophones, which we transcribe using brackets ([ ]). You also have learned that when a group of allophones holds meaning in a language, that group of sounds represents a phoneme. A phoneme is the smallest unit of sound that changes meaning in a language, and phonemes convey meaning as they are sequenced into words. Every language has a distinct set of phonemes that are used to contrast meaning in words. For example, if we exchanged /b/ for /p/ (both phonemes in English) in the word *pack*, we would make a new word—a word with its own unique meaning. Studying how phonemes function in a language is the practice of linguistic phonetics, and it is critical to being able to understand the structure of any language.

As introduced in Chapter 1, phonemes represent abstract underlying mental units, while phones and allophones represent the surface forms of the different articulations of those units. Phonemes are thought to be the underlying sound representations that we have stored in our brains and that we combine to express the words in our language. Whereas changes in phones do not change the meaning of a word, so that we can say ['n̥u.dəl], ['nːu.dəl], or ['n̪u.dəl] and all three productions mean the same thing, changes in phonemes do affect meaning, as in the previous example of *pack* and *back*. Each phonemic symbol, which we transcribe using virgules (/ /), represents a group of sounds, and the allophone that is produced depends on the phonetic context of the production, as well as the rules of the language. These language-specific rules govern how phonemes as abstract units pattern in a language. These patterns result in predictable, surface, and allophonic changes in sounds. Remember that the study of language-specific rules for speech sounds is called phonology, and while intersecting with phonetics, phonology is a separate domain of linguistics.

Phonology is our understanding of how sounds can be combined in a language to create words. For example, can you think of any English words that begin with the consonant cluster [st]? Sure, lots of words begin with the st-cluster, including *stop*, *start*, *sticks*, and *stones*. Now try to think of English words that begin with the consonant cluster [ɹw]. Can you think of any? No English words begin with [ɹw]. Pause for a moment to consider why English doesn't have words that begin with [ɹw]. Thinking articulatorily, nothing prevents us from sequencing the sounds [ɹ] and [w]; however, even though we could, we do not. If production is not holding us back, then why do we not have words that begin with [ɹw]? The reason is that in English phonology these two consonants are not sequenced to form word-initial clusters—it's simply a pattern of our language. Interestingly, we abide by that pattern so faithfully that when we pronounce the name of the East African country *Rwanda*, a word from the Bantu linguistic family, we insert a vowel in-between [ɹ] and [w], producing [ɹə.ˈwɑn.də]—just to avoid making a cluster that violates the phonological patterns of English. If we are to understand how speech sounds function in a language, then we must study the systematic organization of the sounds and the patterns that govern them.

? 7–1. Did You Get It?

Use the following words no more than one time each to complete the following sentences.

physical production, mental representation, phonetic, phonological

1. The language-specific pattern that prohibits words from ending in [h] is part of the English _____ system.

2. Transcribing "p" as [p] signifies a _____.

3. Transcribing "p" as /p/ signifies a _____.

Speech as a Connected Unit

Sometimes our articulation of a consonant or vowel varies because of the physical nature of the articulatory process itself. Imagine you just heard someone say the word *raisin*. If asked, could you name the phones in the word you heard? Absolutely you could. We can name the individual speech sounds that make up a word—and in the order in which they were spoken—because we perceive speech sounds as discrete units of articulation. It is as though we auditorily string together the sequence of individual sounds that we hear, one by one. However, do we *produce* speech in the same way? Do we articulatorily string speech sounds together, one by one, when we talk? Do we articulate idealized target sounds [w ʌ n . s aʊ n d . æ t . ə . t aɪ m]? No, we do not, because speech production is a dynamic, ever-changing event. While we hear words as comprising individual phones, we do not produce speech as discrete units. Instead, we overlap our articulatory gestures, creating movements for one sound that blend into the sounds before and after it. "Speech is not like beads on a string" is an adage that has been repeated from one generation of phonetics students to the next. We repeat it here to emphasize that speech production is dynamic in nature and requires the finessed coarticulation of sounds, a concept that we first introduced in Chapter 1.

Speech is dynamic because the articulatory environments that affect consonants and vowels change from one word to the next. Let's practice, so you can appreciate this important point. Using citation-form speech, say the word *moo* aloud. Now say it again, but this time "freeze" your movements right after producing the initial [m] but before producing the vowel [u]. Without moving your articulators, try to feel the position of your lips. Next, say the word *me* aloud, freezing your movements before you get to the vowel [i], and again, pay attention to the position of your lips. Do this one more time, comparing the position of your lips for the [m] in *moo* versus the [m] in *me*. What you should have felt was a slight puckering of your lips in the production of [m] in *moo*. Did you feel that puckering? If not, practice a few more times until you can feel it. Now try to say the word *me* using the same position your lips were in during your production of *moo*. It feels awkward, doesn't it? Can you think of why we round our lips for [m] in *moo*, but not in *me*? If you hypothesized that because the [u] in *moo* is a lip rounded vowel and that we started to round our lips early, then you are thinking phonetically and you are correct. In this case, the back vowel that followed [m] modified its articulation—it became a lip rounded bilabial nasal consonant, and conversely, the lips are spread to get ready for the [i] in *me*. In our brains, we were anticipating the lip rounding gesture that was coming up in *moo* and the lip spreading gesture that was coming up in *me*, so we started to round and spread our lips early to be able to produce speech sounds that flow smoothly one into the other. We consider these articulatory variants, [mʷ], [m̠], and [m], to be allophones of the phoneme /m/. When a sound's production is modified because of a sound yet to be articulated, as in the case of the [m] in *moo*, we call the phenomenon **anticipatory coarticulation**.

Let us take a moment to examine some other examples of anticipatory coarticulation. Try to identify the articulatory modification of the underlined sounds in the words *sew*, *width*, and *hand*. Say each of these words one at a time, focusing on your articulation of the underlined sounds. What are the anticipatory coarticulation modifications for each of these sounds? Remember that the underlined sounds will be affected by the sound that follows them. Examine those sounds that follow to see what aspect of their production might have affected the preceding sounds. If you are thinking phonetically, you should have identified that the [s] in [soʊ] has lip rounding, because of the lip rounded vowel that follows it; the [d] in [wɪdθ] is dentalized, because of the following interdentalized consonant; and the [æ] in [hænd] is nasalized, because of the following nasal consonant. How might you capture these allophonic productions phonetically? To answer that question, we hope you are recalling your knowledge of diacritical marks. Diacritics, as detailed in Chapter 4, allow us to capture on paper these articulatory modifications, as in [sʷoʊ], [wɪd̪θ], and [hæ̃nd], respectively.

A phone also can be modified by a sound that precedes it. For example, consider the words *look* and *leek*. Say both words slowly, paying particular attention to your articulation of the word-final [k] productions. Can you tell that you produced two different variants of [k]? To help you feel the difference in the production of these two allophones, omit the initial consonant and alternate saying [ʊk] – [ik] several times, again paying attention to the [k] productions. Hopefully you can feel the back of your tongue raised to the velum for the [k] in [ʊk], with the articulation matching the ideal target for this voiceless velar stop phone. However, your articulation of [k] in [ik] should feel more forward in the mouth, forward enough to tell that this velar stop is not produced with the back of the tongue on the velum. The reason? Because the vowel preceding [k]

in the word [lik] is a high front vowel, resulting in the tongue starting high and forward in the mouth, a forward position that also moves the articulation of [k] forward. When a preceding sound affects the production of a sound that follows it, we call it **carryover** (also called perseverative or retentive) **coarticulation**. Carryover coarticulation is when you have just said a sound and you continue to carry over some aspect of that sound into the articulation of a following sound.

Studying a few other examples will further illustrate carryover coarticulation. Try to identify the articulatory modification of the underlined sounds in the words *print* and *clap*. What are these carryover coarticulation variations? Remember that the underlined sounds will be affected by the sound that precedes them. Examine those preceding sounds to see what aspect of their production might have affected the sounds that followed. In the words *print* and *clap*, the liquids [ɹ] and [l] are not voiced, having been affected by the voicelessness of the stop consonants that preceded them. You can feel that devoicing by placing your fingertips lightly on your larynx while slowly saying both words and noticing that voicing does not start until the vowels are produced. Using the voiceless diacritic, we narrowly transcribe the words as [pɹ̥ɪnt] and [kl̥æp]. Allophones created secondary to carryover coarticulation occur in American English less frequently than those resulting from anticipatory coarticulation, but they do occur, so you want to be able to identify this production phenomenon.

? | 7–2. Did You Get It?

Indicate if the allophones described below resulted because of anticipatory or carryover coarticulation.

1. a nasalized vowel in the word *ham*

   _____

2. a dentalized [n] in the word *month*

   _____

3. a nasalized vowel in the word *ring*

   _____

4. a palatal [k] in the word *seek*

   _____

Determining the Status of Speech Sounds in a Language

As we have discussed in previous chapters, certain phonemes in one language might be allophones in another language, and certain allophones in one language might be phonemes in another. To determine if two sounds are (meaning-based) phonemes in a language, we need to begin by identifying pairs of words that differ by only a single consonant or vowel sound. We call such sets of words **minimal pairs**. Minimal pairs are two words that differ only by a single vowel or initial, medial, or final consonant. Let's use an example of the words *cat* and *cot*. Both words begin with [k] and end with [t]; only their vowel sounds differ. Therefore, *cat* and *cot* are a minimal pair. Because both *cat* and *cot* are unique words and differ by only a single sound, we see that if we swap one of the vowels for the other, then we change the meaning of the word. By completing this exercise, we established that /æ/ and /a/ are phonemes in English. Can you think of a minimal pair that would establish "s" and "sh" as phonemes? Examples could include *sun-shun* and *lass-lash*. Can you think of another pair of words with "s" and "sh" in which one of the words is a verb and the other is a pronoun? Yes, *see-she* also is a minimal pair, because the only difference between the words is the initial consonant. If we produce [ʃ] instead of [s] in the verb *see*, we would create the word *she*, and if we produced [s] instead of [ʃ] in *she*, we would produce the word *see*; therefore, this minimal pair establishes that /s/ and /ʃ/ are phonemes in English. When two phonemes occur in minimal pairs that establish them as phonemes, we say that the phonemes are in **contrastive distribution** in the language.

Keep in mind that the sounds that function as phonemes and the sounds that function as allophones differ from one language to another. For example, in English we have a pair of alveolar fricative cognates: [s] and [z]. These sounds are meaning-based units, phonemes, so we cannot interchange them without altering the meaning of words, as in the minimal pairs *sip-zip* and *hiss-his*. However, in some dialects of Latin American Spanish, [s] and [z] are allophones for the phoneme /s/. In these dialects, both of the "s" letters in the word *esposa* (*wife*) are pronounced as [s], as in [es.'po.sa], and even though each of the words *azul* (*blue*), *zapato* (*shoe*), and *paz* (*peace*) is written with the letter "z,"

the "z" letters also are produced as [s], as in [a.'sul], [sa.'pa.to], and [pas].

To exemplify sounds being allophonic in English but phonemic in another language, we can consider vowels of varying durations. In English, we can shorten and lengthen vowel sounds without changing word meaning, because vowel duration variations are allophonic in English. For example, we can say *cookie* using shortened or lengthened vowel sounds, as in ['kŏ.kǐ], ['kŏ.kiː], ['kʊː.kǐ], or ['kʊː.kiː]. Despite the different pronunciations, all four of the productions refer to the same thing: the bakery treats we like to eat. Because vowel length in English can be produced differently in the same contexts, we say that they occur in **free variation** in the language. In Japanese, however, vowel duration does affect meaning. Some Japanese vowels have two forms, a short form and a long form, and those two forms are phonemic. Short and long vowels are designated in the spelling of words in Japanese, as well as in the pronunciation; however, the only articulatory difference between the vowels is duration. For example, the word *here* in Japanese is pronounced as [ko.ko.], with two short [o] vowels. If you lengthened the [o] vowels, as in [koː.koː] you would say the Japanese word for *high school*.

There are a variety of reasons why a speaker might produce a particular allophone in a word at one time, and a different allophone in the same word at another time. In addition to phonetic context, these reasons include factors such as the speaker's dialect or the message they intend to send. Personal speaker factors of age, sex, and class also may affect their articulation of sounds. In addition, speaking contexts such as rate of speech and speaking style can influence speech sound production. While a variety of factors affect speech sound production, sounds in free variation often tend to be predictable once a listener becomes familiar with a given speaker's speaking style.

We have discussed two types of distributions of sounds in a language: sounds in contrastive distribution and sounds in free variation. Sounds in contrastive distribution are established as phonemes because they contrast in minimal pairs. Sounds that we can modify articulatorily one way or another in the same context without changing meaning are called allophones that occur in free variation. There also are allophones that occur in one specific context and only in that specific context, and those allophones are said to be in **complementary**

distribution. Do you remember the articulatory modification called dark-l (i.e., [ɫ]) that we discussed in Chapter 4? When does the [ɫ] allophone occur? It occurs only in post-vocalic position, such as in the words *pal* and *pill*. Speakers do not produce [ɫ] in pre-vocalic position, as in the words *lap* and *lip*, although it would be an interesting experiment for you to try. Say the words *pal* and *pill* using the [ɫ] allophone. Now try to articulate the words *lap* and *lip* using the [ɫ] allophone. It is very difficult to do, isn't it? Because dark-l is a context-dependent allophone, it is said to be in complementary distribution. There are a variety of context-dependent allophones in every language. Later in the chapter, we will explore the pattern-based contexts that affect those consonants. Next, however, we will discuss two other broad concepts that will lay the foundation for your understanding of the patterns that underlie allophonic productions.

?   7–3. Did You Get It?

1. List a minimal pair that establishes [p] and [b] as phonemes.

   _____ and _____

2. List a minimal pair that establishes [i] and [ɪ] as phonemes.

   _____ and _____

Indicate if the sounds described in the examples below are in contrastive, free variation, or complementary distribution.

3. [n] and [t] as phonemes in the minimal pair *spin–spit*

   _____

4. [t] and [tʰ] occurring in the word *hit*

   _____

5. nasalization of [æ] (i.e., [æ̃]) when produced between two nasal consonants

   _____

Syllabicity

Researchers spend a lot of time thinking about how our brains organize speech. We often teach speech

from a phoneme-by-phoneme perspective, assuming that speech development is about learning individual phonemes and then stringing all those individual phonemes together into words. This perspective is common in the beliefs of phonologists who hold to the idea that to understand phonology one must first understand how individual phonemes are stored. Many theories have been developed to try to explain how the patterns for sounds are created. For example, how do we know that [p], [t], and [k] are aspirated in the words *pea*, *tea*, and *key*, and not aspirated in the words *spy*, *sty*, and *sky*? Do we have an underlying phonemic structure to guide our productions? Is that how as speakers we know to do this?

There are also phonologists who suggest that it is not the phoneme but the syllable that is how we organize speech, meaning that instead of having abstract storage of phonemes (or characteristics of phonemes), speech is stored in syllable units. If true, the learning of language would be in syllable productions, that is, combinations of singleton consonants and consonant clusters paired with vowels. Building longer words and utterances would involve putting together these syllables. This would mean that we would have stored units of, for example, voiceless stop + vowel and [s] + voiceless stop + vowel syllables that we would access as we build new words. It also suggests the syllable as a unit of storage for speech, in addition to having individual segments stored. Is there any evidence for this idea? We do have theories of speech development that show the connection of the consonant and vowel in early speech productions. This connection has been observed in babbling and first words, suggesting that simple syllables are the motoric units of speech that are the first ones learned. In addition, when pre-literate children are asked to divide spoken words, they commonly do so by naming syllables, not individual phones. It is not until children begin to read and write that they segment words by phones.

Another potential source of evidence for the syllable as a stored speech unit is the phenomenon of **spoonerisms**. Spoonerisms are a specific type of speech error that is syllable governed. Named for the Reverend William Archibald Spooner, a late nineteenth-century British scholar who purportedly was (in)famous for switching syllables in his word productions, many spoonerisms result in unintentionally funny expressions. One such spoonerism attributed to Spooner was his toast to Queen Victoria that began, "Three cheers for our queer old dean," instead of, "Three cheers for our dear old queen." Oops! Reverend Spooner received renown for supposedly *making these sound switches with great frequency.*

Spoonerisms result from the switching of sounds in words. That is, the order of sounds is changed during the word's production. Analyze the example of "queer old dean" for "dear old queen." Because we are interested specifically in the articulation of those utterances, we need to examine the phonetic transcriptions of those productions.

"queer old dean"   [kwɪɚ oʊld din]

"dear old queen"   [dɪɚ oʊld kwin]

How would you describe the errors you see? We might describe the first error as a substitution of [kw] for [d], and the second error as a substitution of [d] for [kw]. However, that description misses something important in spoonerisms. Examining the errors further, we see that the word-initial consonants in two of the words were switched with one another, that is, the word-initial [d] and the word-initial [kw] switched places with one another. Do the switches in spoonerisms always keep their same place in syllables? Interestingly, the sounds that are switched almost always maintain their same place in a syllable.

While spoonerisms can be fun to decipher, do they contain important information about how speech is organized? We think they do. Spontaneously produced spoonerisms that we hear exhibited by broadcasters, politicians, friends, and others follow the same patterns. The fact that most spoonerisms operate at the syllable level, with sounds continuing to occupy the same place in the new syllable as they did in the original, that is, an onset switches with another onset, a nucleus switches with another nucleus, etc., suggests that we program speech in syllable units—as well as in segmental units. When we mentally retrieve a word that we want to say, we retrieve its segments and its syllables. To be able to speak the word, we will need to send neurological and muscular commands for segments and syllables to our speech production system. The evidence from spoonerisms is an example of speech being mentally stored in syllable units, as well as in speech sound units.

? 7-4. Did You Get It?

Translate the following spoonerisms of common expressions.

1. doored to Beth   _____
2. bings a rell   _____
3. tips of the slung   _____
4. grack to the bind   _____

The Components of Syllables

We have explored the fundamentality of syllables as a core unit in speech. Now we will look at how syllables are structured. We do so by breaking down words into syllables, and then breaking down syllables into their component parts.

Syllables can take on a variety of shapes. Think of the one-syllable words *eye* and *strengths*. Even though these words have significantly different syllable structures, each one is only one syllable long. These two words represent the extremes of syllable length in English: from one phoneme in /aɪ/ to eight phonemes in /stɹɛŋkθs/. Take a moment to think of a few words that have two syllables. Words such as *paper* and *pencil* have two syllables. How many syllables are in the words *eraser*, *fundamental*, and *pentasyllabic*? Three, four, and five syllables, respectively. (By the way, the word *pentasyllabic*, a five-syllable word, describes a five-syllable word!) Hopefully, by now you have become quite good at determining the correct number of syllables in words. In Chapter 4, you also learned that a syllable contains either one vowel or one syllabic consonant. But can you explain what makes a sound or a string of sounds a syllable? In other words, can you define a syllable?

To answer that question, let us return to our examples of *eye* and *strengths*. We determined that despite having very different syllable structures, both words are **monosyllabic**, meaning that they each contain only one syllable. Both words also share the essential element of any syllable: they each contain only one vowel. One vowel equals one syllable and one syllable implies one vowel. Also, remember that diphthongs and triphthongs represent a single vowel. If there are two vowels in a word, that word also has two syllables. Three vowels indicate three syllables, and so on. We call the vowel the **nucleus** of a syllable, and every syllable must have one, but only one, nucleus. In the word *eye*, the syllable structure contains only a nucleus, so its syllable shape is V (vowel).

In addition to having a nucleus, a syllable may also contain one or more consonants. Whereas a vowel is required to designate a syllable, consonants are optional in English. In English, a syllable can contain up to three consonants in syllable-initiating position, and up to four consonants in syllable-arresting position. (In extremely rare instances, a word, such as *angsts*, may contain five syllable-arresting consonants. Because these words are infrequent in occurrence and hardly ever articulated with all five final sounds, we consider them to be extraordinary exceptions to the general pattern.) Can you think of a word that is monosyllabic and has three syllable-initiating consonants and four syllable-arresting consonants? Our previous example of *strengths* satisfies these conditions. Try now to think of a few monosyllabic words that start with three syllable-initiating consonants. The clusters [splʃ] as in *splash*, [spɹ] as in *spray*, [stɹ] as in *street*, and [ʃtɹ] as in loanwords such as *strudel* contain syllable-initiating three-segment clusters. Consonants and consonant clusters in syllable-initial position are said to be in the onset position. The word *eye* would not have a syllable onset, because it does not contain a consonant or cluster in syllable-initiating position. In the word *my*, however, [m] would be the syllable onset and [aɪ] would be the nucleus. In our previous example of the word *strengths*, the [stɹ] cluster would be the syllable onset and [ɛ] would be the nucleus. What about the syllable-arresting cluster [ŋkθs] in *strengths*? How do we categorize those final sounds? If there are syllable-arresting consonants in a word, they are said to be in the **coda** position. In the word *strengths*, the [ŋkθs] cluster is the syllable coda. To review the word *strengths*, [stɹ] is the onset, [ɛ] is the nucleus, and [ŋkθs] is the coda.

There is one additional concept you need to understand to be able to break down syllables: the syllable **rime**. When we begin to analyze a word to determine its sound structure, we first divide it into its syllables. After we have phonetically transcribed each syllable, we then divide each syllable into its onset and rime. The rime is the part of the syllable that contains the nucleus and the coda. In the monosyllabic word *eye*, the rime contains only

the nucleus [aɪ], because there are no consonants in coda position. In the word *mine* ([maɪn]), however, the rime contains the nucleus [aɪ] and the coda [n]. In addition, [m] is the syllable onset.

You are now ready to analyze syllables. Let's review the syllable diagram of the monosyllabic word *I*, which is, of course, the same as for the word *eye*. As you see in Figure 7–1, the word *eye* has one syllable and it is diagrammed as having only a nucleus in the rime, the vowel [aɪ].

Next, let us compare the analysis of *eye* with a variety of phonetically more complex words. As shown in Figure 7–2, the word *lie* is analyzed as having the onset [l] and the rime contains only the nucleus [aɪ]. The word *lime* also contains the onset [l], but the rime contains both the nucleus [aɪ] and the coda [m], as shown in Figure 7–3.

The onset then becomes the more complex sl-cluster when the word *lime* changes to *slime*, as shown in Figure 7–4. And when the word *slime* changes to *slimed*, it is the coda that becomes more complex, as shown in Figure 7–5.

Let's take a moment to review the syllable components for the five monosyllabic words we just analyzed. Refer to Table 7–1 to see the components for the syllables detailed in a table format, which easily permits side-by-side comparisons. Notice how the onsets and codas become more complex as the phonetic complexity of the words increases from one word to the next.

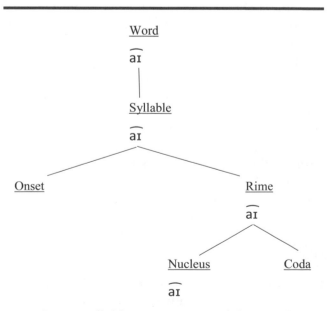

FIGURE 7–1. Syllable components of the word *I*.

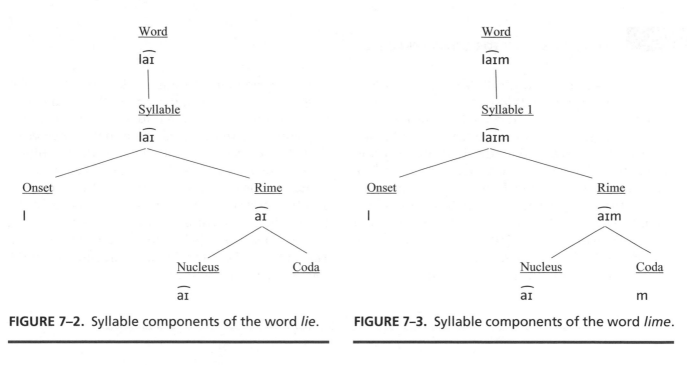

FIGURE 7–2. Syllable components of the word *lie*.

FIGURE 7–3. Syllable components of the word *lime*.

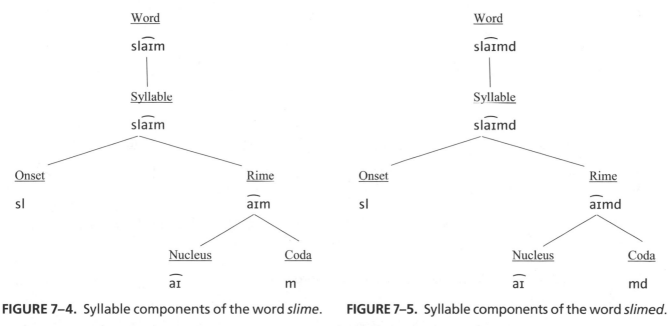

FIGURE 7–4. Syllable components of the word *slime*.

FIGURE 7–5. Syllable components of the word *slimed*.

TABLE 7–1. Syllable Components of Five Monosyllabic Words

Orthographic Word	Phonetic Transcription	# of Syllables	# of Phones	Onset	Rime	Nucleus	Coda
"eye"	[a͡ɪ]	1	1		[a͡ɪ]	[a͡ɪ]	
"lie"	[la͡ɪ]	1	2	[l]	[a͡ɪ]	[a͡ɪ]	
"lime"	[la͡ɪm]	1	3	[l]	[a͡ɪm]	[a͡ɪ]	[m]
"slime"	[sla͡ɪm]	1	4	[sl]	[a͡ɪm]	[a͡ɪ]	[m]
"slimed"	[sla͡ɪmd]	1	5	[sl]	[a͡ɪmd]	[a͡ɪmd]	[md]

We now will create a **disyllabic** word, that is, a word with two syllables. If we change the word *slimed* to *slimy*, we add a second syllable. Remember, we are not diagramming words, but rather, syllables. Therefore, we need to diagram both the first and second syllables in the word, as shown in Figure 7–6. The first syllable of *slimy*, [slaɪ], contains the onset [sl] and the rime [aɪ], which also is the nucleus of the syllable. The second syllable, [mi], has the onset [m] and the rime and nucleus [aɪ]. If the word *slimy* were lengthened to *slimiest*, a **trisyllabic** word, we would need to diagram all three syllables, and so on.

Take a moment to think back to our examples of spoonerisms. How might we use the language of syllable components to explain the speech errors we examined? In the spoonerism that created *queer dean* for *dear queen*, we said that the syllable-initiating consonants switched from one word to the other. Using syllable terms, we can describe the errors as a syllable onset switching with another syllable onset. Indeed, in spoonerisms, it would be very rare for a syllable onset to switch with a coda or vice versa. The integrity of the syllable structure remains intact even in these slips of the tongue.

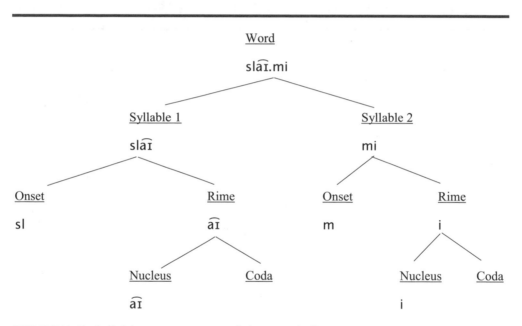

FIGURE 7–6. Syllable components of the word *slimy*.

? 7–5. Did You Get It?

Analyze the syllables in the following words.

1. *flavors*

	Syllable 1	Syllable 2
phonetic transcription	_____	_____
onset	_____	_____
rime	_____	_____
nucleus	_____	_____
coda	_____	_____

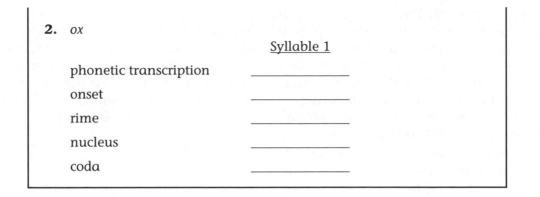

2. *ox*

	<u>Syllable 1</u>
phonetic transcription	_____
onset	_____
rime	_____
nucleus	_____
coda	_____

Patterns for Allophones in Consonant Coarticulation in Typical Speech

As you have learned, phonology covers the rules for how consonant and vowel articulation in a language can be modified in different contexts, in addition to how sounds pattern to form words. These rules connect phonemes to their actual articulations—to the phones and allophones that we produce in specific contexts. Be mindful of how the word "rules" is used in this context: these rules are *descriptive*—not prescriptive—of how speakers of a language modify their articulation of speech sounds in connected speech. We find it helpful to think about phonological rules as sound *patterns*, patterns that may or may not apply to a particular speaker or speaking situation. Understanding these patterns serves as your road map for understanding when these modified variants of phones may be produced, which in turn will help to increase your transcription accuracy.

Some of these sound patterns are descriptions of the articulatory modifications we make in casual speech in various speaking contexts and some occur in different dialects of a language. These patterns provide detail about the contexts in which allophones may be used. You can capture these modifications on paper using the narrow transcription diacritics you learned in Chapter 4. Keep in mind, though, that in speech-language pathology practice, we typically only use diacritics to note when a speaker pronounces a word in an *atypical* manner. As a beginning transcriber, you will first need to learn the typical articulatory modifications, so that later you will be able to identify the atypical ones. Using phonological patterns varies within and across speakers of a language. Every language has its own phonological system, and the patterns change from one language to the next—in some instances, even for the same phoneme. Remember also that articulation results in an acoustic product that has a physical reality. Therefore, we can record on paper what we hear using broad and narrow phonetic transcription, and we also can analyze the resulting acoustic signal using the skills you learned in Chapter 6. Next, we will introduce you to the systematic patterns for consonant allophones in American English. If you find that you have trouble hearing any of the allophonic patterns that follow, we suggest that you use your newly acquired knowledge of acoustics to help you visualize patterns you have difficulty hearing.

To begin to explore when, how, and why speakers vary their articulation of sounds that are in free variation and complementary distribution, we will start by discussing the specific contexts in which typical speakers of American English vary their productions. The types of variations we will study are secondary to systematic conventions for allophones. Nonetheless, variations of phonological patterns abound even for a single language, because of different dialects, individual speaker characteristics, and changing speaking environments. In addition, the same sound produced in different phonetic contexts can result in different articulations (i.e., allophones of a target phoneme). In this section, we hope to show you how the phonetics of sound production and perception can affect the allophonic patterns and sound changes in a language, ultimately influencing its phonology.

We will present the allophonic patterns for consonants in American English as categorized by manner of articulation. We first will discuss the patterns that affect phones as produced with varying degrees of obstruction, including stops, fricatives, and affricates. Because the phones in these three manner classes share the articulatory feature of obstruction, they form the larger class of sounds that we call obstruents. After we discuss the allophonic patterns that describe the obstruent class, we will discuss the patterns that describe nasals, glides, and liquids. These latter three manner classes form the larger class that we call sonorants, because they share the articulatory feature of being produced with a relatively unobstructed airway. (If you think back to earlier readings, we introduced obstruents and sonorants in Chapter 1, and in Chapter 6 we discussed obstruents and sonorants when we talked about the loudness of individual phones.) You will discover that some of the allophonic patterns that affect one manner class of obstruents overlap with another manner class of obstruents. For example, one allophonic pattern that describes stops may also describe fricatives or affricates. Likewise, there is overlap among some of the patterns that describe one manner class of sonorants with another. The reason for grouping different manner classes into the larger categories of obstruents and sonorants is

because each group of sounds shares articulatory and phonological features. Please note that there are many more allophonic patterns used by typical speakers of English than we will discuss. We selected patterns that we hear occurring most frequently in typical, casual, conversational speech across several of the dialects of American English.

Stops

We will discuss 14 allophonic patterns that apply to stop consonants. These modifications change articulatory airflow, place, manner, voicing, duration, and syllable structure. A summary of the 14 patterns can be found in Table 7–2.

Three patterns describe airflow modifications to voiceless stops. As you previously learned, the voiceless stops [p, t, k] are produced with more aspiration than the voiced stops [b, d, g]. The amount of aspiration we produce when articulating stop phones follows predictable contexts because these allophones occur in complementary distribution. The first pattern is the aspirated pattern: when voiceless stops are in the onset position in stressed syllables, they typically are strongly aspirated. Take, for example, the monosyllabic minimal pairs *pay-bay*, *toe-dough*,

TABLE 7–2. Allophonic Patterns Affecting Stop Phones

Pattern	Phone Affected	Description	Allophone	Example	Narrow Transcription
Airflow					
Aspirated	p t k	voiceless stops in onset position in stressed syllables are aspirated	xʰ	pay, toe, coo	pʰeɪ, tʰoʊ, kʰu
Unreleased	p t k	voiceless stops in word-final position can be unreleased	x̚	hop, hot, hock	hap̚, hat̚, hak̚
	p k	first stop in a sequence of two voiceless stops in the same syllable is typically unreleased	x̚	act, hopped	æk̚t, hap̚t
	t	voiceless alveolar stop preceding a syllabic-n can be unreleased	x̚	mitten, button	ˈmɪt̚.n̩, ˈbʌt̚.n̩
Unaspirated	p t k	voiceless stops in s-clusters are not aspirated	x⁼	spy, stew, ski	sp⁼aɪ, st⁼u, sk⁼i

continues

TABLE 7–2. *continued*

Pattern	Phone Affected	Description	Allophone	Example	Narrow Transcription
Place					
Labialized	p b t d k g	stops are rounded before a lip-rounded consonant or vowel	x^w	quack, goofy	k^wwæk, g^wufi
Dentalized	t d	alveolar stops are dentalized before an interdental fricative	x̪	eighth, width	eɪt̪θ, wɪd̪θ
Advanced	k g	velar stops are produced forward in the mouth before a front vowel	k̟	keen, gave	k̟in, ge͡ɪv
		velar stops are produced forward in the mouth after a front vowel	k̟	tack, dig	tæk̟, dɪg
Glottal replacement	t d	alveolar stops are substituted with a glottal stop before syllabic-n	ʔ	mitten, hidden	'mɪʔ.n̩, 'hɪʔ.n̩
Manner					
Nasal release	p b t d k g	stop plosion is released through the nose when the stop precedes a syllabic nasal	x^n	mitten, hidden	'mɪt^n.n̩, 'hɪd^n.n̩
Bilateral release	t d k g	alveolar and velar stop plosion is released over the sides of the tongue in l-clusters	x^l	close, oddly	k^{l}los, 'ad^l.li
Affricated	t d	alveolar stops are affricated in r-clusters	t͡ʃ, d͡ʒ	treat, drip	t͡ʃɹit, d͡ʒɹip
Tap replacement	t d	intervocalic alveolar stops are substituted with a tap before an unstressed vowel	ɾ	attic, middle	'æ.ɾɪk, 'mɪ.ɾəl
Duration					
Shortened	p b t d k g	a stop is shortened when it is doubled	x̚	big guest vs. biggest	bɪg̚.gɛst – 'bɪ.gɛst
Syllable Structure					
Glottal stop inserted	(null)	a glottal stop is inserted between two vowels when one word ends in a vowel and the next word begins with a vowel	ʔ	he eats vs. heats	hi.ʔits – hits
Omitted t	t	voiceless alveolar stop is omitted in word-medial nt-clusters when the syllable containing t is unstressed		enter	'ɛ.nɚ

and *coo-goo*. Say each of these words aloud and feel the stronger bursts of air on the voiceless cognates. Refer to the spectrograms of the words *coo* and *goo* in Figure 7–7 to help you visualize the difference in aspiration. The aspiration of [k] in *coo* is shown in part by the longer voice onset time for the vowel. Hopefully you remember that the diacritic for aspiration is the superscript "h" symbol, as in [pʰeɪ], [tʰoʊ], and [kʰu].

Again, the aspirated pattern has two conditions: the voiceless stop must occupy the syllable-onset position and the syllable must be stressed. In monosyllabic words, the word (syllable) is stressed, as the examples above illustrated. Consider multisyllabic words next. Compare your productions of the words *hated* and *hotel*. Both [t] sounds occupy the onset position in the second syllables; however, you should feel stronger aspiration on the [t] in *hotel*, because it is in the stressed syllable, unlike the [t] in *hated*, which is in the unstressed syllable. Other word pairs you can compare include *attic* versus *obtuse* and *party* versus *atone*, with [t] in a stressed syllable in the second word of each pair.

The articulatory opposite of strongly aspirating a sound is to not release it. There are three contexts in which voiceless stops are unreleased. The first context is when voiceless stops occur in word-final position. Word-final voiceless stops can be released

or not released, so we describe these allophones as being in free variation. This is described as the unreleased pattern. When a word-final voiceless stop is unreleased, it is transcribed using a superscript right angle to the right of the stop, as in [p̚, t̚, k̚]. Practice saying the words *hop*, *hot*, and *hock* first with a released final stop and then with an unreleased final stop. To articulate an unreleased stop, create complete closure for the stop, but do not blow out air at the end of the production. Say the words *hop*, *hot*, and *hock* without blowing out any air at the end of each word. We would transcribe those unreleased productions as [hɑp̚], [hɑt̚], and [hɑk̚]. Figure 7–8 is a spectrogram of productions of [hɑtʰ] and [hɑt̚], where you can see the slight burst of air for the released final [t] in [hɑtʰ], but not in the second, unreleased [t] in the production of [hɑt̚].

There are two other contexts in which voiceless stops tend to be unreleased. Say the word *apt* to see if you can figure out which of the stops, [p] or [t], is not released. The [p] typically is not released in *apt*. When two voiceless stops are abutting in the same syllable, the first one is unreleased, while the second stop typically is aspirated. We would narrowly transcribe *apt* as [æp̚t]. Two other words that exemplify this pattern are *act* and *hopped*, with the unreleased stops transcribed in [æk̚t] and [hɑp̚t]. Figure 7–9 shows a spectrogram of this pattern operating on

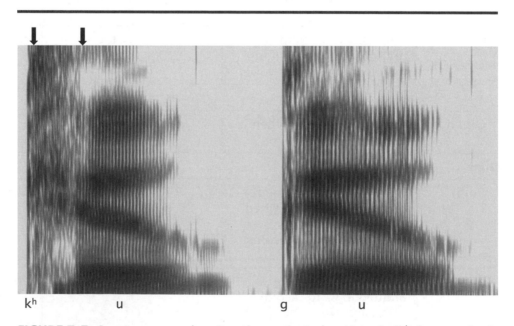

kʰ   u   g   u

FIGURE 7–7. Spectrograms showing the aspirated pattern in [kʰu] versus [gu].

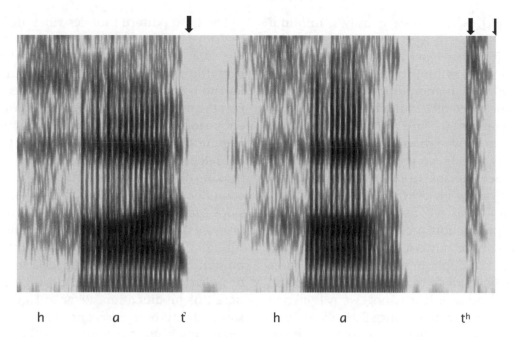

h   *a*   t̚   h   *a*   tʰ

FIGURE 7–8. Spectrograms showing the unreleased pattern in [hat̚] versus [hatʰ].

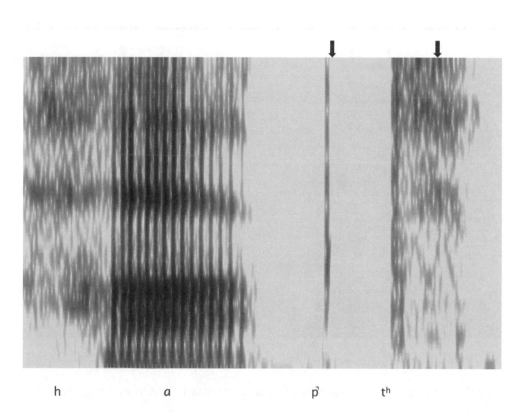

h   *a*   p̚   tʰ

FIGURE 7–9. Spectrogram showing the unreleased pattern in [hap̚t].

the word [hap̚t], where there is only a minimal release on [p]. The last context in which the alveolar voiceless stop [t] is unreleased is when it is followed by the **homorganic** syllabic-n, [n̩], as in the words *mitten* and *button*. A homorganic sound is a sound produced in the same articulatory place as another sound. For example, [t] and [n] are homorganic, because both are alveolar consonants. We would narrowly transcribe these productions as [ˈmɪt̚.n̩] and [ˈbʌt̚.n̩]. See the spectrograms in Figure 7–10 of the productions of an overly articulated production of [ˈmɪ.tʰɪn] versus a causal production of [ˈmɪt̚.n̩], the latter production produced with a syllabic nasal. The use of this pattern largely is dialectal, so it may or may not apply to your speech. Say these three words aloud slowly to determine if this is the pronunciation you use. If it is not, we will discuss two other possible ways to produce these words later in this section and one of them is certain to describe your own production.

The third pattern that describes airflow on voiceless stops is in the clusters [sp, st, sk], as in the words *spy*, *stew*, and *ski*. In this context of s + voiceless stop, the stops are not fully aspirated. Say the following pairs of words: *pie-spy*, *two-stew*, and *key-ski*. Feel the difference in the amount of aspiration from each stop. You should feel less aspiration on the stops in the s-cluster contexts. The stops in s-clusters are released; however, they are not fully aspirated, making them sound a little bit like their voiced cognates [b, d, g]. Most often these unaspirated stops are not transcribed using a diacritical mark because these variations are in complementary distribution and therefore systematic and predictable pronunciations. However, the superscript equal sign, as in [sp͇aɪ], [st͇u], and [sk͇i], can be used to designate this modification. Refer to Figure 7–11 to see spectrograms of *spy*, *pie*, and *bye* to compare the different amounts of aspiration in the three different contexts.

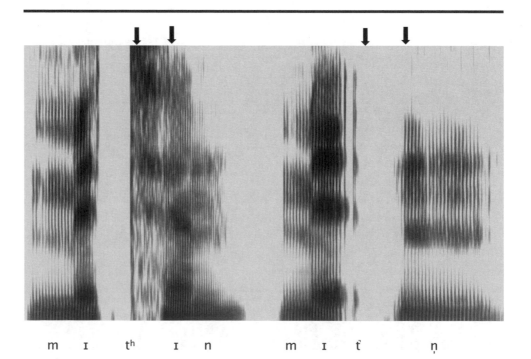

m   ɪ   tʰ   ɪ   n   m   ɪ   t̚   n̩

FIGURE 7–10. Spectrograms showing the unreleased pattern in [ˈmɪ.tʰɪn] versus [ˈmɪt̚.n̩].

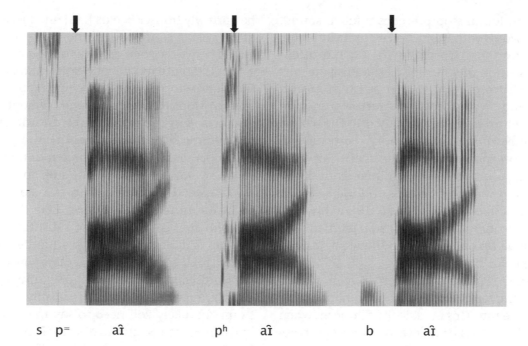

s p⁼   aî   pʰ   aî   b   aî

FIGURE 7–11. Spectrograms showing the unaspirated pattern in [sp⁼aɪ], [pʰaɪ], and [baɪ].

? 7–6. Did You Get It?

1. Indicate which of the three airflow patterns—aspirated, unreleased, or unaspirated—apply to the stops in the following examples.

   keys, caulk, cave   _____

   stove, stem, still   _____

   lick, soak, oink   _____

2. Phonetically transcribe each of the words in number 1, above, using diacritics to illustrate the appropriate allophonic pattern.

   keys, caulk, cave   _____ _____ _____

   stove, stem, still   _____ _____ _____

   lick, soak, oink   _____ _____ _____

The labialized, dentalized, advanced, and glottal replacement allophonic patterns describe place modifications of stops. The first two we will discuss, labialized and dentalized, occur because of anticipatory coarticulation. You hopefully remember the labialized diacritic of superscript "w" that is used to note lip involvement during articulation of a nonlabial stop, and the subscript bridge, or tooth [̪], which denotes a dentalized tongue placement for a nondental stop. The specific context for labialization is when a non-labial stop precedes a labial sound. Examples of words with labialized stops include *coke* and *goofy*. Say these words slowly, paying attention to the position of your lips as soon as you start speaking each word—you should be able to feel a slight rounding of your lips. The narrow transcription of these words is [kʷoʊk] and [gʷufi]. The second modification because of anticipatory coarticulation is dentalization that occurs in the specific context of a stop consonant preceding an interdental [θ] or [ð], as occurs in the words *eighth* and *width*, which would be transcribed narrowly as [eɪt̪θ] and [wɪd̪θ]. During dentalization, the alveolar stop is articulated with the tongue tip on or between the teeth, instead of on the alveolar ridge.

The advanced pattern is when a velar stop is produced by the tongue contacting the hard palate instead of the velum. This modification happens when a front vowel precedes or follows a velar stop; therefore, it is the result of either anticipatory or carryover coarticulation. As you previously learned, the diacritic for an advanced tongue position is the subscript plus sign [₊]. Words exemplifying the anticipatory coarticulatory context include *keen* and *gave*, which would be narrowly transcribed as [ḵin] and [g̱eɪv]. Examples of carryover contexts include *tack* and *dig*, which would be transcribed as [tæḵ] and [dɪg̱].

The last place modification affecting stops involves the glottal stop consonant replacing the alveolar [t] and [d] stops. Glottal stop replacement is dialectal and occurs in the context like an unreleased [t] or [d] before a syllabic-n. When [t] and [d] precede a syllabic-n, as in the words *mitten* and *hidden*, some speakers substitute a glottal stop for the alveolar stop, instead of unreleasing the stop consonant, as in the unreleased pattern. Like the unreleased alveolar stop consonant, the substitution of a glottal stop is dialectal. If your own dialect follows the glottal replacement pattern, then you will produce the words *mitten* and *hidden*, for example, as ['mɪʔ.n̩] and ['hɪʔ.n̩], with a glottal stop substituting the medial stops. You likely will need to say these words slowly and carefully to be able to discern if you produce glottal stops in this context or not, or if you produce the alveolar stop but do not release it, as in the previous examples of ['mɪt̚.n̩] and ['bʌt̚.n̩]. Spectrograms of an overly articulated production of ['mɪ.tʰɪn] versus a production of ['mɪʔ.n̩] are shown in Figure 7–12.

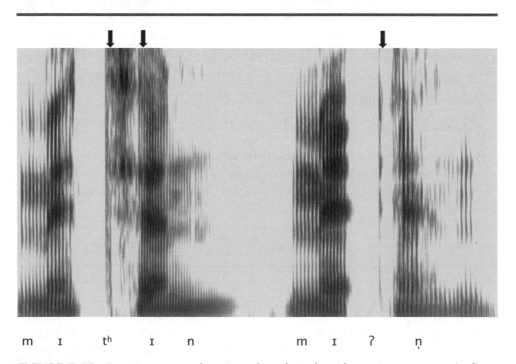

m ɪ tʰ ɪ n   m ɪ ʔ n̩

FIGURE 7–12. Spectrograms showing the glottal replacement pattern in ['mɪ.tʰɪn] versus ['mɪʔ.n̩].

? 7–7. Did You Get It?

1. Indicate the place-related pattern that can apply to the stops in the following examples.

   breadth _____

   key _____

   sudden _____

   goose _____

2. Phonetically transcribe each of the words in number 1, above, using diacritics to illustrate the appropriate allophonic pattern.

   breadth _____

   key _____

   sudden _____

   goose _____

There are four manner-related allophonic patterns that affect stop articulation. The first is called nasal release. This pattern takes effect in similar contexts as the unreleased and glottal replacement patterns: when a stop precedes a syllabic-n. The nasal release allophone results when the stop articulators form the closure, but instead of the plosion releasing through the mouth, it is released through the nose instead. We use the nasal plosion diacritic, the superscript "n," [ⁿ], to transcribe these allophones. For example, productions of *mitten* and *hidden* produced with a nasal release would be transcribed as ['mɪtⁿ.n̩] and ['hɪdⁿ.n̩]. Pay close attention to the direction of the burst as you slowly say each word. Nasal plosion occurs most commonly when the conbsonants are homorganic, as in the two words above, but it also can occur in some other instanbces. Examples of other words that can be produced with a nasal release on the medial stop include *open* ['oʊpⁿ.n̩], *robin* ['ɹɑbⁿ.n̩], *bacon* ['beɪkⁿ.n̩], and *wagon* ['wægⁿ.n̩].

The bilateral release pattern describes alveolar and velar stops released over the sides of the tongue, so that air flows laterally instead of centrally in stop + l word-initial and -medial clusters. Velar stop + l clusters [kl] and [gl] occur in word-initial and -medial positions, as in *clock* and *sunglasses*, whereas alveolar stop + l clusters [tl] and [dl] occur only in word-medial position, as in *antler* and *oddly*. In these contexts, the anticipatory coarticulation of [l] affects the release of the preceding stop. If you say these words slowly enough, you should be able to feel air moving over the sides of your tongue as you release the stop and begin to produce the lateral [l] sound. The tongue feels somewhat flat in the mouth during the release of the stop, permitting air to flow laterally. The diacritic for a bilateral release is a superscript l symbol, as in the narrow transcriptions of *clock* [kˡlɑk] and *antler* ['æntˡ.lɚ].

The affricated pattern describes the articulatory phenomenon of alveolar stops in [tɹ] and [dɹ] clusters sounding like affricates. Say the words *tree* and *drew*. Can you hear the affrication of [t] and [d]? If you do not hear affrication, practice saying the words deliberately with affrication, as in the narrow transcriptions [t͡ʃɹi] and [d͡ʒɹu]. Your typical production will have some degree of affrication. Some people produce stronger affrication, others less. If you begin to carefully listen to your own productions and to those of others, you soon will notice these varying degrees of affrication on tr- and dr-clusters. Figure 7–13 shows two spectrograms of the word *drew*, one produced deliberately without affrication and the other produced naturally with affrication.

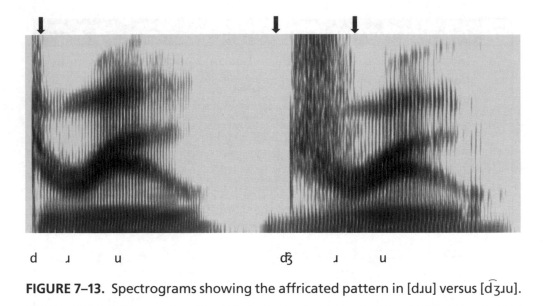

d   ɹ   u   d͡ʒ   ɹ   u

FIGURE 7–13. Spectrograms showing the affricated pattern in [dɹu] versus [d͡ʒɹu].

To capture the affrication in [tɹ] and [dɹ] clusters, we can narrowly transcribe the affricated productions using the [t͡ʃ] and [d͡ʒ] affricate symbols, as in [t͡ʃɹ] and [d͡ʒɹ].

The final pattern affecting the manner of stop articulation that we will discuss is one that you will use frequently, tap replacement, so you want to spend time learning how and when this pattern applies. Tap replacement is when the tap [ɾ] is used as an allophone for [t] or [d]. The contexts in which this allophone occurs is when an alveolar stop is between two vowels, the second of which is unstressed. A consonant occurring between two vowels is said to be the **intervocalic** position. Therefore, we say that for this pattern to apply, [t] or [d] needs to occur intervocalically and before an unstressed vowel.

We can diagram one context in which this pattern applies as 'V.tV (additional consonants and syllables are optional). Let's consider two words: *hotel* and *hated*. Do either of these words fit the context for this pattern to apply? Diagramming *hotel*, we get CV.'tVC, indicating that [t] precedes a stressed vowel, which does not fit the pattern. Therefore, most speakers would not substitute [ɾ] for [t] in the word *hotel*. Diagramming *hated*, we get 'CV.tVC, indicating that [t] is intervocalic and precedes an unstressed vowel, which does fit the pattern. Therefore, when we say the word *hated*, we typically substitute the tap phone for the alveolar stop, as

in ['heɪ.ɾəd]. If you pay close attention, you will be able to tell that even though the word *hated* is spelled with a medial "t," the articulation of that word-medial alveolar consonant is not stop-like, but is more fluid, more dynamic. The latter articulatory characteristic is what indicates tapping. When you're first learning to apply the tap replacement pattern to your transcriptions, practice by saying the word both ways, first with a stop and then with a tap, and that will help you discern which words contain a tap and which words contain a stop. For example, saying the word *hated* as ['heɪ.tʰəd] and ['heɪ.ɾəd] aloud should help you hear that the second production is the most typical one. By examining the spectrograms displayed in Figure 7–14, you will be able to see the differences in [t], [d], and [ɾ] articulation in *writing* ['ɹaɪ.tʰɪŋ], *riding* ['ɹaɪ.dɪŋ], and *writing* ['ɹaɪ.ɾɪŋ]. It is important to realize that the tap consonant in American English is an allophone of /t/ and /d/; however, in some other languages it is a phoneme, which we will discuss in Chapter 9.

There are many words to which the tap replacement pattern applies. If we make a list of words that contain a vowel + "t" + unstressed vowel sequence, we come up with words such as *beauty*, *city*, *biting*, and *visitor*. The tap replacement pattern applies to all of these words, as in ['bju.ɾi], ['sɪ.ɾi], ['baɪ.ɾɪŋ], and ['vɪ.zɪ.ɾɚ], respectively. Words that contain a vowel + "d" + unstressed vowel sequence include *shadow*, *ready*, *lady*, and *medicine*. The tap pattern

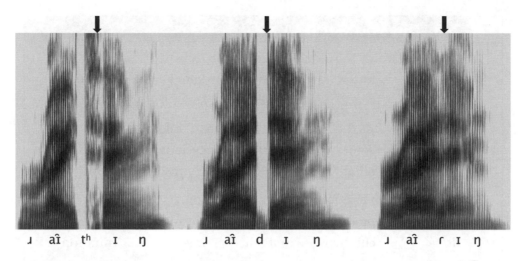

ɹ aɪ̯ tʰ ɪ ŋ   ɹ aɪ̯ d ɪ ŋ   ɹ aɪ̯ ɾ ɪ ŋ

FIGURE 7–14. Spectrograms showing the tap replacement pattern in [ˈɹaɪ̯.tʰɪŋ] versus [ˈɹaɪ̯.dɪŋ] versus [ˈɹaɪ̯.ɾɪŋ].

also applies to all of these words, as in [ˈʃæ.ɹoʊ̯], [ˈɪɛ.ɹi], [ˈleɪ̯.ɹi], and [ˈmɛ.ɹɪ.sɪn], respectively. Alternatively, because of primary stress on the second vowel, the tap replacement pattern does not apply to the words *motel* and *eighteen*. If you produced *motel* with a medial stop instead of a tap, the word would sound more like *modal* than *motel*, and the word *eighteen* would sound more like the name *Adene*. And we would simply ruin the 1968 Beatles song *Obladi-Oblada*, [oʊ̯.bla.ˈdi] [oʊ̯.bla.ˈda], if we replaced the [d] phones with taps!

The tap replacement pattern also applies to some words spelled with double "tt" and "dd," when we produce both sounds. In other words, if both stop phones are articulated, then the tap will not replace either stop. Examples of words that contain the tap allophone for "tt" include *butter*, *lettuce*, and *cottage*. Examples of word that contain the tap allophone for "dd" include *madder*, *muddy*, and *middle*. What about the word *addendum*, which is spelled with three "d" letters—are any of those "d" letters produced as a tap? First, let's divide the word into syllables: V.ˈdVC.dVC. We see that the first [d] sound occurs between two vowels, so it satisfies at least one condition of the pattern. We first see that while there are three "d" letters in the spelling, we produce only two "d" sounds when we say the word. Does it also satisfy the second condition: precedes an unstressed vowel? No, the first [d] precedes a stressed vowel. Therefore, the first [d] does not satisfy both patterns,

so it will be produced as a stop phone. Looking at the second [d], we see that it is preceded by a consonant and not a vowel, so it does not fit the context of the tap pattern either. Therefore, we know that the second [d] also will be produced as a stop and not a tap. The transcription of *addendum* is [ə.ˈdɛn.dəm].

We will finish discussing this pattern by asking you to quiz yourselves on three words: *auditory*, *potato*, and *tomato*. In the first word, *auditory*, we see two potential opportunities for a tap replacement: one [d] and one [t]. Are either of the stops replaced by a tap in pronunciation? Both the [d] and [t] are intervocalic: ˈV.dV.ˌtV.V. Furthermore, the first stop also precedes an unstressed syllable, so the first stop would likely be produced as a tap. The second stop, however, is trickier because while it does not precede the primary stressed syllable, it does precede a syllable that carries secondary stress in this four-syllable word. Therefore, the second stop, [t], is not replaced by a tap. We pronounce *auditory* as [ˈa.ɹɪ.ˌtɔ˞.i]. Let's try another word that has two stops in intervocalic position: *potato*. Does a tap replace either intervocalic [t] in *potato*? Yes, because the second [t] precedes an unstressed vowel, we produce *potato* as [poʊ̯.ˈteɪ̯.ɹoʊ̯]. The third word in our final quiz is *tomato*. We see that *tomato* has one intervocalic stop, the second [t]. Take a moment to narrowly transcribe *tomato*. If you transcribed it as [tʰə.ˈmeɪ̯.ɹoʊ̯], then congratulations, you are on your way to understanding when we typically use this pattern.

? 7–8. Did You Get It?

1. Circle the words that can contain a nasal release.

button	fatten	bottle	kitten	letting
leaden	coddle	madder	sodden	gladden

2. Circle the words that can contain a bilateral release.

class	cows	bicycle	cyclops	clue
angle	gloat	burglar	confusingly	glove

3. Circle the words that can contain affrication.

control	pretty	attract	shrink	country
drive	children	umbrella	freeze	raindrop

4. Circle the words that can contain a medial tap.

bottom	fighter	guitar	gritty	futon
pudding	cadet	cheddar	cedar	teddy

The next pattern, shortened, describes a duration change that affects voiced and voiceless stop consonants that are doubled in a word or abutting words, as in the word *midday* and the phrase *big guest*. In some instances of doubled consonants as orthographically written in English, we produce both; in other instances, we produce only one. We find this pattern to be particularly fun to think about. To begin, say the word *midday* a few times. Did you articulate one [d], or two? Are you certain? To check, say the word two different ways. First, say *midday* with one [d], as in [mɪ.ˈdeɪ]. Next, say *midday* with two [d] phones, as in [mɪd.ˈdeɪ]. You hopefully can hear that the second version is correct, although it should also be clear to you that the first [d] is unreleased—without any plosion—and narrowly transcribed using the unreleased diacritic, as in [mɪd̚.ˈdeɪ]. This narrow transcription is similar to a different stop pattern that we described previously: the unreleased pattern. The unreleased pattern is when the first stop in a sequence of two voiceless stops in the same syllable is not aspirated. While we narrowly transcribe both the unreleased and shortening patterns using the unreleased [̚] diacritic, the two patterns are not identical. Significant differences between the two patterns are that shortening can occur on voiced consecutive stops, as well as across syllables.

Perhaps you are not convinced that there are two stop consonant productions, albeit only one released, in *midday*? We will practice another example. Say the phrase *big guest*. Did you articulate one [g] or two? Again, to help you discern how many [g] phones you produced, practice saying the phrase first with one [g] and then again with two. A single [g] sound would result in a production of [ˈbɪ.gɛst], which is the word *biggest*! Say the word *biggest*, followed by the phrase *big guest*. Can you hear the difference in your stop articulation when you contrast your production of *biggest* with *big guest*? Hopefully you can hear that you produce two stops in the phrase *big guest*, which differentiates it from the word *biggest*. We narrowly transcribe the phrase *big guest* as [bɪg̚.gɛst] (the stress can be on either the first or the second word, depending on which word you emphasize). The difference in the duration of stop articulation in *biggest* versus *big guest* is shown in the spectrograms displayed in Figure 7–15.

We will practice identifying stop lengthening in three final examples before we move to the final pattern affecting stop articulation. For the first example, say the word *happy*. Did you articulate one or two [p] phones? In the word *happy*, we articulate only one [p], [ˈhæ.pi]. Now say the word *lamppost*. Did you articulate this word with one or two [p] phones? In *lamppost*, you articulated the gesture

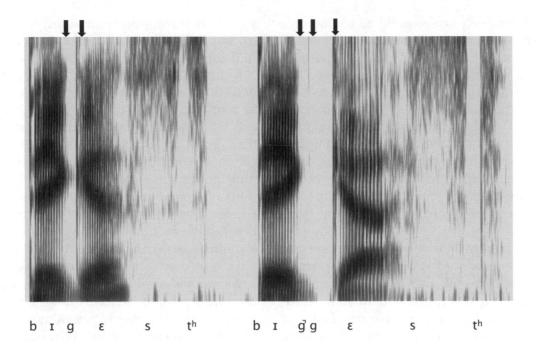

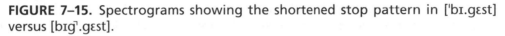

b ɪ g   ɛ   s   tʰ   b   ɪ g̚g   ɛ   s   tʰ

FIGURE 7–15. Spectrograms showing the shortened stop pattern in [ˈbɪ.gɛst] versus [bɪg̚.gɛst].

for both [p] phones; however, you did not release the first [p], as in *lamp + post*, [lamp̚.poʊst]. If you had not articulated the first [p] gesture, your production would have sounded more like *lamb + post*. Last, say the phrase *stop Pete*. How many [p] phones did you articulate? In this phrase, you also produced an unreleased [p] phone, as in [stap̚.pit]; otherwise, the phrase would have resembled the consonants in the phrase *stop it*, which contains only a single [p] phone. Contrast those two phrases, *stop Pete* and *stop it*, to help you hear the difference in the medial stop articulations. If you could figure out the examples above, then you are on your way to understanding this pattern. If you continue to have difficulty hearing repeated consonant articulations, it will become easier with practice, so do not give up.

There are two contexts in which stop production can affect syllable structure. The first is when an additional stop is added to a syllable, and the second is when a stop is deleted from a syllable. The glottal stop insertion pattern applies when one word ends in a vowel and the next word begins with a vowel and a glottal stop is inserted in-between the two vowels. For example, practice saying aloud the phrase *he eats*. Do you insert a glottal stop? Many speakers insert a glottal stop in-between the two vowels, producing [hi ʔits]. If producing a glottal stop in-between the two vowels is not in your dialect, practice saying the utterance until you can produce the glottal stop insertion. If you do not insert a glottal stop, you likely insert a glide in-between the two vowels, as in [hi jits]. If we did not insert a glottal

---

? 7–9. Did You Get It?

1. Circle the phrases that contain an unreleased articulation of the first stop in doubled stop consonants.

lob balls	climbed down	lamb bleats	white teeth
ask kindly	sing good	cheap pen	big goose

stop (or a glide), the phrase would be produced as [hits], as in the word *heats*. Alternate between saying *heats* and *he eats* until you can produce and hear a glottal stop insertion in the phrase. Figure 7–16 displays spectrograms of *heats* and *he eats* to help you visualize the glottal stop that is inserted in the spoken phrase. You also can alternate saying the phrases *say yay* and *say ABC* to produce and hear a glottal stop inserted in the second phrase. Last, alternate saying the phrases *say yahoo* and *say achoo*. In which phrase did you insert a glottal stop? The phrase *say achoo* would contain a glottal stop, transcribed as [seɪ.ʔa.t͡ʃu].

The second pattern that affects syllable structure is when a stop consonant is omitted from a word. This pattern is dialectal, and it may or may not apply to your own speech. [t] is omitted in word-medial nt-clusters when the syllable containing [t] is unstressed, as in the word *enter*. The citation form of *enter* is [ˈɛn.tɚ], with a *strong*-weak stress pattern. However, in casual connected speech some people pronounce *enter* as [ˈɛ.nɚ]. Compare the spectrograms of [ˈɛn.tɚ] and [ˈɛ.nɚ] in Figure 7–17. Before

you say that you never pronounce *enter* without the [t], use a casual speech style to say a few phrases that contain *enter*. For example, say the utterance, "I'll enter using the back door," being certain to pronounce *enter* as [ˈɛ.nɚ]. Does it feel at all natural to your own casual style of speaking? Most people exhibit this casual production at least some of the time, but it predominates in some dialects. It is so commonly used by some individuals that these pronunciations have creeped into spelling. Can you think of a popular song by 1980s pop singer Cyndi Lauper that is the result of this pattern? Yes, it is *Girls Just Wanna Have Fun*. The phrase *want to*, which contains both an nt-cluster and a double consonant, often is reduced to *wanna* in casual speech.

A few other words in which the [t] in an nt-cluster is omitted include *incentive* [ɪn.ˈsɛ.nɪv] and *intersection* [ˈɪ.nɚ.sɛk.ʃən]. Words that do not fit the pattern include *interrogate* and *intern*. Why does [t] need to be produced in the latter two words? Because [t] precedes the stressed vowel in *interrogate* and *internment*; it is the onset in the primary stressed syllable. We transcribe these words as [ɪn.ˈtɛɚ.ə.geɪt] and [ɪn.ˈtɚn.mənt].

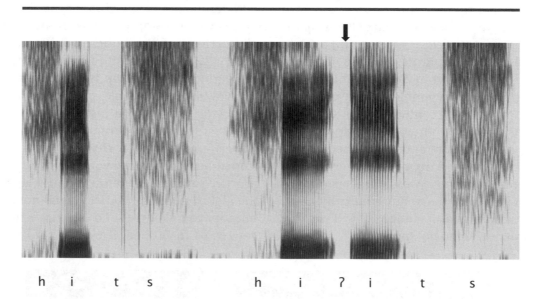

FIGURE 7–16. Spectrograms showing the glottal stop inserted pattern in [hits] versus [hi.ʔits].

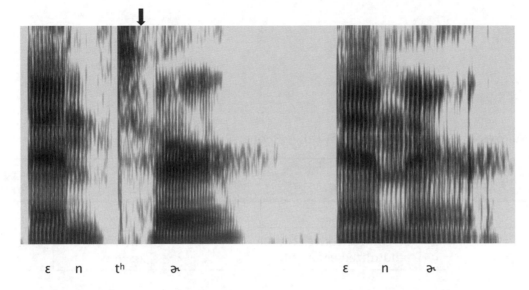

ɛ   n   tʰ   ɚ   ɛ   n   ɚ

FIGURE 7–17. Spectrograms showing the [t] omission pattern in [ˈɛn.tɚ] versus [ˈɛ.nɚ].

? 7–10. Did You Get It?

1. Circle the phrases that can contain a glottal stop insertion.

   she exited   flee early   I ached   we left   they admitted

2. Circle the words in which [t] can be omitted.

   banter   pontificate   scented   contact   winter

Fricatives

We will discuss six allophonic patterns that apply to fricative consonants. The patterns involve changes in articulatory place, voicing, duration, and syllable structure. A summary of the six patterns can be found in Table 7–3.

The first phonetic context in which a fricative can be modified that we will discuss involves a change in articulatory place. This pattern is called palatalized [s] and [z], and it occurs secondary to anticipatory coarticulation. When [s] or [z] precedes [j], the artic-

ulatory place of the alveolar fricatives moves closer to the place of articulation for [j], which is palatal. If we palatalize the alveolar fricatives, which pair of fricatives (produced further back in the mouth) would those productions sound like? Yes, [s] would be produced as [ʃ], and [z] would be produced as [ʒ]. Let's practice saying some examples so you can hear the palatalization. In the phrases *bless you* and *miss you*, we see that [s] precedes [j]; therefore, this pattern could apply. If this allophonic pattern describes your own speech, then your production of /blɛs.ju/ would be articulated as [blɛ.ʃu], and /mɪs.ju/ would

TABLE 7–3. Allophonic Patterns Affecting Fricative Phones

Pattern	Phone Affected	Description	Allophone	Example	Narrow Transcription
Place					
Palatalized	s z	alveolar fricatives can be palatalized before [j]	ʃ, ʒ	bless you, as you	ˈblɛ.ʃu, ˈæ.ʒu
Voicing					
Voiceless	v	voiced labiodental fricative can be voiceless when followed by a voiceless consonant	v̥	have to vs. have	ˈhæv̥.tu – hæv
Voiced	θ	voiceless interdental fricative can be voiced when followed by a voiced consonant	θ̬	with many vs. with	wɪθ̬.ˈmɛ.ni – wɪθ
Voiced	s	s as a morphosyntactic morpheme is voiced when following a voiced consonant	z	heeds vs. heats	hidz – hits
Duration					
Lengthened	f v θ ð s z ʃ	a fricative is lengthened when it is doubled	xː	miss, sing! vs. missing	mɪsː.ɪŋ – ˈmɪs.ɪŋ
Syllable Structure					
Omitted *h*	h	[h] can be omitted in unstressed environments		give him a book vs. give HIM a book	gɪv.ɪm.ə.bʊk – gɪv.ˈhɪm.ə.bʊk

be articulated as [mɪ.ʃu]. In the phrases *as you like it* and *he's young*, your careful production of [æz.ju.laɪk.ɪt] would be articulated casually as [æ.ʒu.laɪk.ɪt], and [hiz.jʌŋ] would be articulated as [hi.ʒʌŋ]. Not everyone palatalizes [s] and [z] in this context, but many people do. Spectrograms of the casually produced articulations of *azure* and *as you're* are displayed in Figure 7–18. Analyze the spectrograms to see the differences in the fricatives articulated in these two productions.

Three of the patterns describe changes to voicing of fricatives. The first pattern is devoicing of [v] when it occurs in word-final position and is followed by a word that begins with a voiceless consonant. One frequently occurring example of this pattern is the phrase *have to*, as in *I have to go*. As you can see, the word *have* ends in [v] and the word *to* begins with [t]; this is the context in which [v] could be devoiced. If [v] were devoiced, what would it sound like? It would sound like [f]. Try saying the phrase *have to* by substituting [f] for [v], as in [hæf.tu]. Does the phrase sound natural to you? For most people, it is a natural production. In fact, the phrase *have to* is so commonly produced with devoicing of [v] that in slang it is spelled as *hafta*. In a narrow transcription, we would use the devoicing diacritic to denote this articulatory modification, as in [hæv̥.tu]. Another example is the phrase *have some*, as in, *I'd like to have some, too*. In this phrase [v] also could be devoiced, resulting in [hæv̥.sʌm]. Figure 7–19 shows spectrograms of *have* and *have to*. Compare the spectrograms for the voicing of [v] in *have* and the devoicing of [v] in *have to*. Remember to look at the vowel durations as indicators of voicing.

The second pattern is voicing of [θ] when it occurs in word-final position and is followed by a word that begins with a voiced consonant or vowel. This pattern largely is restricted to certain words and phrases. One word in which voicing of [θ] occurs frequently in these contexts is *with*, as in the phrases *with many* and *with a*. . . . Coarticulation of the sounds in these phrases often results in [θ] becoming voiced because of the voiced phone that follows it. We would use the voiced diacritic to narrowly transcribe the productions as [wɪθ̬.ˈmɛ.ni] and [wɪ.θ̬ə]. A word in which voicing of [θ] frequently occurs is *without*, spoken as [wɪ.ˈθ̬aʊt]. Can you hear the voicing component? If not, then try exaggerating a production as [wɪ.ˈðaʊt]. Be certain not to apply the voiced [θ] pattern when [θ] precedes a voiceless consonant, because you could say, for example, the word [ˈwɪ.ðɚ] (*wither*) when you mean the phrase [wɪθ.hɚ] (*with her*). One other context in which voicing of [θ] is common is when the -ing verb marker is added to nouns ending in "th." Examples of these words include *teething*, *clothing*, *breathing*, and *mouthing*. All these words

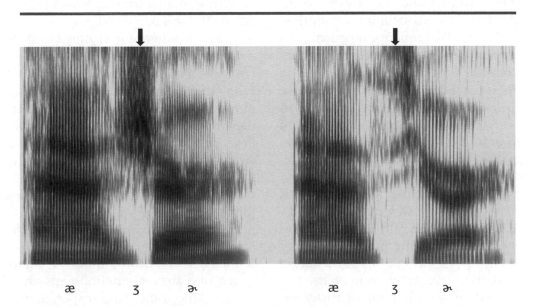

æ   ʒ   ɚ   æ   ʒ   ɚ

FIGURE 7–18. Spectrograms showing the palatalized [s,z] pattern in *azure* [ˈæ.ʒɚ] and *as you're* [ˈæ.ʒɚ].

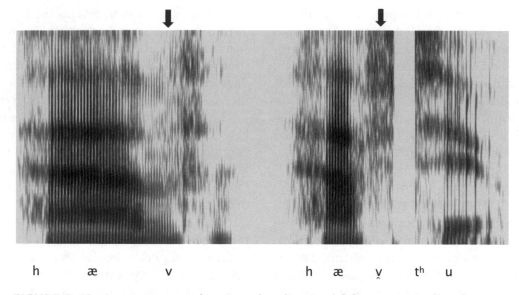

| h | æ | v | | h | æ | v̥ | tʰ | u |

FIGURE 7–19. Spectrograms showing the devoiced [v] pattern in [hæv] versus [hæv̥.tu].

typically are articulated with the voiced variant [θ̬] instead of the voiceless phone [θ]. In broad phonetic transcription, you would transcribe the voiced [θ] as [ð].

Another pattern that affects voicing is when "s" is used as a morphosyntactic marker. When preceding a voiced consonant, [z] is produced as an allophone. We first discussed this phenomenon in Chapter 4 when we provided transcription advice for words that end in the letter "s" as a linguistic marker. When "s" is used to mark a language function, such as plurality, possessiveness, or verb tense, it is only produced as voiceless [s] if the sound before it also is voiceless. When the sound before "s" is voiced, we continue voicing and produce [z]. For example, in the word *heats*, "s" is used to mark verb tense, and the sound before "s" is [t], which is voiceless. Therefore, we pronounce the ts-cluster as [ts]. However, in the word *heeds*, another word in which "s" is used to mark verb tense, the sound before "s" is [d], which is voiced. Therefore, in this case we pronounce the ds-cluster as [dz]. Remember, this pattern only applies when "s" serves as a linguistic marker. In other words that end in "s" (or "se" or "ce"), the target sound may be [s], as in *face*, or [z], as in *phase*.

The next pattern is lengthening of fricatives. Lengthening in fricatives occurs when fricatives are doubled, as in the word *misspell* and the phrase *this seat*. In both the word and phrase, the [s] sounds are doubled and both are articulated by the lengthening of one of them. We can transcribe them using the lengthened diacritic. This phenomenon is similar to the one affecting stop consonants; however, fricatives are continuant sounds, so we can describe the doubling of fricatives as lengthening. The word *misspell* would be transcribed as [mɪsː.ˈpɛl] and the phrase *this seat* as [ðɪsː.it].

The final pattern for fricatives that we will discuss involves a change in syllable structure. This pattern is omission of [h] when [h] is in an unstressed environment. For example, when we casually say the phrase *give him a book*, if the word *him* is not stressed, then we are likely to omit the word-initial [h] in *him*, producing [gɪv.ɪm.ə.bʊk]. However, if the target was *give HIM a book*, then we are less likely to omit the [h] in *him*. We also may omit more than one word-initial [h] sound if none of the words beginning with [h] are stressed in an utterance. For example, we may casually produce the phrase *if he could have his way* as [ɪf.i.kʊ.dæ.vɪz.weɪ], with overlapping of sounds across word boundaries. Again, when [h] occurs in a stressed environment and/or when we are speaking using careful speech, we typically do not omit target [h] sounds.

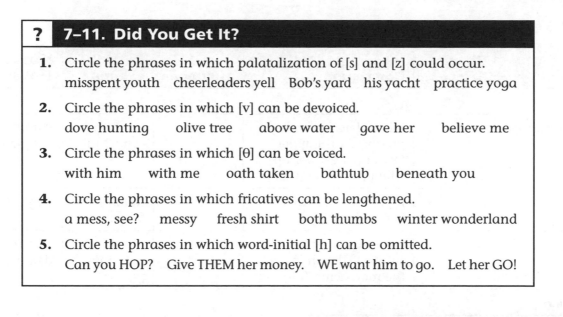

? 7–11. Did You Get It?

1. Circle the phrases in which palatalization of [s] and [z] could occur.
   misspent youth   cheerleaders yell   Bob's yard   his yacht   practice yoga

2. Circle the phrases in which [v] can be devoiced.
   dove hunting   olive tree   above water   gave her   believe me

3. Circle the phrases in which [θ] can be voiced.
   with him   with me   oath taken   bathtub   beneath you

4. Circle the phrases in which fricatives can be lengthened.
   a mess, see?   messy   fresh shirt   both thumbs   winter wonderland

5. Circle the phrases in which word-initial [h] can be omitted.
   Can you HOP?   Give THEM her money.   WE want him to go.   Let her GO!

Affricates

We will discuss only one allophonic pattern that impacts affricates: labialization. See Table 7–4 for a summary of this pattern. This pattern describes a change in secondary place of articulation in [t͡ʃ] and [d͡ʒ]. When an affricate precedes a rounded back vowel, the affricate is produced with additional lip rounding. To help you understand this pattern, say the minimal word pair *cheese-choose*. Because the word *choose* has a rounded vowel, you should be able to feel and see more lip rounding on the [t͡ʃ] that precedes the [u]. Another word pair that can help you understand this pattern is *jack* and *joke*. You should be able to feel and see more lip rounding on [d͡ʒ] in *joke* because it also contains a rounded vowel. We narrowly transcribe the rounded allophones of [t͡ʃ] and [d͡ʒ] using a superscript [ʷ], as in [t͡ʃʷuz] for *choose* and [d͡ʒʷoʊk] for *joke*.

? 7–12. Did You Get It?

1. Circle the words in which [t͡ʃ] can become [t͡ʃʷ].
   cheek   chill   choke   chew   chunk

2. Circle the words in which [d͡ʒ] can become [d͡ʒʷ].
   jukebox   jump   juicy   jubilant   justice

Nasals

We will discuss six allophonic patterns that describe nasal consonants. Three of the patterns involve articulatory place, one involves duration, and two involve syllable structure. A summary of the phonological patterns for nasals can be found in Table 7–5.

TABLE 7–4. Allophonic Pattern Affecting Affricate Phones

Pattern	Phone Affected	Description	Allophone	Example	Narrow Transcription
Place					
Labialized	t͡ʃ d͡ʒ	affricates are typically produced with additional lip rounding when preceding a rounded back vowel	xʷ	choose, joke	t͡ʃʷuz, d͡ʒʷoʊk

TABLE 7–5. Allophonic Patterns Affecting Nasal Phones

Pattern	Phone Affected	Description	Allophone	Example	Narrow Transcription
Place					
Labiodentalized	m	bilabial nasal can be produced with upper teeth on the lower lip when preceding [f] or [v]	m̪	comfort, come forth	ˈkʌm̪.fɚt, ˈkʌm̪.fɔ͡ɚθ
Velarized	n	[n] is velarized when before [k] or [g]	ŋ	thank, finger	θæŋk, ˈfɪŋ.gɚ
N-replacement	ŋ	velar nasal can be substituted with [n] in the morpheme "ing"	n	runnin', jumpin'	ˈɹʌ.nɪn, ˈd͡ʒʌm.pɪn
Duration					
Lengthened	m n	a nasal is lengthened when it is doubled	x:	mean Ness, meanness	minː.ɛs, ˈminː.ɛs
Syllable Structure					
Syllabic nasal	m n	[m] or [n] in word-final position in an unstressed syllable takes on the weight of the syllable	x̩	chasm, mitten	ˈkæ.zm̩, ˈmɪtˈ.n̩
Stop inserted	(null)	a voiceless homorganic stop can be inserted in nasal + voiceless fricative clusters preceding an unstressed vowel	p t	something, fence	ˈsʌmp.θɪŋ, fɛnts

The first three patterns that we will discuss involve a change in the articulatory place for nasal consonants. As you already know, English has one bilabial nasal, one alveolar nasal, and one velar nasal. Could you imagine having a labiodental nasal, too? We do have a pair of labiodental fricatives, [f] and [v], but is it even possible to produce a labiodental nasal? Try it by placing your upper teeth on your lower lip, lowering your velum, and vibrating your vocal folds to create sound that will flow through your nose. Hopefully you discovered that it is possible to produce a labiodental nasal. In fact, the labiodental nasal is a phoneme in some languages. In English it is not a phoneme, but are there any phonetic contexts in which speakers produce a labiodental nasal allophone of [m]? As it turns out, yes, there is one specific context in which this allophone occurs because of anticipatory coarticulation. We produce the labiodental allophone of [m] in word-medial and -final mf-clusters. When you say the words *pamphlet* and *triumph*, freeze your movements during articulation of [m]. You should feel your upper teeth on your lower lip when articulating [m], in preparation of the very next sound, [f]. This pattern also applies across word boundaries. Alternate between saying *comfort* and *come forth*; you should be able to feel the labiodental allophone produced in the word and in the phrase. The diacritic we use to denote the labiodentalized pattern is the tooth, [̪]. A narrow transcription of the word *pamphlet* is [ˈpæm̪.flɛt] and *triumph* is [ˈtɹɑɪ.əm̪f].

The second pattern is velarized [n]. Velarization of [n] occurs in the contexts of "nk" and "ng" clusters in word-medial and -final positions. Examples of words include *thank* and *finger*. In each of these words, the velar nasal [ŋ] is substituted for [n], as in [θæŋk] and [ˈfɪŋ.gɚ]. As illustrated by these examples, nk-clusters become [ŋk]-clusters and ng-clusters become the cluster [ŋg].

The third pattern that affects nasal place of articulation is [n] as a substitute for [ŋ] in the -ing morphosyntactic context. When -ing is used to denote an inflected form of a verb, as in *shaking* ("shake" +" ing") and *trying* ("try"+"ing"), the -ing verb ending is produced in citation-form speech as [ɪŋ]. In casual speech, however, this verb ending often is produced as [n], as in *shakin'*, [ˈʃeɪ.kɪn] and *tryin'*, [ˈtɹaɪ.ɪn]. Surely, you have used this [n] for [ŋ] substitution in your own speech many times and have heard many other people use it, too.

The next pattern we will discuss is the lengthened pattern, which affects duration. The lengthened pattern that affects nasals is identical to the lengthening pattern that affects fricatives. This pattern is the lengthening of a nasal that is doubled in a word or phrase. Examples of this pattern affecting nasals include the word *meanness* and the phrase *mean Ness*. Articulation of *meanness* and *mean Ness* each include a lengthened medial [n], which would be narrowly transcribed as [ˈminː.ɛs]. If these productions contained only a single [n], then they would sound like [ˈmi.nɛs], a production that would sound

similar to *Venus* ([ˈvi.nəs]). Practice alternating saying *meanness* and *Venus*, and *mean Ness* and *Venus* to hear the lengthened [n] in the first word/phrase of each pair. Compare the spectrograms of productions of *Venus* and *mean Ness* in Figure 7–20, paying attention to the duration of the medial consonants in both utterances.

The last two patterns involving nasals affect syllable structure. The first is when [m], as in *chasm*, and [n], as in *hidden*, become syllabic. Previously we talked about words containing syllabic nasals, but this is the first time we are discussing the contexts in which syllabic nasals can be created. When [m] or [n] is in an unstressed syllable in word-final position, the unstressed vowel can be omitted, making the nasal sound syllable-like. In these cases, we call the nasals syllabic and transcribe them using the syllabic diacritic [ˌ]. For example, *chasm* would be narrowly transcribed as [ˈkæ.zm̩] and *open* as [ˈoʊ.pn̩].

One mistake that beginning transcribers often make is to overapply the syllabic pattern. Remember that for this pattern to be able to apply, the nasal consonant must be at the end of the word and it must occur in an unstressed syllable; therefore, a word that is a potential context must be multisyllabic. Words such as *pen*, *tan*, and *sun* are not contexts for applying the syllabic nasal pattern. In addition, if the syllable containing the nasal consonant

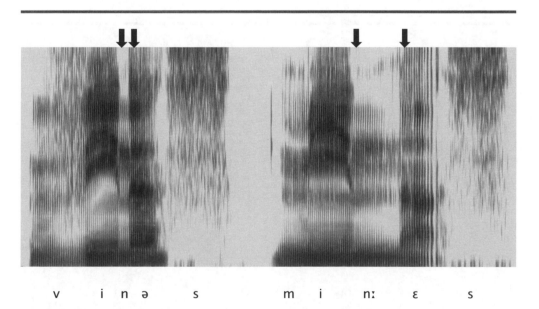

v   i   n   ə   s   m   i   nː   ɛ   s

FIGURE 7–20. Spectrograms showing the nasal lengthening pattern in [ˈvi.nəs] and [ˈminː.ɛs].

is fully articulated, it will be transcribed with the unstressed vowel and without the syllabic consonant. For example, the word *chasm* articulated with two vowels would be transcribed as ['kæ.zəm], while a more casual articulation without the unstressed vowel and with a syllabic nasal would be transcribed as ['kæ.zm̩]. Refer to the spectrograms of both forms of the word *chasm* as shown in Figure 7–21.

The second syllable structure pattern describes adding a sound when none is shown in the spelling of a word, which is called **epenthesis**. In nasal + fricative clusters that precede an unstressed vowel, we typically insert a homorganic (same place of articulation) stop, because of overlapping speech gestures. When the fricative in the cluster is voiceless, we insert a voiceless homorganic stop. For example, casually speak the words *something* and *fence*. The fricatives in both clusters, [θ] and [s], are voiceless. Can you hear a voiceless stop phone articulated before each fricative, even though no stops are in either spelling? In the first word, *something*, we sometimes insert [p] in-between the [mθ]-cluster, as in ['sʌmp.θɪŋ]. Which voiceless stop consonant do you hear in the ns-cluster when you say *fence*? Yes, the stop that is inserted is the alveolar [t], as in [fɛnts]. Hopefully you also noticed that the stops inserted in both words were homorganic to the clusters. In English, the second pattern that involves alveolar consonants, as in *fence*, is stronger than the one involving labials. To help you to discern the insertion of [t], practice saying the word pairs *prince–prints*, *mince–mints*, and *hence–hints*. The cluster in each pair of words is pronounced the same, even though the words are spelled differently. Respectively, the consonants in each pair of words would be transcribed the same way, as [pɹɪnts]–[pɹɪnts], [mɪnts]–[mɪnts], and [hɛnts]–[hɪnts].

Similarly, in alveolar nasal + voiced fricative clusters that precede an unstressed vowel, we typically insert a voiced homorganic (alveolar) stop. For example, casually speak the word *buns*. The fricative is voiced [z], so its homorganic voiced stop is [d]. Can you hear [d] inserted in your production of *buns*, as [bʌndz]? If you're not convinced, alternate saying the words *mines* and *minds*. Hopefully you can hear that despite having different spellings, both words are produced the same way, as [maɪndz]. To contrast the voiceless and voiced stop insertions, practice saying the word pairs *bunts–buns*, *wince–winds*, and *once–ones*. Respectively, these words would be transcribed [bʌnts]–[bʌndz], [wɪnts]–[wɪndz], and [wʌnts]–[wʌndz].

To see spectrograms of the words *prince* and *mines*, see Figure 7–22. Both words were spoken naturally by a speaker who did not see the phonetic transcription of either word. Using your knowledge of acoustic analysis, examine the spectrograms for evidence of the stop insertions. Hint: look for the stop closures.

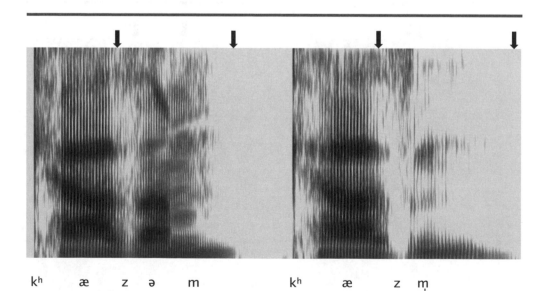

kʰ   æ   z   ə   m   kʰ   æ   z   m̩

FIGURE 7–21. Spectrograms showing the syllabic nasal pattern in ['kæ.zəm] versus ['kæ.zm̩].

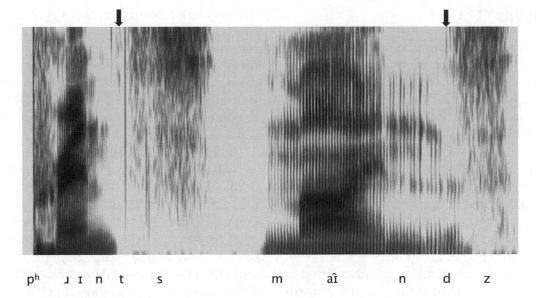

pʰ   ɹ   ɪ   n   t   s   m   aɪ̯   n   d   z

FIGURE 7–22. Spectrograms showing the stop insertion pattern in *prince* [pɹɪnts] and *mines* [maɪndz] spoken by a naïve speaker.

? | 7–13. Did You Get It?

1. Circle the words that can contain a labiodental nasal consonant.
   dolphin   symphony   amphetamine   uphill   lymph
   emphasis   harrumph   homophone   amphibian   hyphen

2. Circle the words in which [n] can be an allophone of [ŋ].
   ring   running   hurrying   thing   falling
   laughing   sing   writing   singing   sting

3. Circle the words in which [n] can be lengthened.
   brownnoser   unnerve   tenderness   planned   unnatural
   thinness   penny   suddenness   openness   annex

4. Circle the words in which [m] can become a syllabic consonant.
   blossom   rhythm   exam   requiem   calcium

5. Circle the words in which [n] can become a syllabic consonant.
   frighten   begun   sudden   again   hidden

6. Circle the words in which a voiceless homorganic stop can be inserted in nasal + voiceless fricative clusters that precede an unstressed vowel.
   pence   ounce   since   cons   hansom cab

7. Circle the words in which a voiced homorganic stop can be inserted in nasal + voiced fricative clusters that precede an unstressed vowel.
   pans   wonder   fins   whines   hams

Approximants

The same allophonic patterns that apply to glides also apply to liquids, because the sounds in these two manner classes share articulatory features, as well as phonological functions. Because of these similarities in articulation and function, as we discussed in Chapter 4, glides and liquids can be grouped into a larger category called approximants. In American English, the approximants include [w, j, l, ɹ]. We will discuss five phonological patterns that describe modifications of approximant consonants. The patterns involve articulatory place, voicing, duration, and syllable structure. A summary of the five patterns can be found in Table 7–6.

The first pattern affects place of articulation of [l]. In Chapter 2, you learned this allophone as the dark-l. Dark-l occurs in post-vocalic position, in words such as *yell* and *spill*, when the tongue body is farther back in the mouth than for articulation of the alveolar [l], with the tongue body raised toward the hard palate. The symbol for transcribing dark-l is the [l] phonetic symbol with a tilde [~] through the middle of it, as in [ɫ]. The narrow transcription of *yell* is [jɛɫ] and *spill* is [spɪɫ].

Devoicing of approximants is the next pattern we will discuss. All four of the approximants are devoiced when they follow a voiceless stop in syllable-initial clusters. Clusters that are permissible in English include /p/ + /j, l, ɹ/, as in *pew*, *place*, and *price*; /t/ + /w, ɹ/, as in *between* and *train*; and /k/ + /w, j, l, ɹ/, as in *quick*, *cute*, *clap*, and *cry*. Can you remember the voiceless diacritic from Chapter 4? It is the open "o" symbol placed below the phonetic

TABLE 7–6. Allophonic Patterns Affecting Approximant Phones

Pattern	Phone Affected	Description	Allophone	Example	Narrow Transcription
Place					
Dark-l	l	[l] is produced with tongue tip and body back and raised toward hard palate when post-vocalic	ɫ	yell vs. low	jɛɫ vs. loʊ
Voicing					
Devoiced	w j l ɹ	approximants are devoiced when in voiceless stop + approximant clusters	x̥	quick, cute, clap, cry	kw̥ɪk, kj̥ut, kl̥æp, kɹ̥aɪ
Duration					
Lengthened	l	[l] is lengthened when it is doubled	lː	smell Lee vs. smelly	smɛlː.i–ˈsmɛ.li
Syllable Structure					
hw-replacement	w	[w] produced as [hw] in words spelled with "wh"	hw	whether vs. weather	hwɛðɚ–wɛðɚ
Syllabic-l	l	[l] in word-final position in an unstressed syllable takes on the weight of the syllable	l̩	handle, bagel	ˈhæn.dl̩, ˈbeɪ.gl̩

consonant symbol. The words *quick, cute, clap*, and *cry* are narrowly transcribed as [kwɪk], [kjut], [kl̥æp], and [kɹ̥aɪ], respectively.

The next pattern we will discuss affects the duration (i.e., lengthening) of [l] in double consonant contexts. Like the lengthening patterns describing fricatives and nasals, double [l] in one word or across two words is lengthened. Examples of [l] lengthening can be found in the phrases *smell Lee* and *yell loudly*. These productions are narrowly transcribed as [smɛlː.i] and [jɛlː.aʊd.li]. Contrast productions of *smell Lee* with the word *smelly*, which has only a single [l] articulation. Then contrast productions of *yell loudly* with the word *yellow*, which also has only a single [l] articulation. The words *guileless* and *soulless* also would be produced with a lengthened [l], as in [ˈgaɪlː.ɛs] and [ˈsoʊlː.ɛs]. If *guileless* and *soulless* did not contain two [l] sounds, then *guileless* would sound more like the phrase *guy less* and *soulless* would sound a little like the word *solace*.

One pattern applies exclusively to the approximant [w] when it occurs at the beginning of a word that is spelled with "wh," as in the word *which*. This pattern of speech is dialectal and you may or may not use it in your own speech. Say the words *which* and *witch* aloud. Do you say both words the same way, as [wɪtʃ]? If so, then you likely do not employ the pattern. But if you pronounce *which* as [hwɪtʃ] and *witch* as [wɪtʃ], then this pattern, the hw-pattern, applies to your speech. It describes the production of words spelled with "wh" articulated with an h-like fricative before the [w]. Some other minimal word pairs that you can say aloud to help you discern if you follow this pattern or not include *whether* and *weather*, *whee* and *we*, and *what* and *watt*. If this pattern does describe your speech, then you will say the first word in each pair by articulating [hw] instead of [w] in word-initial position.

The last approximant allophonic pattern that we'll discuss applies to only one approximant, [l], and it is a pattern that we previously discussed as applying to stops and nasals. Like syllabic-m and -n, syllabic-l describes a change in syllable structure when [l] occurs in an unstressed syllable in word-final position and the preceding unstressed vowel is omitted, making the liquid syllable-like. For example, *hassle* would be narrowly transcribed as [ˈhæ.sl̩] and *axel* as [ˈæk.sl̩]. However, the words *excel, cartel*, and *personnel* would not contain a syllabic-l because each [l] is in a stressed syllable.

?   7–14. Did You Get It?

1. Circle the words in which [l] can become [ɫ].
   full   puddle   follow   peaceful   lengthen

2. Circle the words in which an approximant can become devoiced.
   tackle   clock   trick   please   police

3. Circle the phrases in which [l] can become lengthened.
   awful lamp   love life   idyll lion   final lap   small ladder

4. Circle the phrases in which [w] can become [hw].
   who   what   where   when   how

5. Circle the words in which [l] can become a syllable.
   aerial   vinyl   angel   sell   muscle

Phonological Patterns in Consonant Coarticulation in Disordered Speech

As we discussed above, allophonic patterns can be used to capture regularities in consonant variations produced by typical speakers of a language or dialect. Phonological patterns also are helpful to describe the speech of individuals with speech sound disorders, as well as the speech of individuals learning a second language. These patterns typically are systematically used by an individual, appearing to be rule governed. Identifying phonological patterns in atypical speech is in the domain of clinical phonetics, which we introduced to you in Chapter 1. Speech-language pathologists classify speech errors into four different types, easily remembered by the acronym SODA: substitutions (when one sound is replaced by another sound, for example, someone saying ['tʊ.ti] for ['kʊ.ki]); omissions (when a sound is not produced, for example, someone saying [tap] for [stap]); distortions (when a sound is imprecisely articulated, for example, someone producing a slurred [st], as in [st̪a˞] for [sta˞]); and additions (when a sound is added, for example, someone saying ['kʌ.tə] for [kʌt]). It is critical that speech-language pathologists know the phonetic, allophonic, and phonological patterns of the speaker's language and dialect, so that actual speech errors can be determined; otherwise, the speech-language pathologist may incorrectly label a pronunciation as incorrect, when in fact, it is an acceptable production in the individual's language or dialect. The presence of systematic types of errors—of incorrect phonological patterns—indicates that the individual has formed incorrect rules for sound production and usage. Speech-language pathologists use this information to help guide their clinical decision making in intervention, as they determine which errors to address, and in which order and how to address them.

? 7–15. Did You Get It?

1. Describe each misarticulation using the correct classification of substitution, omission, distortion, or addition.

   a. The type of error exhibited in the production of [haʊ̯ts] for [haʊ̯s] is a(n) _____.

   b. The type of error exhibited in the production of [bæt] for [bæθ] is a(n) _____.

   c. The type of error exhibited in the production of [θæk.ju] for [θæŋk.ju] is a(n) _____.

   d. The type of error exhibited in the production of a lateralized [s], as in [sˡʌn] for [sʌn], is a(n) _____.

Putting It All Together

We covered a variety of topics in this chapter that were related to the study of linguistic phonetics and phonology. We discussed the role of the phonologist in studying the sounds of a language to understand which of its sounds hold meaning and which are articulatory modifications that do not hold meaning. We also discussed how those sounds can be combined into words. We discussed the overlapping nature of speech production and the effects of anticipatory and carryover coarticulation as resulting in allophones. Minimal pairs were discussed as tools phonologists use to differentiate phones and allophones from phonemes. We also discussed syllables as being planned and programmed as units of speech that we string together to form utterances. Last, we described a wide variety of the phonetic and phonological contexts in which we modify consonant production to create allophonic variations. In clinical phonetics, we use our skill of being able to identify phonological patterns in typical speech to help us find patterns in an individual's misarticulations. So far, we have discussed patterns in consonants only. In the next chapter, we will explore the phonology of English vowels.

Applied Science: Revisited

Summary

A second-grade child, Luis, was referred to his school diagnostic team by his classroom teacher with concerns of a possible speech disorder. Luis is bilingual, speaking Puerto Rican Spanish at home and English at school. Luis's monolingual English-speaking speech-language pathologist noted that Luis inconsistently produced [s] in the middle of words. In some words, he correctly produced [s], but in other words he substituted [h] for [s]. The speech-language pathologist wondered whether a formal speech evaluation was warranted.

One Step at a Time

1. The speech-language pathologist noted that Luis substituted the aspirated [h] for [s] in four out of eight words containing a word-medial [s], as well as in the one word in which [s] was word-final.

2. Comparing the phonetic contexts of the correct and incorrect productions, the speech-language pathologist noticed a pattern: [s] was correctly articulated when it was syllable-initial, but [h] was substituted for [s] when [s] was syllable-final. For example, Luis correctly articulated [s] in the word *pencil*. In the word *pencil*, [s] is syllable-initial: [ˈpɛn.səl]. However, when [s] was syllable-final, as in the word *baseball*, [ˈbeɪs.bɔl], Luis consistently substituted [h] for [s]. The speech-language pathologist discovered a more distinct and consistent pattern to Luis's misarticulations.

3. Once the speech-language pathologist figured out that Luis had a consistent substitution pattern of [h] for [s] in syllable-final contexts, she wanted to understand if there was an underlying explanation for Luis's substitution pattern.

4. Because Luis is not a native English speaker, she decided to research Luis's native language of Puerto Rican Spanish and its typical dialectal features. The speech-language pathologist specifically wanted to see if a substitution of [h] for [s] in syllable-final position occurs in any typical dialects of Puerto Rican Spanish.

5. The speech-language pathologist discovered many dialectal patterns within Puerto Rican Spanish related to fricatives, including syllable-final [h] for [s] substitution, where [s] may become replaced by the aspirated [h] following the vowel.

6. The speech-language pathologist suspected that Luis's errors in English may be consistent with the typical dialectal pattern from his home language. To discern whether the family spoke a dialect of Puerto Rican Spanish that had this substitution pattern, the speech-language pathologist talked with Luis's parents. The speech-language pathologist discovered that Luis's parents did speak in a dialect characterized by this substitution pattern.

Answer

Based on the information the speech-language pathologist gathered from Luis's parents regarding his home language, no further articulation testing was warranted.

Science Applied

Looking beneath the surface, we often can discover patterns to speech sound production that we initially may have thought were isolated or random errors. Sometimes those patterns are due to dialectal differences, other times to acquisition delays or disordered speech. As clinical speech-language pathologists, we need to examine speech production for patterns of errors, and then try to discern why such patterns exist for an individual.

Interest Piqued?

Recommended materials to further your understanding of topics covered in this chapter.

Print Resources

Chomsky, N., & Halle, M. (1968). *The sound structure of language.* New York, NY: Harper & Row.

Davis, B. L., & MacNeilage, P. F. (1995). The articulatory basis of babbling. *Journal of Speech, Language, and Hearing, 38,* 1199–1211.

Gick, B., Wilson, I., & Derrick, D. (2013). *Articulatory phonetics.* Malden, MA: Wiley-Blackwell.

Ladefoged, P., & Maddieson, I. (1996). *The sounds of the world's languages.* Hoboken, NJ: Wiley-Blackwell.

MacNeilage, P. F., & Davis, B. L. (1990). Acquisition of speech: Frames, then content. In M. Jeannerod (Ed.), *Attention and performance XIII: Motor representation and control* (pp. 453–476). Hillsdale, NJ: Lawrence Erlbaum.

Silverstein, S. (2005). *Runny babbit: A silly hook.* New York, NY: Harper Collins.
This is a fun children's book written in spoonerisms.

Online Resources

http://www.asha.org/Practice-Portal/Clinical-Topics/Speech-Sound-Disorders-Articulation-and-Phonology/Selected-Phonological-Processes/
Web page of the American Speech-Language-Hearing Association where you can find phonological patterns of disordered speech.

http://clas.mq.edu.au/speech/phonetics/phonology/syllable/syll_structure.html
Diagramming syllable components: onsets, rimes, nuclei, and codas.

https://swphonetics.com/coarticulation/whatcoart/
Examples of connected speech production.

https://www.youtube.com/watch?v=McO4Bcfk3zc
Instruction on phonological rules as applied to typical speech in American English.

https://www.youtube.com/watch?v=Qj6f_wxz4YI
A short video of someone explaining the difference between phonetics and phonology.

https://www.youtube.com/watch?v=1Up5hSm7LYI
Here you will find someone inventing his own language, and the steps he is taking to do so.

You can find many examples of spoonerisms on the Internet, including Archie Campbell's renditions of classic fairytales in spoonerisms, such as *Rindercella* (*Cinderella*) and *The Pee Little Thrigs* (*The Three Little Pigs*).

ANSWER KEY

7–1.

Use the following words no more than one time each to complete the following sentences:

physical production, mental representation, phonetic, phonological.

1. The language-specific pattern that prohibits words from ending in [h] is part of the English <u>phonological</u> system.

2. Transcribing "p" as [p] signifies a <u>physical production</u>.

3. Transcribing "p" as /p/ signifies a <u>mental representation</u>.

7–2.

Indicate if the allophones described below resulted because of anticipatory or carryover coarticulation.

1. a nasalized vowel in the word *ham*
   <u>anticipatory</u>

2. a dentalized [n] in the word *month*
   <u>anticipatory</u>

3. a nasalized vowel in the word *ring*
   <u>anticipatory</u>

4. a palatal [k] in the word *seek*   <u>carryover</u>

7–3.

1. List a minimal pair that establishes [p] and [b] as phonemes.
   <u>answers will vary; could include pie-buy, tap-tab, etc.</u>

2. List a minimal pair that establishes [i] and [ɪ] as phonemes.
   <u>answers will vary; could include he's-his, beat-bit, etc.</u>

Indicate if the sounds described in the examples below are in contrastive,

free variation, or complementary distribution.

3. [n] and [t] as phonemes in the minimal pair *spin–spit*
   <u>contrastive distribution</u>

4. [t] and [tʰ] occurring in the word *hit*
   <u>free distribution</u>

5. nasalization of [æ] (that is, [æ̃]) when produced between two nasal consonants
   <u>complementary distribution</u>

7–4.

Translate the following spoonerisms of common expressions.

1. doored to Beth   <u>bored to death</u>

2. bings a rell   <u>rings a bell</u>

3. tips of the slung   <u>slips of the tongue</u>

4. grack to the bind   <u>back to the grind</u>

7–5.

Analyze the syllables in the following words.

1. *flavors*

	Syllable 1	Syllable 2
syllable transcription	fleɪ	vɚz
onset	fl	v
rime	eɪ	ɚz
nucleus	eɪ	ɚ
coda		z

2. *ox*

syllable transcription	ɑks
onset	
rime	ɑks
nucleus	ɑ
coda	ks

7–6.

1. Indicate which of the three airflow patterns—aspirated, unreleased, or unaspirated—apply to the stops in the following examples.

keys, caulk, cave	aspirated
stove, stem, still	unaspirated
lick, soak, oink	unreleased

2. Phonetically transcribe each of the words in number 1, above, using diacritics to illustrate the appropriate phonological pattern.

keys, caulk, cave	[kʰiz]	[kʰɔlk]/[kʰɑlk]	[kʰeɪv]
stove, stem, still	[st˭oʊv]	[st˭ɛm]	[st˭ɪl]
lick, soak, oink	[lɪk̚]	[soʊk̚]	[ɔɪŋk̚]

7–7.

1. Indicate the place-related allophonic pattern that can apply to the stops in the following examples.

breadth	dentalized
key	advanced
sudden	glottal stop insertion
goose	labialized

2. Phonetically transcribe each of the words in number 1, above, using diacritics to illustrate the appropriate phonological pattern.

breadth	[bɹɛd̪θ]
key	[k̟i]
sudden	[ˈsʌʔn̩]
goose	[gʷus]

7–8.

1. Circle the words that can contain a nasal release.

   <u>button</u>   <u>fatten</u>   bottle   <u>kitten</u>   letting
   <u>leaden</u>   coddle   madder   <u>sodden</u>   <u>gladden</u>

2. Circle the words that can contain a bilateral release.

   <u>class</u>   cows   bicycle   <u>cyclops</u>   <u>clue</u>
   angle   <u>gloat</u>   <u>burglar</u>   confusingly   <u>glove</u>

3. Circle the words that can contain affrication.

   <u>control</u>   pretty   <u>attract</u>   shrink   <u>country</u>
   <u>drive</u>   <u>children</u>   umbrella   freeze   <u>raindrop</u>

4. Circle the words that can contain a medial tap.

   <u>bottom</u>   <u>fighter</u>   guitar   <u>gritty</u>   futon
   <u>pudding</u>   cadet   <u>cheddar</u>   <u>cedar</u>   <u>teddy</u>

7–9.

1. Circle the phrases that contain an unreleased articulation of the first stop in doubled stop consonants.

   <u>lob balls</u>   <u>climbed down</u>   lamb bleats   <u>white teeth</u>
   <u>ask kindly</u>   sing good   <u>cheap pen</u>   <u>big goose</u>

7–10.

1. Circle the phrases that can contain a glottal stop insertion.

   <u>she exited</u>   <u>flee early</u>   <u>I ached</u>   we left   <u>they admitted</u>

2. Circle the words in which [t] can be omitted.

   <u>banter</u>   pontificate   <u>scented</u>   contact   <u>winter</u>

7–11.

1. Circle the phrases in which palatalization of [s] and [z] could occur.

   misspent youth   <u>cheerleaders yell</u>   <u>Bob's yard</u>   <u>his yacht</u>   <u>practice yoga</u>

2. Circle the phrases in which [v] can be devoiced.

   <u>dove hunting</u>   <u>olive tree</u>   above water   <u>gave her</u>   believe me

3. Circle the phrases in which [θ] can be voiced.

   with him   <u>with me</u>   oath taken   bathtub   <u>beneath you</u>

4. Circle the phrases in which fricatives can be lengthened.

   <u>a mess, see?</u>   messy   <u>fresh shirt</u>   <u>both thumbs</u>   winter wonderland

5. Circle the phrases in which word-initial [h] can be omitted.

Can you HOP?   <u>Give THEM her money.</u>   <u>WE want him to go.</u>   Let her GO!

7–12.

1. Circle the words in which [t͡ʃ] can become [t͡ʃʷ].

cheek   chill   <u>choke</u>   <u>chew</u>   chunk

2. Circle the words in which [d͡ʒ] can become [d͡ʒʷ].

<u>jukebox</u>   jump   <u>juicy</u>   <u>jubilant</u>   justice

7–13.

1. Circle the words that can contain a labiodental nasal consonant.

dolphin   <u>symphony</u>   <u>amphetamine</u>   uphill   <u>lymph</u>
<u>emphasis</u>   <u>harrumph</u>   homophone   <u>amphibian</u>   hyphen

2. Circle the words in which [n] can be an allophone of [ŋ].

ring   <u>running</u>   <u>hurrying</u>   thing   <u>falling</u>
<u>laughing</u>   sing   <u>writing</u>   <u>singing</u>   sting

3. Circle the words in which [n] can be lengthened.

<u>brownnoser</u>   <u>unnerve</u>   tenderness   planned   <u>unnatural</u>
<u>thinness</u>   penny   <u>suddenness</u>   <u>openness</u>   annex

4. Circle the words in which [m] can become a syllabic consonant.

<u>blossom</u>   <u>rhythm</u>   exam   <u>requiem</u>   <u>calcium</u>

5. Circle the words in which [n] can become a syllabic consonant.

<u>frighten</u>   begun   <u>sudden</u>   again   <u>hidden</u>

6. Circle the words in which a voiceless homorganic stop can be inserted in nasal + voiceless fricative clusters that precede an unstressed vowel.

<u>pence</u>   <u>ounce</u>   <u>since</u>   cons   <u>hansom cab</u>

7. Circle the words in which a voiced homorganic stop can be inserted in nasal + voiced fricative clusters that precede an unstressed vowel.

<u>pans</u>   wonder   <u>fins</u>   <u>whines</u>   hams

7–14.

1. Circle the words in which [l] can become [ɫ].

full   <u>puddle</u>   follow   <u>peaceful</u>   lengthen

2. Circle the words in which an approximant can become devoiced.

tackle   <u>clock</u>   <u>trick</u>   <u>please</u>   police

3. Circle the phrases in which [l] can become lengthened.

<u>awful lamp</u>   love life   <u>idyll lion</u>   <u>final lap</u>   <u>small ladder</u>

4. Circle the phrases in which [w] can become [hw].

who   <u>what</u>   <u>where</u>   <u>when</u>   how

5. Circle the words in which [l] can become a syllable.

<u>aerial</u>   <u>vinyl</u>   <u>angel</u>   sell   <u>muscle</u>

7–15.

1. Describe each misarticulation using the correct classification of substitution, omission, distortion, or addition.

   a.   The type of error exhibited in the production of [ha͡ʊts] for [ha͡ʊs] is an <u>addition</u>.

   b.   The type of error exhibited in the production of [bæt] for [bæθ] is a <u>substitution</u>.

   c.   The type of error exhibited in the production of [θæk.ju] for [θæŋk.ju] is an <u>omission</u>.

   d.   The type of error exhibited in the production of a lateralized [s], as in [sˡʌn] for [sʌn], is a <u>distortion</u>.

8

LINGUISTIC PHONETICS AND PHONOLOGY OF VOWELS

Learning Objectives

By reading this chapter, you will learn:

1. typical phonological patterns for English vowels
2. allophonic patterns for stressed and unstressed vowels in multisyllabic words
3. allophonic patterns for nonphonemic diphthong reduction
4. allophonic patterns for tense and lax vowels
5. allophobnic patterns for vowels
6. the concept of vowel reduction in citation versus conversational speech
7. differences between rhotic and nonrhotic dialects of English

Applied Science: Difference or Disorder in the Production of Rhotic Vowels

As a speech-language pathologist in the schools, you are assessing the speech and language skills of 8-year-old Elise. Elise and her family recently moved from Australia. According to her parents, Elise received speech-language therapy in Australia for a literacy disorder. While her reading, spelling, and decoding skills have improved since she started therapy, her parents think her overall literacy development is still behind her peers.

You conduct a comprehensive assessment of Elise's speech and language to evaluate her skills. The results of your testing confirm her delay in literacy development. Testing results indicate that Elise has a speech disorder, corresponding to the slightly unintelligible speech you observed during her assessment. Curiously, neither the previous speech-language pathologist nor her family had reported speech difficulties.

To understand Elise's speech errors, you review the single words that Elise produced in a picture naming task. All of her errors are in the production of rhotics. On closer examination, you discover that Elise produces initial [ɹ] accurately in words and her errors are on rhotic monophthongs, diphthongs, and triphthong vowels. She deletes some rhotic vowels but not all of them.

The single word speech assessment did not provide enough information to fully understand Elise's inconsistent [ɝ] productions. To see if there is a pattern to her speech errors, you transcribe sentences from Elise's storytelling task that contain rhotic vowels. Your first observation was correct: Elise produces [ɹ] correctly in syllable onset position but is inconsistent with rhotics in other places in the word. Elise's errors do not seem consistent, since you see differences in rhotic vowel production across sentences, even when she is using the same word. You also note that Elise produces [ɹ] in some words when there is not an "r" in the word.

Below are some of the sentences you transcribed from Elise's speech sample, sorted into three groups: correct production, deletion of "r," and insertion of rhotics. The target words are underlined. Note that the transcriptions focus on rhotic qualities only and do not include diacritics

to capture dialectal differences between GAE and Australian English vowels.

Rhotic Vowel Produced Correctly

My teacher only speaks to us in Spanish.
[maɪ ˈti.t͡ʃɚ ˈoʊn.li spiks tə ʌs ɪn ˈspæ.nɪʃ]

My dad's car is being fixed.
[maɪ dædz kaɚ ɪz ˈbi.ɪŋ fɪkst]

Did you hear a truck honking?
[dɪd ju hɪɚ ə tɹʌk ˈhɑŋ.kɪŋ]

The butter is on the table.
[ðə ˈbʌ.tɚ ɪz ɑn ðə ˈteɪ.bəl]

Rhotic Vowel Deletion

The child can hear his dad.
[ðə t͡ʃaɪld kæn hɪə hɪz dæd]

I would like a new car. [aɪ wʊd laɪk ə nu kaə]

My teacher praised my project.
[maɪ ˈti.t͡ʃə pɹeɪzd maɪ ˈpɹɑ.d͡ʒɛkt]

He eats peanut butter with jelly.
[hi its ˈpi.nət ˈbʌ.tə wɪð ˈd͡ʒɛ.li]

Rhotic Insertion

We had pasta and meatballs last night.
[wi hæd ˈpɑs.tə ɹæn ˈmit.bɑls læst naɪt]

Sofia is my best friend. [soʊ.ˈfiə ɹɪz maɪ bɛst fɹɛnd]

I want a cookie after lunch.
[aɪ wɑnt ə ˈkʊ.ki ˈɹæf.tə lʌnt͡ʃ]

You find these results confusing. Elise does not appear to have a consistent pattern for when she produces rhotics and when she does not. However, you have never worked with a person who speaks Australian English. Before diagnosing Elise with a speech disorder, you want to make sure you are not considering a difference in her speech as a disorder. To fully understand Elise's speech, you research Australian English to see if there are different patterns for rhotic vowels that may explain Elise's rhotic errors.

As you read this chapter, consider Elise's rhotic errors. Do you think Elise's errors indicate a speech disorder? Is it possible that Elise exhibits a speech disorder in American but not Australian English? Or is there a phonological pattern to Elise's errors that can be explained by dialect differences?

Vowel Phonological Patterns

In Chapter 3, you learned about English vowel phonemes, including English monophthongs, diphthongs, and triphthongs, and their defining articulatory properties, such as tongue height, tongue advancement, lip posture, and tenseness. You have learned how vowels are contrasted by moving our articulators to change sound quality. And you know how this articulatory information is conveyed to the listener through distinct acoustic cues.

Chapter 7 introduced you to patterns for consonant allophone production in English. This chapter explores allophonic vowel patterns in General American English (GAE). Many of these vowel patterns relate to the length of the vowel. They are frequently observed in unstressed syllables in longer words and in conversational speech. Other common allophonic patterns result from coarticulation. Before we examine these patterns, though, we explore how vowel phonology differs from that of consonants.

If two phoneticians compare their transcriptions of conversational speech, they are more likely to differ subtly in how they transcribe vowels than consonants. In general, vowels tend to be harder to transcribe than consonants. There are a number of reasons for this transcription difficulty. Some distinctions between vowel phonemes are difficult to hear, especially in longer words and in unstressed syllables. And vowel phonemic boundaries are trickier to define due to the continuous nature of vowels. There are clearer boundaries between consonant phonemes than there are vowel phonemes. For example, there are clear distinctions in voicing between [p] and [b], and clear differences in consonant manner, such as between the voiceless alveolar fricative [s] and stop [t]. In contrast, the articulatory difference between vowels is less clear. If you raise the mandible with the tongue carriage forward and the vocal folds vibrating, you produce the vowel [i]. While producing [i], slowly lower your jaw while continuing to phonate. As your jaw lowers, the [i]

becomes [ɪ], then [ɛ], and finally [æ]. While one can hear the shift from one phonemic category to the next when the vowels are produced continuously, distinctions are harder to transcribe if a borderline vowel is produced in isolation. In fact, it can be difficult for two different transcribers to agree 100% on vowel transcription, especially if vowels are distorted or are reduced.

You learned about vowels produced in citation form in Chapter 3. We rarely speak this clearly and deliberately, tending to speak faster, coarticulating sounds and producing vowels with less extreme articulatory postures than we do in citation speech. Casual speech has a greater impact on vowel than consonant phoneme quality, also contributing to the difficulty of transcribing vowels.

Vowels differ more than consonants between English dialects, with differing patterns for dialect-specific vowel production and allophonic patterns across dialects. For example, New Zealand dialect differs from GAE in vowel phonemes, so the phrase, *Every little bit can help*, sounds more like [ˈɪv.ɹi ˈlə.ɾəl bət kʌn hɪlp]. For a bilingual speaker of American English, first language influences on English are often observed in the vowel productions, with overlap in vowel categories observed at times.

As a clinician, it tends to be easier to teach someone with a speech sound disorder how to produce a consonant than a vowel. It is easier to describe where and how to place the articulators for most consonants, as well as to point out major acoustic differences between correct and incorrect consonant productions. The articulatory description of vowel differences is subtler, as are the techniques for teaching vowel production.

Lastly, there are differing underlying properties for English vowel and consonant phonemes. In particular, all English vowel phonemes are voiced and oral—there are neither /voiced/voiceless nor oral/ nasal contrasts for English vowel phonemes. Because there are no phonemic contrasts in voicing or orality in English, we do not refer to these characteristics when describing vowels. However, the lack of phonemic contrast does not mean we never produce voiceless or nasal vowels, because we do. English vowels have voiceless and nasal allophones. For example, vowels are voiceless in whispers and in some unstressed syllables and nasalized vowels are acceptable in English in certain contexts as a result of coarticulation. We will learn patterns for nasal and voiceless vowel allophones later in this chapter.

Vowel Allophones in Multisyllabic Words

Unlike citation speech, in conversational and casual speech, some vowel phonemes are not typically produced in their full phonemic form, but instead, are reduced. While there are some common patterns for vowel reduction, these reduced vowel allophones are not required, but occur in free variation. In other words, we do not have to reduce them in these contexts, we just tend to do so.

As you learn about allophonic vowel productions, say the words aloud to yourself to hear the vowel changes. Be careful not to overemphasize words, though. If you do, you probably will not reduce any vowels. So say words as naturally as possible to hear the difference between citation vowels and their vowel allophones.

Stressed Versus Unstressed Syllables

Vowels in longer words change because of English stress patterns in multisyllabic words. In citation speech, we overenunciate and produce full vowels like [ʌ] or [aɪ] in stressed and unstressed syllables. To hear this difference, say the word *enthusiastically* in hyperarticulated form, with stress on each vowel. If you say this word slowly and overenunciate, you will say something like [ˈɛn.ˈθu.ˈzi.ˈæs.ˈtɪ.ˈkʌ.ˈli]. In natural speech, we alter our stress patterns, stressing some vowels and reducing some unstressed vowels. It sounds much more natural to say *enthusiastically* as [ən.θu.ˈzjæ.stə.kli], with two vowels reduced and two deleted.

Stressed [ʌ] Versus Unstressed [ə]
We start our exploration of allophonic vowel variations by returning to the schwa, [ə], the most common allophonic production of a vowel. [ə], the allophonic

unstressed counterpart of stressed [ʌ], appears frequently in English, occurring in the majority of two-syllable English words and often multiple times in words that are three syllables or longer. In addition to the allophonic production for [ʌ], [ə] replaces many vowel phonemes in unstressed syllables in longer words. For example, the word *decline* is pronounced [di.ˈklaɪn]. In the word *declination*, however, [aɪ] is no longer in a stressed syllable. It is much shorter and typically produced as a schwa. *Declination* is often pronounced [ˌdɛ.klə.ˈneɪ.ʃən]. All six written English vowels—"a, e, i, o, u, y"—can be produced as [ə] in longer words. Hard to believe? Say the following words aloud and see whether you produce a schwa for the underlined vowels: *catalyst, review, imagine, autograph, successful, bicycle*. How would you transcribe these words?

You are not alone if you find it difficult to distinguish between [ʌ] and [ə]. While you can differentiate schwa or wedge based on articulatory information, the distinction is slight and can differ between transcribers. While there are slightly different qualitative properties (the mouth is more open during [ʌ] than [ə] production), most transcribers differentiate these allophones based on stress patterns, only using [ʌ] in stressed syllables and [ə] in unstressed syllables. The distinction between schwa and wedge is easier to learn and more straightforward if you differentiate these vowels based on word stress.

To correctly identify [ʌ] and [ə], determine whether a sound in a word is stressed or unstressed. When we transcribe a one-syllable word such as *cup*, we use [ʌ], transcribing the word as [kʌp] because there is only one vowel and it is stressed. Similarly, *shush* is transcribed [ʃʌʃ]. In the two-syllable word *about*, the first syllable is unstressed so the "uh" sound is transcribed with the schwa: [ə.ˈbaʊt]. In contrast, in *prefer*, the second syllable is stressed so the schwa is in the first syllable: [pɹə.ˈfɝ]. *Above* contains unstressed and stressed mid central vowels, with stress on the second syllable. *Above* is transcribed [ə.ˈbʌv].

In sentences, single-syllable words can be transcribed with [ə] if a word is reduced and unstressed. This is often the case with closed class parts of speech, such as determiners, pronouns, and prepositions. This means that words like *the* are often said as [ðə] in running speech. Say the sentence, *The dog was chewing on a bone.* If you said this sentence quickly, it is likely that both *the* and *was* were produced with the unstressed schwa. These reduced vowels are captured in the transcription [ðə ˈdɑg wəz ˈtʃu.ɪŋ an ðə boʊn]. Does this transcription of this sentence match how you said it? If not, did you produce other vowels as unstressed? How would you transcribe your production?

As you have learned, there are articulatory differences between [ə] and [ʌ], with the mandible raised slightly higher for [ə]. The difference in articulatory placement is very slight and it is difficult to differentiate these vowels solely based on tongue height. Can you hear the difference between these two vowels? They occur frequently in English and it can take time for a new phonetician to distinguish them.

Say the words from the last paragraph that contain [ʌ]: *cup, shush*; then the words with unstressed [ə]: *about, prefer*; then *above*, which has a schwa and wedge in it. And finally listen to how you say each *the* in *The dog is chewing on the bone*. Remember to say all of these words at a natural rate of speech and not in citation form. Did you hear a difference in the wedge and the schwa? How would you describe the differences? The listener is paying attention to acoustic differences and not whether they were produced differently. Acoustically, the differences are in loudness and length: the stressed [ʌ] is louder and longer in duration than the unstressed [ə].

A spectrogram shows clearly the vowel length distinctions between [ə] and [ʌ]. Figure 8–1 is a spectrogram of the word *above*, with stress on the second syllable. This word is 0.72 seconds in length and the distance between each vertical dotted line is 0.05 seconds in length. Can you figure out how we know these length measurements? Remember, time is marked in the bottom-right corner of the spectrogram. And if you count the dotted vertical lines, you will find 14 of them. These lines are equidistant apart, dividing the 0.72-second-long spectrogram into a little over 14 segments. Determine the length difference between the stressed [ʌ] and the unstressed [ə]. The first vowel, [ə], is approximately one third the length of the vowel [ʌ]. [ə] is 0.1 seconds in length, whereas the [ʌ] is 0.23 seconds in length.

Figure 8–2 is a spectrogram of the word *bucket*, with stress on the first syllable. *Bucket* was pronounced [ˈbʌ.kət]. The stressed [ʌ] is 0.11 milliseconds in length and the unstressed [ə] is 0.06 milliseconds in length. If you compare Figure 8–1 and Figure 8–2, you see how relative length difference between the vowels differentiates [ʌ] and [ə].

Figure 8–3 is a spectrogram of the word *believe*, transcribed [bə.ˈliv]. In this word, the [ə] syllable is about one third of the length of [i] in the second syllable. Did you measure the actual length of each vowel?

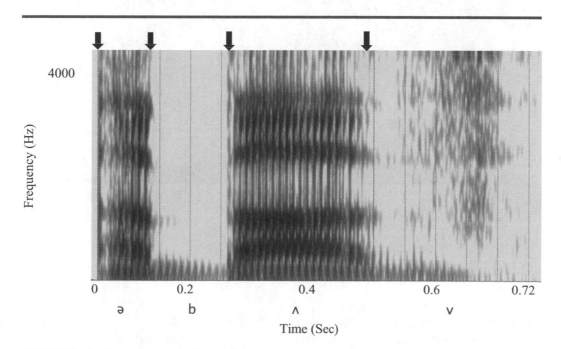

FIGURE 8–1. Spectrogram of the word *above*.

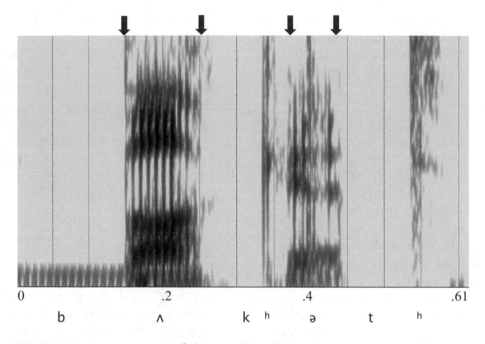

FIGURE 8–2. Spectrogram of the word *bucket.*

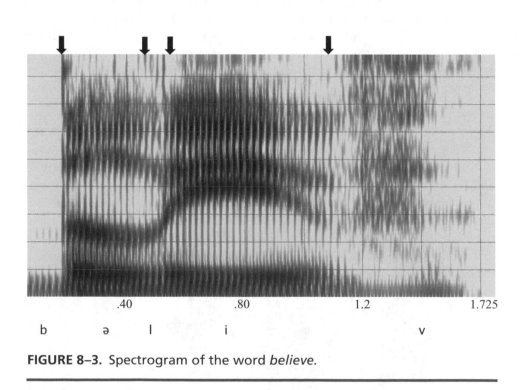

FIGURE 8–3. Spectrogram of the word *believe.*

Spectrograms have visually verified the length difference, a key acoustic distinction between [ʌ] and [ə]. To transcribe accurately, you must hear the distinction between stressed and unstressed syllables. For some people, hearing stressed syllables comes easily and for others, it is a skill that is only learned after a lot of practice. Tapping out syllables as you say words in your head can help if you tap the rhythm pattern with loudness contrasts. To do so, think the word *conversational* while tapping out the word's rhythm. Do not say the word aloud but think saying it while you tap. If you capture the stress pattern accurately, you would have tapped *soft-soft-LOUD-soft-soft* to capture the stress on the third syllable of *conversational*. Another way to determine stress patterns is to say the word quickly and multiple times. By repeating the word fast, you are less likely to overemphasize the word and lose natural stress patterns.

Stressed [ɝ] Versus Unstressed [ɚ]

Like /ʌ/, the rhotic monophthong /ɝ/ has stressed and unstressed allophonic variations. The stressed [ɝ] is a mid central rounded tense vowel; the unstressed [ɚ] allophone tends to be produced with slightly less rounding. Articulatory differences are very slight; in fact, some speakers do not make a distinction in vowel rounding.

There are parallel distinctions between the stressed [ɝ] and unstressed [ɚ] and the stressed [ʌ] and unstressed [ə]. Length is the primary distinction be-tween the two: [ɝ] is longer in duration than [ɚ]. Figure 8–4 is a spectrogram of the word *perturbed,* transcribed [pɚ.'tɝbd]. *Perturbed* is typically produced with an unstressed [ɚ] in the first syllable and a stressed [ɝ] in the second syllable. Figure 8–4 shows that the second syllable is longer than the first. The vertical lines are 0.05 seconds apart. Measure the two /ɝ/ allophones to compare the unstressed and stressed vowel lengths. Notice that in this figure, the dotted lines are 0.1 seconds apart. Did your measurements show that the unstressed [ɚ] was 0.07 seconds and [ɝ] was 0.24 seconds?

Figure 8–5 is a spectrogram of the word *perhaps,* [pɚ.'hæps], with the unstressed /ɚ/ in the first syllable. Measure the length of both vowels in this word. What did you find? Did your measurements confirm that the unstressed /ɚ/ is shorter in length than the stressed vowel?

? 8–1. Did You Get It?

Each word below is typically produced with [ə], [ʌ], or both of them. Underline the syllable (or syllables) that contain a wedge or a schwa. Put a check in the appropriate column if the word contains a schwa, wedge, or a schwa and a wedge. Then transcribe the word, marking the stressed vowel with the apostrophe diacritic at the beginning of the syllable.

Identifying and Transcribing Stressed and Unstressed Schwa and Wedge

	Word	[ə]	[ʌ]	Phonetic Transcription
1	review			
2	cupboard			
3	ugly			
4	aluminum			
5	funny			
6	phonetics			
7	extra			
8	seventy			

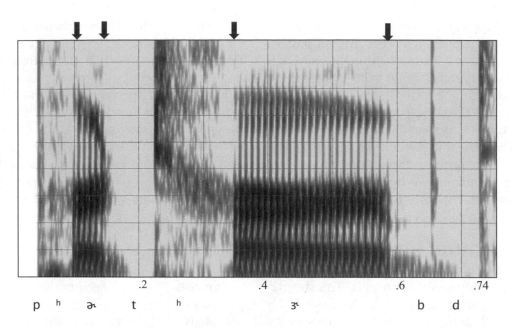

FIGURE 8–4. Spectrogram of the word *perturbed*.

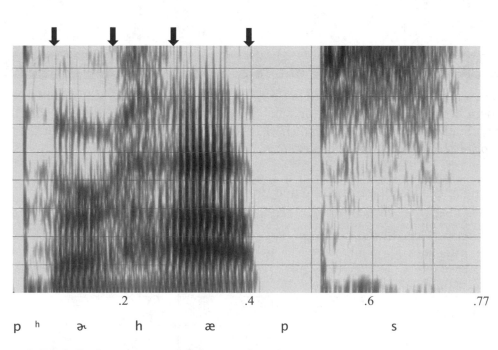

FIGURE 8–5. Spectrogram of the word *perhaps*.

Nonphonemic Diphthongs

/o/ and /e/ are frequently produced as the nonphonemic diphthongs [oʊ] and [eɪ] in GAE. For that reason, we have presented these mid vowels as nonphonemic diphthongs throughout this book. Some phoneticians do not note the diphthong quality of nonphonemic vowels in their transcription, transcribing them as the monophthongs [e] and [o] regardless of allophonic differences. However, the diphthong is quite pronounced in these two mid vowels and the lack of diphthongal quality tends to distinguish dialects of English.

There are contexts where you are more likely to produce these vowels as monophthongs and certain contexts where you are more likely to produce them as diphthongs. In general, the phonemes /e/ and /o/ are produced as the diphthongs in stressed syllables. Thus [eɪ] and [oʊ] are the typical production for most stressed monosyllabic words. This results in the production of diphthongs in monosyllabic words that are stressed, as well as the diphthong production in stressed syllables in longer words, such as vacation: [və.ˈkeɪ.ʃən].

The production of [eɪ] and [oʊ] as monophthongs in shorter words is often a sign of someone learning English as a second language, since many languages, such as Spanish and Vietnamese, do not have this allophonic diphthong pattern and only produce the tense mid vowels as the monophthongs [e] and [o].

Try comparing the diphthongs [oʊ] and [eɪ] and nondiphthong [o] and [e] allophones. Say the word *go*, lengthening the word and prolonging the vowel for a few seconds before you end the word. Notice that your articulators change position during the vowel, ending the word with lip rounding. While you can say *go* without the rounding at the end (try it), it has an unfinished abrupt quality that is not typical American English. Now say the word *goat*. Do you also feel the articulator movement during the vowel? You should feel your jaw raising, moving from a mid back to a high back position. Both *go* and *goat* are typically produced with the diphthong [oʊ]. Say *may*, again lengthening the vowel and noting the articulatory movement during [eɪ]. Prolong the vowel in *make* as well, exaggerating the transition from the mid to high front components in [eɪ].

Nonphonemic diphthongs are produced as monophthongs when followed by a rhotic vowel. As we have seen, there is not a tense/lax phonemic contrast between the nonphonemic diphthongs [oʊ] and [eɪ] and their lax counterparts [ɛ] and [ɔ] when followed by a rhotic vowel. The diphthong quality that was apparent in the nonrhotic vowel is gone in this context, as is the extreme articulatory production and length of tense vowels. Hence we pronounce words such as *or* and *air* as [ɔɚ] and [ɛɚ], not [oʊɚ] or [eɪɚ]. While you can say these tense rhotic triphthongs, they are allophonic versions of rhotic diphthongs with lax vowels, confirming the loss of the meaningful tense/lax distinction in the rhotic context.

Some English monophthongs are produced as nonphonemic diphthongs in single-syllable words. For example, /i/ and /u/ are often produced with an offglide as nonphonemic diphthongs. To observe these diphthong offglides, say the word *see*. If you elongate the vowel, do you notice your tongue placement changing slightly? You might capture this longer vowel as [iɪ]. What about if you say the word *who* very slowly—can you feel a change in the position of the lips in the offglide? This could be transcribed [uʊ]. While these offglides are frequently produced, very few clinical scientists capture the diphthong quality in transcription, because the off-glide results from a very slight movement of the articulators and does not result in a vowel height change. In contrast, both nonphonemic diphthongs [oʊ] and [eɪ] change vowel height, gliding from mid to high vowel properties.

? 8–2. Did You Get It?

Each multisyllabic word below is produced with a stressed [ɝ] or unstressed [ɚ], or both. Underline the syllable (or syllables) that contains a stressed or unstressed schwar. Put a check in the appropriate column if the word contains a stressed [ɝ], an unstressed [ɚ], or one of each. Then transcribe the word.

Identifying and Transcribing Stressed and Unstressed Schwar

	Word	[ɝ]	[ɚ]	Phonetic Transcription
1	courageous			
2	discerning			
3	nourishment			
4	cupboard			
5	further			
6	encouragement			
7	feather			
8	burger			

Tense Versus Lax Vowels

There are four English vowel cognates that differ only in tenseness. Tense vowels are often described as having greater articulatory tension and greater tongue root advancement than their lax vowel counterparts. However, articulatory differences between tense and lax vowels are not universally agreed on, especially for the back vowel pairs. While there may be some differences in muscular tension, the most important distinction between lax and tense vowels is how they pattern phonologically. The greatest acoustic difference between tense and lax vowels is their duration, or length. With all else being equal, speakers will tend to produce longer tense vowels than lax vowels. More than vowel quality differences, it is this difference in length that listeners pay attention to when they distinguish tense from lax vowels.

The spectrogram in Figure 8–6 compares tense/lax length differences by contrasting the words with high front vowels: *beat* and *bit*. The start and endpoints of each vowel is marked with a dark arrow. Measure the length of each vowel. Did you find that the tense vowel [i] is about 0.35 seconds, longer than the lax counterpart [ɪ] in [bɪt], which is approximately 0.13 seconds?

In addition to length differences, tense and lax vowels differ in syllable types. Tense vowels can occur in open or closed syllables; lax vowels do not occur in stressed open syllables, but do occur in closed syllables. Can you think of a situation that demonstrates this pattern? English has many CV words that end with the high front tense vowel /i/. Some examples include *bee, key, he, she, tree, ski, plea*. But we do not have words that end in /ɪ/ in most English dialects, nor words that end in lax vowels, such as /ɛ/ and /ʊ/. Try for yourself. Come up with a list of words that end in the tense vowel [eɪ] and another list with words that end in [u]. Probably not too hard, right? Can you come up with any words that end with the lax phones [ɛ] or [ʊ]? While you may find an exception, there are extremely few of these.

Phonological Patterns for Vowels

We have explored differing vowel allophones as well as how tense and lax vowels contrast. Now we will

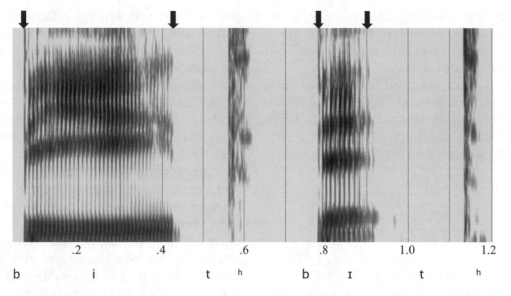

FIGURE 8–6. Spectrogram of the words *beat* and *bit,* comparing vowel length in tense and lax vowels.

Vowel Length

We use vowel length information to increase clarity of our communication in many ways. Speakers change vowel length and stress in patterned ways, as we saw in the tense/lax vowel length differences in the previous section. In addition, vowel length differences signal phonemic and phonotactic differences. The same vowel tends to differ in length depending on whether it occurs in open or closed syllables; one-, two-, three- or more syllable words; whether the syllable is stressed or unstressed; and as you have learned, whether the vowel is tense or lax. Vowel length differences also indicate whether the final consonant is voiced or voiceless. As we explore vowel length differences, remember that they are relative, requiring a contrasting vowel to indicate long or short.

Below we present three vowel length patterns and explain the context in which they occur. As we explore vowel length patterns, you will want to differentiate between long, medium, and short vowel durations using the diacritics you learned in Chapter 4. Remember that the diacritic for marking a long vowel is a colon (ː). If we transcribe *shoe* and want to indi-

cate that the [u] is long, we transcribe the word as [ʃuː]. The diacritic for marking a short vowel is [˘]. If we want to compare three vowels, we can use the vowel length diacritic (·) for the vowel that is not long or short. Because what we are discussing in this chapter are patterns that are inherent to typical speech, most of the time we do not mark these length differences with a diacritic; instead, it is just assumed. We will use the diacritics in this chapter to emphasize these length distinctions as you learn about them.

Besides explaining patterns for relative length of vowel production, we can use diacritics to capture individual differences in vowel production. For example, if you wanted to capture that a vowel stood out for the production length, you could use the diacritic for a slightly longer or medium-length vowel: the single raised dot (·). This diacritic would be used to transcribe *speech* as [spi·tʃ], to capture that the [i] was a little longer than expected.

Within-Syllable Vowel Length Differences

The first vowel length pattern applies to single syllables and one-syllable words. This pattern is:

If everything else is equal, a vowel is (a) longest in an open syllable, (b) next longest in a syllable that ends with a voiced consonant, and (c) shortest if the syllable ends with a voiceless consonant.

In other words, any vowel has three length possibilities within a syllable, depending on whether there is a consonant in the coda and whether that final consonant is voiced or voiceless.

To test this pattern, we need to compare words where everything but the coda is the same. Therefore, we need to compare words that have the same sounds in the onset and nucleus but differ in the coda. The set of words below fits these conditions:

see	seed	seat
/si/	/sid/	/sit/
CV	CVC	CVC

Say these words to yourself. Can you hear the differences in vowel length? How would you capture the

differences in transcription? These words are transcribed using narrow and broad phonetic transcription in Table 8–1. Note that vowel length differences are captured only in narrow transcription, with the single dot noting medium vowel length.

Like the narrow transcription of consonants, we rarely use diacritics to mark allophonic vowel differences that occur in typical speech. While you may hear these vowel length differences, compare them on a spectrogram to verify their differences. *See, seed,* and *seat* are shown in a spectrogram in Figure 8–7. Looking at the vowels in the spectrogram should show you that the vowels get increasingly shorter in the three words. Now measure the vowel /i/ in all three words. What measurements did you come up with? Your measurements should confirm this within-syllable vowel length pattern.

TABLE 8–1. Phonetic Transcription of Vowel Length in the Words *see, seed, seat,* Contrasting Length in an Open Syllable, a Syllable Closed by a Voiced Consonant, and a Syllable Closed by a Voiceless Consonant

Word	Word Shape	Broad Phonetic Transcription	Narrow Phonetic Transcription	Vowel Context
see	CV	[si]	[siː]	Ends in vowel
seed	CVC	[sid]	[siˑd]	Ends in voiced consonant
seat	CVC	[sit]	[sĭt]	Ends in voiceless consonant

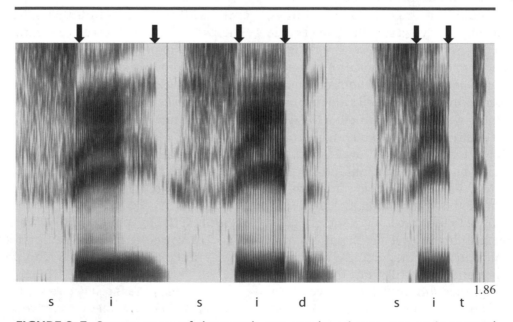

1.86

s   i   s   i   d   s   i   t

FIGURE 8–7. Spectrogram of the words *see, seed,* and *seat,* comparing vowel length in words ending in a vowel, voiced consonant, and voiceless consonant.

Here is one more set of vowels that differ in vowel length. Say the words *play, played,* and *plate* aloud. Can you hear the vowel length differences? How would you transcribe the differences? Table 8–2 compares the narrow transcription of these vowels to capture the vowel lengths of each word type. Figure 8–8 is a spectrogram of the three words for you to measure length differences.

Vowel Length and Syllable Stress
The second vowel length pattern occurs in multisyllabic words. It states:

> *If everything else is equal, vowels are longer in stressed syllables.*

In other words, the length of a vowel in the same syllable changes dependent on whether the syllable is stressed or unstressed. Similar to the first pattern, if a vowel is stressed it will be longer than the same vowel in unstressed or secondarily stressed syllables.

To test this stressed vowel length pattern, we need words that have the same two syllables but one word is stressed on the first syllable and the other word is stressed on the second syllable. Below are two sets of words that fit this stress change pattern. Say the words aloud, first in the sentence and then in isolation. Can you hear the differences between them? Do you hear the vowel length differences in each pair of words? Table 8–3 shows the broad and narrow transcription for each of the word pairs.

TABLE 8–2. Phonetic Transcription of Vowel Length in the Words *play, played, plate,* Contrasting Length in an Open Syllable, a Syllable Closed by a Voiced Consonant, and a Syllable Closed by a Voiceless Consonant

	Word Shape	**Broad Phonetic Transcription**	**Narrow Phonetic Transcription**	**Vowel Context**
play	CCV	[pleɪ]	[pʰleɪː]	Ends in vowel
played	CCVC	[pleɪd]	[pʰleɪ·d]	Ends in voiced consonant
plate	CCVC	[pleɪt]	[pʰlĕɪt]	Ends in voiceless consonant

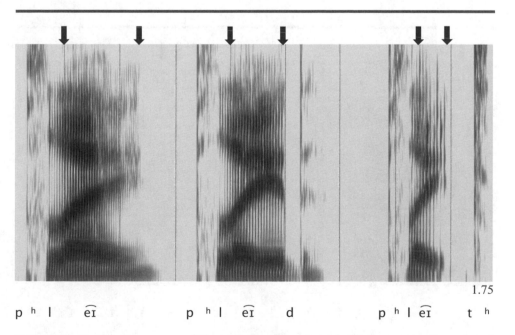

1.75

pʰ l eɪ   pʰ l eɪ d   pʰ l eɪ t ʰ

FIGURE 8–8. Spectrogram of the words *play, played, plate,* comparing vowel length in words ending in a vowel, voiced consonant, and voiceless consonant.

permit (noun) *My brother got his driver's PERmit yesterday.*

permit (verb) *I cannot perMIT him to drive.*

decrease (noun) *There has been a DEcrease in the price of cellphones.*

decrease (verb) *We need to deCREASE the cost of our shoes.*

While you should be able to hear vowel length differences in unstressed and stressed syllables, Figure 8–9 shows the contrast in a spectrogram of the noun and verb words *permit*. The difference between these words is in stress, indicated by vowel length. Measure the length difference between the stressed and unstressed vowels. First, compare the vowel [ɝ] in both syllables. How long is each [ɝ]? Now measure and compare the two stressed and unstressed productions of [ɪ]. How do these two vowels compare in duration?

In many unstressed syllables, the vowel quality reduces to a schwa. In those cases, this rule does not apply, because the actual vowel has changed and you cannot compare this reduced vowel to the vowel in a stressed syllable. Therefore, the condition of *all other things equal* no longer applies.

Vowel Length in Words

The third vowel length pattern describes how vowels change as words get longer. It states:

TABLE 8–3. Phonetic Transcription of Vowel Length Differences of the Same Syllable in Stressed and Unstressed Contexts

Word	Part of Speech	Stress Pattern	Broad Transcription	Narrow Transcription
the permit	noun	strong-weak	['pɝ.mɪt]	['pʰɝː.mɪ̆t]
to permit	verb	weak-strong	[pɚ.'mɪt]	[pʰɚ.'mɪːt]
the decrease	noun	strong-weak	['di.kɹis]	['diː.kʰɹɪ̆s]
to decrease	verb	weak-strong	[di.'kɹis]	[dɪ̆.'kʰɹiːs]

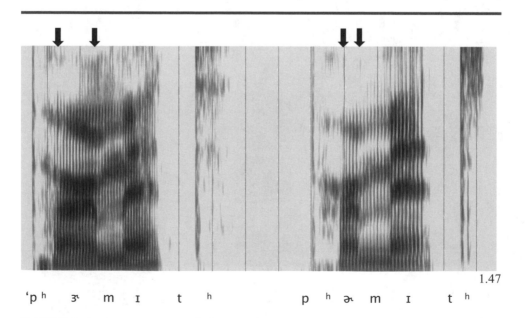

1.47

ˈpʰ   ɝ   m   ɪ   t   ʰ   pʰ   ɚ   m   ɪ   t   ʰ

FIGURE 8–9. Spectrogram of the word *permit* produced twice: first as a noun and then as a verb.

If everything else is equal, a stressed vowel is (a) longest in a monosyllabic word, (b) next longest in a two-syllable word; and (c) shortest in a word that is three or more syllables.

Thus, vowels get shorter as words get longer. This pattern interacts with others. For example, a vowel in an open syllable will be longer than a vowel in a closed syllable but will be relatively shorter if it is produced in an unstressed syllable and even shorter if that unstressed syllable is in a three-syllable word. And stressed vowels in the same syllable will get shorter as the word gets longer.

To test this length pattern, compare identically stressed syllables in longer and longer words. Consider the syllable [spid], which is stressed in the words *speed*, *speedy*, and *speedily*. Another example is [wɪl], which is stressed in the words *will*, *willing*, *willingly*, and *unwillingly*. Say these words aloud. You should hear that the syllable [spid] in the first sequence and the syllable [wɪl] in the second sequence of words is stressed. In each series, the stressed syllable gets shorter as the words get longer. Narrow transcription can be used to compare these distinctions as shown in Table 8–4.

The words *speed*, *speedy*, and *speedily* are shown in the spectrogram in Figure 8–10. First, find the syllable

TABLE 8–4. Phonetic Transcription of Vowel Length Differences by Word Length

Word	# Syllables	Broad Phonetic Transcription	Narrow Phonetic Transcription
speed	1	[spid]	[spiːd]
speedy	2	[ˈspi.di]	[ˈspiˑ.di]
speedily	3	[ˈspi.də.li]	[ˈspĭ.də.li]
will	1	[wɪl]	[wɪːɫ]
willing	2	[ˈwɪ.lɪŋ]	[ˈwɪˑ.lɪŋ]
willingly	3	[ˈwɪ.lɪŋ.li]	[ˈwĭl.ɪŋ.li]

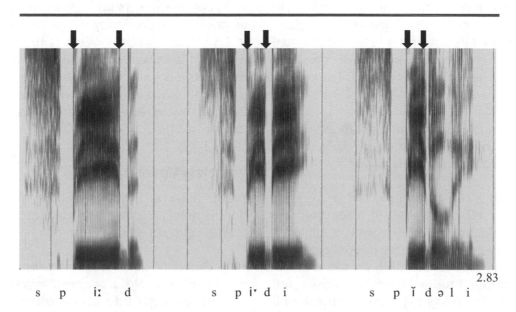

2.83

s p iː d   s p iˑ d i   s p ĭ d ə l i

FIGURE 8–10. Spectrogram comparing stressed vowel length in the words *speed, speedy, speedily.*

[spid] in each word. Then measure the length of each [i]. Did you confirm these vowel length distinctions?

You have now learned three phonological patterns of English that affect vowel length. When we produce vowel length differences in open and closed syllables that end with voiced or voiceless consonants, in stressed and unstressed syllables, and in multisyllabic words, the vowel length patterns interact. It is amazing that we as speakers convey such subtle vowel length differences to increase intelligibility in every word we produce without even thinking about them. Although they are unconscious, we are quite adept at manipulating this information. For instance, pay attention to what you do if someone does not understand something you say. Did you emphasize the length differences, without even thinking about it?

To further your understanding of these vowel length patterns, try recording some words yourself to contrast length contexts. You can record and analyze words to compare these vowel length differences using one of the free acoustic software programs suggested at the end of this chapter.

Vowel Reduction in Unstressed Syllables

In Chapter 5, you learned that in longer words and phrases in English, some vowels lose their stress, giving English its characteristic intonation pattern. These stressed syllables are longer than unstressed syllables. In many cases, the unstressed vowels are produced as reduced vowels. Most vowels of English can be reduced in running speech, in patterned ways. In English, as syllables are added, vowels in unstressed syllables tend to be reduced. The pattern for this is:

Stressed syllables are said at approximately regular intervals, and unstressed syllables are reduced to fit this rhythm.

Thus, most vowels can be reduced. While [ʌ, ɝ, eɪ, oʊ] are transcribed as [ə, ɚ, e, o] when they are reduced, the reduction of other vowels is captured differently. If the vowel phoneme does not change, you can indicate vowel reduction by using a diacritic. For example, produce the words *exploit* and *exploitation*. Was the vowel [ɔɪ] shorter in the second

word? This vowel length change results from the changes in stress and word length. We can capture the vowel length differences with narrow transcription: [ɛks.ˈplɔɪt] versus [ɛks.plɔɪ̆.ˈteɪ.ʃən], with the [˘] diacritic describing the shorter diphthong.

Vowel reduction occurs as the rate of speaking increases or as stress on a vowel is decreased. In general, the reduced vowel's duration decreases and the vowel is produced in a more centralized manner. If a vowel in an unstressed syllable changes its vowel quality, the reduced vowel is typically [ə] in most tertiary or less stressed syllables. For example, the [oʊ] in *phone* changes quality when the primary word stress shifts in the word *phonetics*. We would capture the vowel change by transcribing with a schwa: [fə.ˈnɛ.ɾɪks]. Reduced vowels are also transcribed with [ɪ].

Vowel alternations are frequent in words as they get longer. In *explain*, pronounced [ɛk.ˈspleɪn/, both vowels are reduced when the word becomes *explanation* and the third vowel receives primary stress: [ĕk.splə.ˈneɪ.ʃən].

Vowel reduction also occurs in monosyllable words in longer sentences. Figure 8–11 is a spectrogram of the sentence *We saw you pet the cat,* pronounced [wi sa ju pɛt ðə kæt]. Segment the spectrogram to find the vowels. Now compare duration of the vowels in *the* and in *cat*. How long is the vowel in each word? You should find that the vowel in *the* is much shorter in length than the vowel in *cat*.

As our speech gets faster, we tend to reduce most unstressed vowels. Many vowels eventually reduce to [ə] if the vowel phoneme is in a multisyllabic word and is an unreduced vowel. In addition to [ə], many vowels reduce to [ɪ] in unstressed syllables. If you transcribe reduced vowels with [ɪ], remember that this unstressed vowel is shorter in duration than the stressed [ɪ].

Voiceless Vowels

You have learned that vowels are voiced by definition. However, reduced vowels may be voiceless in certain contexts. This pattern can be described as:

Reduced vowels are often voiceless between two voiceless stops, or after a voiceless stop or voiceless stop cluster in an unstressed syllable.

Voiceless vowels are frequent when unstressed reduced vowels occur between voiceless stops at the beginning of the word, or when a reduced vowel occurs before a stressed syllable. Some speakers only produce a voiceless vowel when the reduced vowel is between two voiceless sounds.

Figure 8–12 is a spectrogram of the words *pecan* and *picky*, contrasting the vowels in the first syllable.

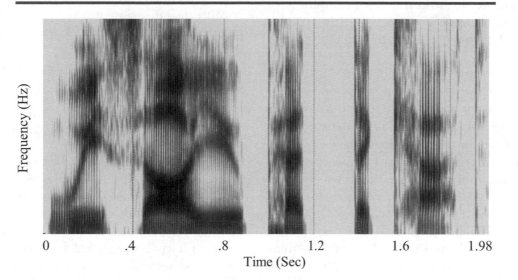

FIGURE 8–11. Spectrogram of the sentence. *We saw you pet the cat.*

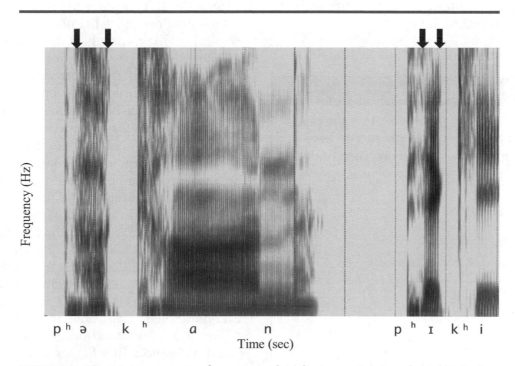

FIGURE 8–12. Spectrograms of *pecan* and *picky* to contrast reduced voiceless and voiced vowels.

In *pecan,* the first syllable is unstressed and follows the voiceless aspirated [pʰ]. Note that the first vowel is voiceless, while in the second word, *picky,* the first vowel is stressed and voiced. Can you see the difference on the spectrograms? The first word, narrowly transcribed as [pʰə̥.ˈkan], does not have a voicing bar at 100 Hz, confirming the voiceless quality of this vowel. In contrast, the first vowel in [ˈpʰɪː.ki] has a voicing bar that continues through the vowel's production.

At times, a reduced vowel is deleted. The easiest way to determine whether a reduced vowel is voiceless or deleted is by counting syllables. A voiceless vowel is a placeholder for a syllable; it ensures that the word with a reduced vowel does not lose its syllable shape. To demonstrate this, say the word *suppose* quickly. You probably did so in one of two ways. If you say *suppose* quickly with two syllables, there will be a voiceless schwa in the first syllable: [sə̥.ˈpʰoʊːz]. You can also say *suppose* quickly as a one-syllable word, [spoʊːz]. Notice how the different productions result in the application of different allophonic consonant patterns. If you say *suppose* as a two-syllable word with a voiceless vowel, [p] is aspirated. If you delete the first vowel, you create an /sp/ cluster, and [p] is no longer aspirated as a result of the stop consonant cluster rule that applies.

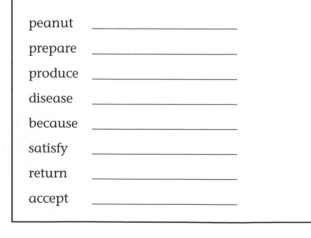

? | 8–3. Did You Get It?

Look at the list of words below. Circle the words that could have a voiceless reduced vowel in them. Then narrowly transcribe each of these words.

peanut   _____

prepare   _____

produce   _____

disease   _____

because   _____

satisfy   _____

return   _____

accept   _____

Vowel Nasalization

All English vowel phonemes are oral (that is, non-nasal). But we do produce nasal vowels allophonically in English since vowels are nasalized as a result of coarticulation in certain contexts. In English, vowel nasalization is allophonic, not phonemic, because nasalization serves no contrastive role in meaning. In some languages, such as French, nasalized vowels are phonemic.

The context for when vowels can become nasalized in English is:

> *Vowels are nasalized in syllables*
> *closed by a nasal consonant.*

This pattern only applies to vowels followed by a nasal consonant. If the syllable begins with a nasal consonant, the vowel is not nasalized. Vowel nasalization results from coarticulation. Because nasalizing the vowel does not affect intelligibility or the vowel that will be perceived, English vowels are typically nasalized if there is a nasal consonant that follows them. Table 8–5 compares broad and narrow transcription for vowels, showing nasalization for vowels that fit this coarticulatory pattern.

Figures 8–13 compares the words *can* versus *cat* in a spectrogram. Note the nasal bar in the [n]. Do you see how the formants in the two [æ] vowels differ? Can you see the nasal bar in the vowel in *can,* as well as the faded nasal formants?

If a syllable starts with a nasal, the following vowel is less likely to be nasalized. A nasalized vowel is likely in *can,* but less likely in *knack.* Say the words *nap* and *pan* aloud, elongating the vowels in both productions. Do you hear the oral vowel in *nap* and the nasal vowel in *pan*? If you remember our discussion of coarticulation in Chapter 7, producing the nasal vowel in the word *pan* is an example of anticipatory coarticulation, which is the most common type of coarticulation in English.

While the nasalization pattern applies to vowels followed by a nasal consonant, some individuals nasalize vowels if they are preceded by a nasal consonant; such nasalization would be an example of carryover coarticulation. There also are individual differences in whether vowels followed by some word-medial nasals are nasalized. For example, some people nasalize the vowel in *funny,* pronounced [ˈfʌ̃.ni], and others do not.

TABLE 8–5. Vowel Nasalization Transcription

Word	Ends with Nasal Consonant?	Broad Phonetic Transcription	Narrow Phonetic Transcription
beat	no	[bit]	[bit]
bean	yes	[bin]	[bĩn]
son	yes	[sʌn]	[sʌ̃n]
song	yes	[saŋ]	[sã̃ŋ]
knock	no	[nɑk]	[nɑk]
hymn	yes	[hɪm]	[hɪ̃m]
map	no	[mæp]	[mæp]

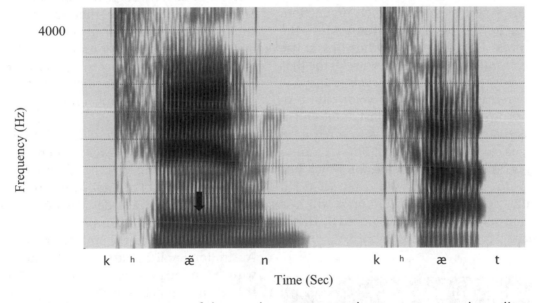

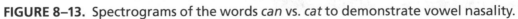

FIGURE 8–13. Spectrograms of the words *can* vs. *cat* to demonstrate vowel nasality.

? **8–4. Did You Get It?**

In the list of words below, underline the words that have a nasal vowel in them. Then transcribe those words.

queen _____

messy _____

tempo _____

men _____

bench _____

notch _____

Vowel Retraction

In Chapter 7, we learned the pattern for allophonic productions of syllable-final /l/ as a velar l, [ɫ]. The velarization of [l] affects vowels. The context is:

Vowels are retracted before syllable final [ɫ].

The velarization of syllable-final [l] affects the vowel preceding it due to anticipatory coarticulation. As a result of this coarticulation, vowels are produced with the root of the tongue retracted, resulting in a farther-back production for the vowel than in other environments.

As we hope you remember from Chapter 4, the diacritical mark for a retracted vowel is a lower level underline: [x̠].

To compare retracted and nonretracted vowel productions, say the words *see, seal,* and *seat* slowly, elongating the vowel as you say each production. Is your tongue farther back in *seal* than it is in the other two words? Be sure to note what [l] you are producing: you will only retract the vowel if the [l] is velarized. Narrow transcription of *seal* is [sḭɫ].

Vowels are retracted if there is a velarized-l produced in the coda of a syllable, not just at the end of a word. Thus *call* can be produced with a retracted vowel, [kɑ̠ɫ], as can *calling:* [kɑ̠ɫ.lɪŋ]. This is because [l] in *calling* is ambisyllabic. And *health,* which has [ɫθ] in the coda, is produced with a retracted [ɛ]: [hɛ̠ɫθ]. Finally, nonphonemic diphthongs will lose their diphthong quality preceding velarized [l]. Hence *sail* is produced [sḛɫ] and even [sɛ̠ɫ], but not [seɪɫ].

| **?** | **8–5. Did You Get It?** |

In the list of words below, underline the words that could have a retracted vowel in them. Then transcribe those words.

ball   _____

melted   _____

lamp   _____

cattle   _____

hapless   _____

chalk   _____

Rhotic Versus Nonrhotic Dialects of English

We conclude our introduction to English vowel patterns with a larger vowel allophonic pattern, the difference between rhotic and nonrhotic dialects of English. GAE is a rhotic dialect of English. This means that in GAE, rhotic vowels contrast meaning. Other rhotic dialects of English include Canadian, Irish, and Scottish English. Most dialects of English throughout the world are nonrhotic; in fact, rhotic vowels are some of the rarest vowels in any language. Most British English dialects are nonrhotic, as are Australian, New Zealand, and South African English. In the U. S., there are also nonrhotic English dialects, including some variations of African American Vernacular English and New England dialects.

That nonrhotic English dialects have consonant /ɹ/ but many do not have monophthong /ɝ/ or diphthong vowels ending in [ɚ] emphasizes the difference between consonant and vowel rhotics. Just as with rhotic English dialects, in nonrhotic dialects of English, consonant /ɹ/ is phonemic and it would be considered a speech error if syllable-initial /ɹ/ were not produced.

In general, nonrhotic dialects of English do not have rhotic vowels. However, there are allophonic exceptions. Rhotic vowels are produced in some nonrhotic dialects of English when a word ending in a rhotic vowel precedes a word that begins with a vowel, as in, for example, the utterance *My ear aches.* This is called the **linking-r.** For example, in Australian English, the word *fear* would be produced with "r" in the phrase, *my fear is.* . . . This "r" makes the distinction between the two vowel phones clear, much like the linking-n does in the a/an contrast, for example, we say *a cookie* but **an ice cream.**

Intrusive-r also occurs in some nonrhotic dialects. Intrusive-r can be produced when a word ending in a vowel is followed by a word that starts with a vowel. Like linking-r, intrusive-r serves to clearly differentiate two consecutive vowel phonemes. Intrusive-r would be produced in the phrase *The sofa is red,* transcribed [ðə ˈsoʊ.fə ɹɪz ɹɛd].

Nonrhotic dialects of English illuminate the underlying differences between the consonant and vowel rhotics. Many nonrhotic dialects appear to have had but then lost the vocalic "r" phoneme over time, while rhotic dialects retain final "r" as a vocalic "r", combining the rhotic property with the preceding vowel. The distinction between consonant and vowel rhotics in different dialects parallels the distinction between consonant and vowel rhotics in English, suggesting that the rhotics that occur in syllable nuclei are phonologically distinct from the consonant "r" in syllable onset.

Putting It All Together

You have now learned the most frequent vowel patterns for GAE. These vowel patterns include the allophones that exist in free variation in English for [ɝ, ʌ, eɪ, oʊ]. In addition, you have learned pho-nological patterns that underlie allophonic vowel productions in English in particular contexts. Table 8–6 summarizes these phonological patterns for vowels and provides examples of when they can occur.

You now know how to capture many of the different English vowel sounds using phonetic symbols and diacritics. Study the information regarding the production of vowels, as well as the phonetic symbols that represent them so that you can become adept at the skill of transcribing and hearing these distinctions. While the differences are subtle, the lack of the allophonic distinctions can decrease the intelligibility of a speaker; therefore, they are important to be aware of.

TABLE 8–6. Summary of Vowel Phonological Patterns

Vowel Pattern	Example Occurrence	
	Word(s)	**Narrow Transcription**
A vowel is (a) longest in an open syllable, (b) next longest in a syllable that ends with a voiced consonant, and (c) shortest if the syllable ends with a voiceless consonant.	shoe	[ʃuː]
	shoed	[ʃuˑd]
	shoot	[ʃŭt]
Vowels are longer in stressed syllables.	abduct	[əbˈ.dʌːkt]
	adduct	[æːˈdəkt]
Stressed vowels are (a) longest in a monosyllabic word, (b) next longest in a two-syllable word; and (c) shortest in a word that is three or more syllables.	leave	[liːv]
	believe	[bəˈliˑv]
	unbelievable	[ən.bəˈlĭv.ə.bəl]
Stressed syllables are said at approximately regular intervals, and unstressed syllables are reduced to fit this rhythm.	anesthesiology	[ˌæn.əz.θi.ˈzja.lə.dʒi]
	internationalization	[ɪ.nɚ.ˌnæ.ʃə.nəl.aɪ.ˈzeɪ.ʃən]
Reduced vowels are often voiceless after a voiceless stop or voiceless stop cluster in an unstressed syllable.	catastrophe	[kə̥ˈtæ.stɹə.fi]
	topography	[tə̥ˈpɑ.gɹə.fi]
Vowels are nasalized in syllables with a nasal consonant in the coda	queen	[kwĩn]
	hanger	[ˈhæ̃ŋ.ɚ]
Vowels are retracted if followed by /ɫ/ in the coda	poll	[pọɫ]
	wealth	[wɛ̣ɫθ]

Applied Science: Revisited

Summary

We began this chapter wondering if 8-year-old Elise had a speech sound disorder. Elise had recently moved from Australia to the United States. Her speech-language pathologist was concerned because Elise produced rhotics inconsistently. At least we thought she did when we applied the patterns for rhotic vowel production in General American English. As you have learned, though, phonological patterns apply to vowels and can change their phonetic realization. You also learned that dialects of English differ in their patterns for rhotic vowels. The final "r" in General American English is produced as a rhotic vowel in monophthongs, diphthongs, and triphthongs. In Australian English, the written "r" is not produced in word-final position, unless the word following the final "r" begins with a vowel. You also learned that Australian English has an intrusive-r: a rhotic inserted between words where no "r" is written if the first word ends with a vowel and the second word begins with a vowel.

One Step at a Time

Below we re-examine the sentences produced by Elise in her speech sample

Answer

Group A: Rhotic Vowel Produced Correctly

My teacher only speaks to us in Spanish.
[maɪ 'ti.tʃɚ 'oʊ.nli spiks tə ʌs ɪn 'spæ.nɪʃ]

My dad's car is being fixed.
[maɪ dædz kaɚ ɪz 'bi.ɪŋ fɪkst]

Did you hear a truck honking?
[dɪd ju hɪɚ ə tɹʌk 'haŋ.kɪŋ]

The butter is on the table.
[ðə 'bʌ.tɚ ɪz an ðə 'teɪ.bəl]

We find that the above rhotic productions fit the linking rule of Australian English. In every case, when Elise produces a rhotic vowel it is before another vowel.

Group B: Rhotic Vowel Deletion

The child can hear his dad.
[ðə tʃaɪld kæn hɪə hɪz dæd]

I would like a new car.
[aɪ wʊd laɪk ə nu kaə]

My teacher praised my project.
[maɪ 'ti.tʃə pɹeɪzd maɪ 'pɹa.dʒɛkt]

He eats peanut butter with jelly.
[hi its 'pi.nət 'bʌ.tə wɪð 'dʒɛ.li]

The deletion of rhotic "r" follows the Australian English rule for final rhotics. In every word that is spelled with word-final "r", Elise did not produce the rhotic vowel. If she were an American English speaker, we would consider this a rhotic vowel reduction, but for an Australian English speaker, the final "r" is just a written letter that is not produced, like the "gh" in *though*.

Group C: Rhotic Insertion

We had pasta and meatballs last night.
[wi hæd 'pas.tə ɹæn 'mit.bals læst naɪt]

Sofia is my best friend. ['soʊ.'fi.ə ɹɪz maɪ bɛst fɹɛnd]

I want a cookie after lunch.
[aɪ want ə 'kʊ.ki 'ɹæf.tə lʌntʃ]

Finally, we look at the words where "r" was inserted. In these phrases, Elise is applying the rule for intrusive-r, producing [ɹ] to divide two vowel productions.

Science Applied

We are glad that we researched Australian English vowel patterns before inappropriately diagnosing Elise with a speech disorder. We find that Elise is producing rhotic vowels accurately according to Australian English rules for rhotic vowel production. While it took extra research to learn the Australian English rhotic vowel patterns, the discovery that Elise's speech pattern was a difference in dialect and not a sign of disordered speech was an important one. It is not enough to know how to capture sounds phonetically, it is also important to know how those speech sounds are used in a language. Applying our knowledge of phonological rules to the errors in Elise's speech was critical to differentiating difference from disorder in her speech.

Interest Piqued?

Recommended materials to further your understanding of topics covered in this chapter.

Print Resources

Bragg, M. (2015). *The adventure of English: The biography of language.* New York, NY: Arcade.

Bryson, B. (2001). *The mother tongue: English and how it got that way.* New York, NY: William Morrow.

Katz, J. (2016). *Speaking American: How y'all, youse, and you guys talk: A visual guide.* Boston, MA: Houghton-Mifflin.

? Did You Get It?

ANSWER KEY

8–1.

Each word below is typically produced with [ə], [ʌ], or both of them. Underline the syllable (or syllables) that contain a wedge or a schwa. Put a check in the appropriate column if the word contains a schwa, wedge, or a schwa and a wedge. Then transcribe the word, marking the stressed vowel with the apostrophe diacritic at the beginning of the syllable.

Identifying and Transcribing Stressed and Unstressed Schwa and Wedge

	Word	[ə]	[ʌ]	Phonetic Transcription
1	re<u>view</u>	X		[ɹə.ˈvju]
2	<u>cu</u>pboard		X	[ˈkʌ.bɚd]
3	<u>ug</u>ly		X	[ˈʌg.li]
4	<u>a</u>lumi<u>num</u>	X		[ə.ˈlu.mɪ.nəm]
5	<u>fun</u>ny		X	[ˈfʌ.ni]
6	<u>pho</u>netics	X		[fə.ˈnɛ.tɪks]
7	ex<u>tra</u>	X		[ˈɛk.strə]
8	se<u>ven</u>ty	X		[ˈsɛ.vən.ti]

8–2.

Each multisyllabic word in the table below is produced with a stressed [ɝ] or unstressed [ɚ]. Underline the syllable (or syllables) that contains a stressed or unstressed schwar. Put a check in the appropriate column if the word contains a stressed [ɝ], an unstressed [ɚ], or one of each. Then transcribe the word.

Identifying and Transcribing Stressed and Unstressed Schwar

	Word	[ɝ]	[ɚ]	Phonetic Transcription
1	<u>cou</u>rageous		X	[kɚ.ˈeɪ.d͡ʒ.əs]
2	dis<u>cer</u>ning	X		[dɪ.ˈsɝ.nɪŋ]
3	<u>nou</u>rishment	X		[ˈnɝ.ɪʃ.mənt]
4	cup<u>board</u>		X	[ˈkʌ.bɚd]
5	<u>further</u>	X	X	[ˈfɝ.ðɚ]
6	en<u>cou</u>ragement	X		[ɛn.kɝ.əd͡ʒ.mənt]
7	fea<u>ther</u>		X	[ˈfɛ.ðɚ]
8	<u>burger</u>	X	X	[ˈbɝ.gɚ]

8–3.

Look at the list of words below. Underline the words that could have a voiceless reduced vowel in them. Then narrowly transcribe each of these words.

peanut

<u>prepare</u>   [pɹ̥ə̥.ˈpe͡ɚ]

<u>produce</u>   [pɹ̥ə̥.ˈdus]

disease

because

satisfy

return

accept

8–4.

In the list of words below, underline the words that have a nasal vowel in them. Then transcribe those words.

<u>queen</u>   [kwĩn]

messy

<u>tempo</u>   [ˈtẽm.po͡ʊ]

<u>men</u>   [mẽn]

<u>bench</u>   [bɛnt͡ʃ]

notch

8–5.

In the list of words below, underline the words that have a retracted vowel in them. Then transcribe those words.

<u>ball</u>   [bɑɫ]

<u>melted</u>   [mɛɫ.təd]

lamp

<u>cattle</u>   [ˈkæ.ɾəɫ]

hapless

chalk

9

BEYOND GENERAL AMERICAN ENGLISH
Speech Possibilities Within and Across Languages

Learning Objectives

By reading this chapter, you will learn:

1. information about languages of the world
2. the concepts of languages and dialects
3. different types of dialects, including dialects of English
4. different uses of the speech mechanism in other languages
5. different uses of the respiratory system in the production of speech
6. differences in VOT across languages
7. different uses of the phonatory system in other languages
8. differences in consonant manner and place categories across languages
9. different ways vowels are contrasted
10. differences in stress and intonation patterns across languages
11. differences in syllables across languages
12. general principles to consonant and vowel inventories in languages

---

Applied Science

Thirteen-year-old Geovany has been referred to you, a middle school speech-language pathologist, by his history teacher. His teacher explains that Geovany is extremely hard to understand, making sounds that are quite distracting when he speaks. To get a better sense of Geovany's speech, you observe Geovany in the cafeteria speaking with friends. As Geovany speaks, you do notice some unusual sounds, perhaps best described as back of the throat as well as popping noises. You also notice a breathy, nasal quality to Geovany's speech. It is also clear that he has not been speaking English for very long.

In preparation for your speech assessment, you review Geovany's school records. You learn that Geovany came to the United States from Guatemala 10 months ago and that he had only learned a little English before he arrived. School records indicate that Geovany speaks K'iche and Spanish at home. Although you know nothing about K'iche, you suspect that the unusual sounds in Geovany's English are influenced by sounds from K'iche. With strong multicultural training as a speech-pathologist, you suspect that Geovany's unusual speech may be a result of a difference rather than a disorder. In other words, you wonder if the atypical sounds in Geovany's English are being carried over from Spanish or K'iche.

You begin your full speech evaluation of Geovany. You will fully review his school records and learn more about his background and developmental history from his parents. You will request a K'iche-Spanish speaking interpreter to assist you in the assessment process of understanding Geovany's speech in all three languages. You will then meet with Geovany to gather speech samples from him, transcribing what sounds he produces in English, Spanish, and K'iche. You also realize you must learn more about K'iche and Spanish before concluding that Geovany's speech differences are not a disorder. As you read this chapter, think about what information you will need to correctly make this determination.

Speech Possibilities

This final chapter expands on your knowledge of phonetics by exploring ways languages and dialects can and do differ in speech production. You have learned how humans contrast meaning with sounds through consonant, vowel, word structure, and suprasegmental differences, as well as ways these phonetic properties can vary allophonically without changing meaning. To simplify these topics initially, this text has focused on the phonological properties of the dialect of English this book was written in: General American English. Focusing on GAE has given you a clear foundation for the principles of phonetics. However, the phonetic properties of GAE do not provide you with a full picture of the ways the human vocal tract can be used to contrast meaning across languages. There are also many ways sounds differ across dialects of languages, including English.

In this final chapter, we explore differences across languages and the many ways humans manipulate the speech mechanism to communicate by providing an overview of the impressive range and number of languages and dialects around the globe. We then introduce possibilities for speech that are not exploited in GAE, including other ways of manipulating the airstream, articulating consonants and vowels, phonating, and contrasting stress, intonation, and length. This deeper knowledge of speech potential prepares you to work with clients from a variety of linguistic backgrounds, including **bilingual** (user of two languages), **multilingual** (user of more than two languages), and non-English speaking individuals. It also provides research and clinical tools that can assist you as you encounter different ways people speak English, including accented, developing, and disordered speech.

As you learned in Chapter 1, the field of phonetics allows us to describe and classify speech sounds that occur in all spoken languages. The goal of the International Phonetic Association was a symbol system that captured all the sounds of languages with as few symbols as possible. There are IPA symbols for the most common sounds, and diacritics adding additional information for less common sounds. However, the IPA tends to describe the sounds of Indo-European languages better and with fewer diacritics than the sounds of many Asian, African, and American languages that have more complex consonant and vowel systems.

The World's Languages and Speakers of Them

The world's languages can be organized hierarchically into language families, languages, and dialects. Before we examine these, it is important to recognize how fluid language categories are. While you can find counts of languages, the numbers reported differ dramatically among linguists. There cannot be exact counts of languages, because what constitutes a language can be defined in multiple ways. **Dialects**, defined as mutually intelligible variants of a language, are categorized in different ways by linguists as well. For this reason, all of the language family, language, and dialect counts presented below are approximates.

Language families are groups of related languages that share linguistic properties. Comparative linguists study the shared features, attempting to trace back the languages of a language family to a **proto-language**, a hypothesized single language that shares properties with and is considered the predecessor connecting the current languages in the language family. Frequently, languages in a language family share phonological features that are not observed in other language families. There are 18 agreed upon language families, although some linguists define even more. English and 440 other languages belong to the Indo-European language family, as do other Germanic languages. Romance languages, which include Italian and Spanish, are another branch of the Indo-European language family, as are Armenian and Hellenic. Niger-Congo is the world's largest language family, comprising ~1,500 or almost 20% of the world's languages. At the other end of the continuum are **language isolates** like Basque, spoken in Spain. Language isolates, do not belong to a language family and do not share a proto-language with any other language in the world today.

Even though many Americans can go days without hearing any language except English, English is only one of approximately 7,000 living languages. The native language of the most people in the world is Mandarin, spoken by over a billion people. There are also languages that have only a few speakers, and every year a few languages are lost as the final speaker of these languages dies. From most to least number of native speakers, the top 10 languages in the world are Mandarin Chinese, Spanish, English, Hindi/Urdu, Arabic, Portuguese, Bengali, Russian, Japanese, and Javanese. If we count languages by the number of native and non-native people who speak them, English is spoken by the most people in the world, followed by Mandarin Chinese, Hindi/Urdu, Spanish, Russian/Belarusian, Arabic, Bengali, Malay, Portuguese, and Japanese.

English is the official or de facto language of roughly 100 countries in the world. English is the de facto language of the United States because there is not an officially recognized language. Other languages spoken in many countries include Arabic (60 countries), French (50), Spanish (30), and Russian and Portuguese, both spoken in 11 countries. English and other widely spoken languages often serve as a **lingua franca**, a language used to communicate between individuals who do not share the same first language. In fact, many countries recognize English as an official language, even when only a minority of people in the country speak it. For example, English is one of two official languages of India, even though over 40% of Indians do not speak English.

Dialect Versus Language

A **language** can be defined as a community's shared communication system of words and the rules for combining and producing those words. **Dialects** are variants of a language that are mutually intelligible but differ in linguistic properties and are spoken by a subgroup. It is typical for one dialect of a language to be given "language" status, but understand the limitations of such status. Every dialect of a language has equal standing as a communication system. Nonetheless, it is true that at any point in time, the language with the arbitrary higher status tends to be referred to as the language, which results in the other variants being considered lesser. From a linguistic perspective, *any* dialect could be the dialect with language status. But from a sociological perspective, the language with the most power—political, economic, prestige—tends to be referred to and thought of as the language. Regardless, in no way is that particular dialect better or more correct. It just got lucky.

It is not simple to distinguish languages and dialects. Linguists differ on what they consider to be a language and how they define distinctions and "mutual intelligibility." Importantly, speakers of languages do not always agree with linguists. There are no absolutes for dialects, or for languages. Most frequently, whether the communication system of a specific group has language or dialect status has more to do with politics and power than it does linguistic properties. For example, Danish, Swedish, and Norwegian are considered different languages and are spoken in different countries. However, Danish, Swedish, and Norwegian speakers can carry on trilingual conversations, with each person speaking his/her own language. The three languages are so similar that speakers will have little difficulty understanding each other (McWhorter, 2016). In contrast, Italian is often referred to as a language, even though there are 25 different "dialects" of Italian, many of which are not mutually intelligible, and these dialects come from Romance, Germanic, and Slavic branches of the Indo-European language family.

There is no systematic and error-proof way to measure mutual intelligibility. Factors that play into whether two communication systems are dialects or languages are affected by multiple elements, including whether one group has greater value or greater power, one subculture is valued more than the other, the two spoken languages share a writing system, or the language groups share the same religion or country, among other factors. Linguist Max Weinrich is credited with the statement, "a language is a dialect with an army and a navy." There are many examples of civil wars bringing about or exacerbating existing political, religious, and cultural divisions that result in subgroups of people who were considered to speak the same language prior to the conflict, but who purported to no longer understand one another afterwards. A fairly recent example of the shift from dialects to distinct languages took place when the former Yugoslavia became seven distinct countries. Prior to Yugoslavia's dissolution, the country's language was considered Serbo-Croatian, of which there were many dialects. Now it depends on political and cultural views as to whether the language is referred to as Serbo-Croatian or as Bosnian, Croatian, Montenegrin, Serbian, or another language. Even linguists differ on whether they consider Serbo-Croatian to be onelanguage with many dialects, or many separate languages.

Dialects are further broken down by their geneses. **Regional dialects** are variants of a language that can be traced to the geographic region of the speakers or their ancestors. **Social dialects** are not geographically based but tend to be shared by individuals identifying as a subgroup of a community. Social dialects result from shared identities related to ethnic, cultural, religious, social class, and age groups. Dialects are further differentiated by the age of the speaker, what they are talking about, where they are talking about it (e.g., home?, work place?, with friends?, etc.), and social status.

Before we proceed, we want to caution you in generalizing about a particular dialect, or language, for that matter. Dialects and languages are on a continuum, and even within dialects there are continua of phonological and linguistic properties. Languages and sound systems are alive and constantly evolving. We want to describe, rather than prescribe, how people talk.

English

Now that you have a familiarity with the concepts of dialects, languages, and language families, we will look a little more closely at English. The English people colonized many parts of the world and left behind a widespread linguistic influence. There are approximately 30 dialects of English spoken in England, 14 in Ireland, 20+ in India, and 5 to 8 in Australia. There are other English dialects spoken in Scotland, Wales, Northern Ireland, Isle of Man, Gibraltar, South Africa, Nigeria, Kenya, Swaziland, Tanzania, Bahamas, and Guyana, as well as in many other countries. Thus, there are individuals from all over the world whose first language is a dialect of English or who grew up learning English and other languages simultaneously. It can be shocking for Nigerians or Guyanese to come to the United States and be told by an uninformed American that they are doing a great job learning English when they speak their own English dialect perfectly!

While there are many people in the U.S. who speak English only, many of them are bi-dialectal and all of them are exposed to individuals who speak different dialects of English, whether the dialect is different because of the region of the United States the people are from, the country they learned English in, the social group they identify with, or the context in which they communicate with each other. As a college student, you have likely had experience with people from all four groups!

U.S. social dialects that are identified with cultural groups include African American Vernacular English (AAVE), Cajun Vernacular English, and Chicano English. These social dialects tend to be used by individuals who identify with specific ethnic groups. While cultural dialects tend to be spoken by ethnic groups, that is not always the case. For example, there are many African Americans who do not speak AAVE and there are people who do not identify as African American who do. AAVE shares many phonological properties with rural Southern dialects of English. AAVE can differ in vowels, such as monophthongization of diphthongs; consonant differences, with /ð/ pronounced as [d] or [t] word-initially and [v] or [f] word-finally; and phonotactic differences, including cluster reductions and deletion of some final consonants. Many of these phonological patterns are shared with regional dialects of English, such as U.S. Southern dialects and dialects in England. There are dialects that are both social and regional, such as Pennsylvania Dutch English, spoken in some older Amish and Mennonite communities in the Northeast of the U.S.

United States dialects of English tend to differ more in vowel properties than consonants. There are dialects in which speakers produce /æ/ in words like *bag*, producing a vowel much closer to [ɛ] than [æ]. There are speakers of dialects that do not phonemically contrast /ɪ/ and /ɛ/. There are also many American English dialects where diphthongs are monophthongized, such as *oil* produced as [ɔl] instead of [ɔɪl], as in a West Texas dialect, or *hi* produced as [ha] rather than [haɪ] in Appalachian English. In addition, there are many nonrhotic varieties of American English, such as a New York dialect and some variations of AAVE.

We must admit to being hypocrites. We have just warned you not to overgeneralize dialects. However, throughout this textbook we simplified vowel contrasts in GAE to two versions, one dialect that has a phonemic contrast between /ɑ/ and /ɔ/ and one that considers [ɑ] and [ɔ] as allophones of /ɑ/. By doing so, we have oversimplified GAE, because some dialects of English have only /ɔ/, not /ɑ/. There are other dialects that produce the /ɑ/ phoneme as [a], or raised, more rounded, and backed versions of the [a] vowel, with other regions of the country producing the [ɑ] vowel more like [ʊ]. We hope that you are beginning to grasp the complexities of languages and dialects.

While not as frequent, consonants can also differ across English dialects, with, for example, some regional and social dialects differing in substitution of [t] for /θ/. This occurs in regional dialects in New England and in social dialects such as AAVE.

Bilingualism

Most people in the world are bilingual and many are trilingual. Many speakers of English in the Western hemisphere are monolingual English speakers, especially in England, the U.S., New Zealand, and Australia. But monolingualism in the U.S. is exaggerated. The U.S. Census Bureau estimates the number of languages spoken in the U.S. at around 350. Only one of those languages is English. Over 20% of the U.S. population speaks more than one language at home. And many other people in the United States may not speak another language at home, but speak two or more languages well enough to use the second language at work, with extended family and friends, or in social or other environments. Many people have learned English as a second language. That means many people in the U.S. are bilingual—knowing the phonology for more than one language—or are exposed to adults who speak two languages and likely speak English with influences from their first language(s). As people learn a second language, their first language can influence it, and as clinical scientists we need to be aware of how segmental and phonotactic properties of one language can influence these properties in a second language. There may be subtle differences from monolingual speakers in sounds and phonological patterns. Individuals who are exposed to Spanish, for instance, will be familiar with a language that does and one that does not make phonemic tense/lax vowel distinctions. In English, some Spanish speakers will indicate tense/lax distinctions exclusively or primarily with vowel length distinctions. This difference in use of the vowel space can affect English production.

Communities worldwide have developed a remarkable number of languages and dialects to communicate with each other. The variety of sounds in these languages reflects the human capacity to create sounds with the vocal tract. English has capitalized on only a few of these sound contrasts. Thank goodness you have gained a strong foundation of the ways sound can be manipulated in the vocal tract, as well as phonetic symbols and transcription skills to be able to describe and transcribe this larger variety of sounds.

? 9–1. Did You Get It?

1. Variants of a language that are mutually intelligible are called _____.

2. Which type of dialect is Chicano English? _____

3. Which type of dialect is Appalachian English? _____

4. Languages that share a protolanguage are called a _____.

5. If people who speak two different languages share a third language to speak to each other, that shared language is called a _____.

Speech Sounds Across Languages

Learning about English has provided you with an exposure to many of the most common ways of producing speech sounds. English has quite a few vowels, a variety of consonants, complex syllable and word shapes, and different ways of manipulating suprasegmentals to convey distinct meanings. While you have the building blocks for transcribing other languages, there are many ways languages contrast sounds that are not utilized in English. As clinical scientists, it is important to know all the possible ways to articulate consonants and vowels and manipulate the airstream, phonation, and intona-

tion. This information is useful for understanding how different sounds are made and for transcribing new languages, different dialects of English, non-English, and even disordered speech.

Up until now you have been transcribing with a subset of possible phonetic symbols. To capture new sounds, you need to use the full IPA, shown in Figure 9–1. Take a moment to familiarize yourself with this chart. You will see many phonetic symbols and diacritics you know well, as well as some unfamiliar ones. You may also notice some differences in the chart from how we have transcribed and categorized sounds in this textbook. New symbols and diacritics will be introduced in the following sections of this chapter. As you explore these new sounds, we encourage you to visit many of the websites we have listed at the end of this chapter. Doing so will familiarize you with the sounds of these phonetic symbols, as well as the phonemic contrasts in other languages that contain them.

Consonants

English has 24 consonants. To uniquely define the consonants of English we have needed three properties: place of articulation, manner of articulation, and voicing. However, there are about 600 different consonants that have been identified in the world's languages! English has a moderate-sized consonant inventory compared with many languages, and most consonants of English are common in other languages of the world. That is, places of articulation such as bilabial, alveolar, and velar are used phonemically in many languages, as are the manner classes of stops, nasals, fricatives, and glides. The sounds of GAE that are infrequent in other languages are /θ, ð, ɹ/. English consonants also use the most common phonation types and airstream. Let's build on the information we know about English consonants to understand how at least some of those other 576 consonants are produced.

Place and Manner of Articulation
English consonants make use of many of the possibilities for place and manner obstruction. There are a few new place and manner categories that exist for sounds in other languages and there are ways to combine these categories to make unique sounds that do not exist in English.

THE INTERNATIONAL PHONETIC ALPHABET (revised to 2015)

CONSONANTS (PULMONIC)

© 2015 IPA

	Bilabial	Labiodental	Dental	Alveolar	Postalveolar	Retroflex	Palatal	Velar	Uvular	Pharyngeal	Glottal
Plosive	p b			t d		ʈ ɖ	c ɟ	k ɡ	q ɢ		ʔ
Nasal	m	ɱ		n		ɳ	ɲ	ŋ	ɴ		
Trill	ʙ			r					ʀ		
Tap or Flap		ⱱ		ɾ		ɽ					
Fricative	ɸ β	f v	θ ð	s z	ʃ ʒ	ʂ ʐ	ç ʝ	x ɣ	χ ʁ	ħ ʕ	h ɦ
Lateral fricative				ɬ ɮ							
Approximant		ʋ		ɹ		ɻ	j	ɰ			
Lateral approximant				l		ɭ	ʎ	ʟ			

Symbols to the right in a cell are voiced, to the left are voiceless. Shaded areas denote articulations judged impossible.

CONSONANTS (NON-PULMONIC)

Clicks	Voiced implosives	Ejectives
ʘ Bilabial	ɓ Bilabial	ʼ Examples:
ǀ Dental	ɗ Dental/alveolar	pʼ Bilabial
ǃ (Post)alveolar	ʄ Palatal	tʼ Dental/alveolar
ǂ Palatoalveolar	ɠ Velar	kʼ Velar
ǁ Alveolar lateral	ʛ Uvular	sʼ Alveolar fricative

OTHER SYMBOLS

ʍ Voiceless labial-velar fricative

w Voiced labial-velar approximant

ɥ Voiced labial-palatal approximant

ʜ Voiceless epiglottal fricative

ʢ Voiced epiglottal fricative

ʡ Epiglottal plosive

ɕ ʑ Alveolo-palatal fricatives

ɺ Voiced alveolar lateral flap

ɧ Simultaneous ʃ and x

Affricates and double articulations can be represented by two symbols joined by a tie bar if necessary.

t͡s k͡p

VOWELS

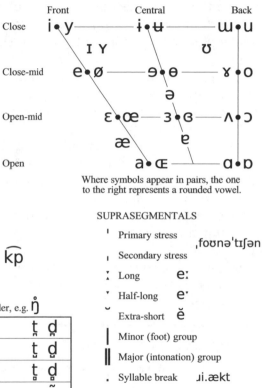

Where symbols appear in pairs, the one to the right represents a rounded vowel.

SUPRASEGMENTALS

ˈ	Primary stress	ˌfoʊnəˈtɪʃən
ˌ	Secondary stress	
ː	Long	eː
ˑ	Half-long	eˑ
˘	Extra-short	ĕ
ǀ	Minor (foot) group	
‖	Major (intonation) group	
.	Syllable break	ɹi.ækt
‿	Linking (absence of a break)	

DIACRITICS Some diacritics may be placed above a symbol with a descender, e.g. ŋ̊

̥ Voiceless	n̥ d̥	̤ Breathy voiced	b̤ a̤	̪ Dental	t̪ d̪
̬ Voiced	s̬ t̬	̰ Creaky voiced	b̰ a̰	̺ Apical	t̺ d̺
ʰ Aspirated	tʰ dʰ	̼ Linguolabial	t̼ d̼	̻ Laminal	t̻ d̻
̹ More rounded	ɔ̹	ʷ Labialized	tʷ dʷ	̃ Nasalized	ẽ
̜ Less rounded	ɔ̜	ʲ Palatalized	tʲ dʲ	ⁿ Nasal release	dⁿ
̟ Advanced	u̟	ˠ Velarized	tˠ dˠ	ˡ Lateral release	dˡ
̠ Retracted	e̠	ˤ Pharyngealized	tˤ dˤ	̚ No audible release	d̚
̈ Centralized	ë	̴ Velarized or pharyngealized	ɫ		
̽ Mid-centralized	e̽	̝ Raised	e̝ (ɹ̝ = voiced alveolar fricative)		
̩ Syllabic	n̩	̞ Lowered	e̞ (β̞ = voiced bilabial approximant)		
̯ Non-syllabic	e̯	̘ Advanced Tongue Root	e̘		
˞ Rhoticity	ɚ a˞	̙ Retracted Tongue Root	e̙		

TONES AND WORD ACCENTS

LEVEL			CONTOUR		
e̋ or ˥	Extra high		ě or ˩˥	Rising
é or ˦	High		ê or ˥˩	Falling
ē or ˧	Mid		e᷄ or ˦˥	High rising
è or ˨	Low		e᷅ or ˩˨	Low rising
ȅ or ˩	Extra low		e᷈ or ˧˦˧	Rising-falling
ꜜ Downstep			↗ Global rise
ꜛ Upstep			↘ Global fall

FIGURE 9–1. Full chart of the IPA. *Source:* Copyright © 2015 International Phonetic Association. Available under a Creative Commons Attribution-Sharealike 3.0 Unported License.

As a review, in English we constrict or obstruct air in many locations in the oral tract, resulting in phoneme place categories of bilabial, labiodental, interdental, alveolar, post-alveolar, alveopalatal, palatal, velar, and glottal. We also constrict air in different ways, including differing ways for oral and nasal stops, glides, fricatives, affricates, and liquids. Because there are even more ways to constrict air in the oral cavity, in this chapter we will call stops by their more technical term: plosives. Figure 9–2 is a subset of phonetic symbols from the IPA phonetic symbol chart that shows only pulmonic egressive speech sounds; that is, those consonants that can be made with the place categories described above on exhaled airflow from the lungs. We will explore these broader place and manner categories next.

Active and Passive Articulators. As we learn new places of articulation, we need to identify the role each articulator is playing in the constriction or obstruction. In consonant production, there is typically one **active** and one **passive** articulator. The active articulator moves to touch or approximate the passive articulator. As an example, if you produce [d], your tongue tip moves to briefly touch the alveolar ridge; therefore, the tongue tip is the active articulator and the alveolar ridge is the passive articulator.

Active articulators are typically lower surface articulators. The only exception is the upper lip, because both lips move to produce bilabial sounds; therefore, the upper lip is an active articulator. Figure 9–3 illustrates all active articulators. From front to back, the active articulators are the lips, underside of the tongue (for retroflex sounds), tongue tip, tongue blade, tongue front, and tongue back. These active articulators are used for English sounds. Think of sounds produced using an active articulator. Again, the only upper surface articulator that is active is the upper lip, which moves to meet the lower lip (which is also active) for bilabial sounds. The tongue back is an active articulator in velar sounds, where it is raised to the soft palate. Figure 9–3 introduces you to two new active articulators as well: the tongue root and the epiglottis. Both the tongue root and the epiglottis can move to approximate the pharyngeal wall during consonant production.

The passive articulators are primarily upper surface articulators. Figure 9–4 illustrates the passive articulators. The passive upper surface articulators are, from front to back, the upper teeth, alveolar ridge, post-alveolar region, hard palate, soft palate, and uvula. If you remember from Chapter 2, the uvula is the fleshy extension of the soft palate. You can see the uvula hanging down at the back of your mouth if you open your mouth wide while looking into a mirror. The uvula is the only upper surface articulator that is not used in English. Additionally, the pharyngeal wall serves as a passive articulator for consonants in many languages.

CONSONANTS (PULMONIC)   © 2015 IPA

	Bilabial	Labiodental	Dental	Alveolar	Postalveolar	Retroflex	Palatal	Velar	Uvular	Pharyngeal	Glottal
Plosive	p b			t d		ʈ ɖ	c ɟ	k g	q ɢ		ʔ
Nasal	m	ɱ		n		ɳ	ɲ	ŋ	ɴ		
Trill	ʙ			r					ʀ		
Tap or Flap		ⱱ		ɾ		ɽ					
Fricative	ɸ β	f v	θ ð	s z	ʃ ʒ	ʂ ʐ	ç ʝ	x ɣ	χ ʁ	ħ ʕ	h ɦ
Lateral fricative				ɬ ɮ							
Approximant		ʋ		ɹ		ɻ	j	ɰ			
Lateral approximant				l		ɭ	ʎ	ʟ			

Symbols to the right in a cell are voiced, to the left are voiceless. Shaded areas denote articulations judged impossible.

FIGURE 9–2. Pulmonic egressive consonants. *Source:* Copyright © 2015 International Phonetic Association. Available under a Creative Commons Attribution-Sharealike 3.0 Unported License.

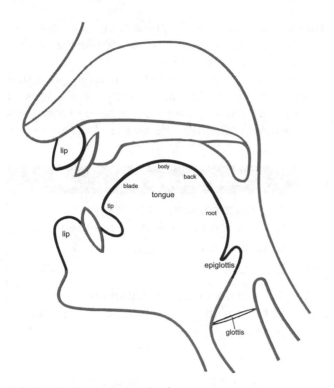

FIGURE 9–3. Active articulators.

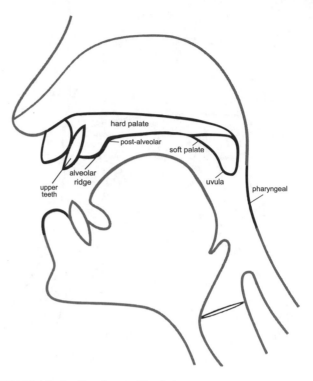

FIGURE 9–4. Passive articulators.

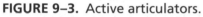

? 9–2. Did You Get It?

1. As an articulator for speech sounds, the hard palate is:
   a. a passive lower surface structure
   b. an active lower surface structure
   c. a passive upper surface structure
   d. an active upper surface structure

2. The following is a passive articulator:
   a. the uvula
   b. the tip of the tongue
   c. the back of the tongue
   d. the lower lip

Place of Articulation. Figure 9–5 shows the possible places of articulation. The arrows indicate the movement of the active articulator to the passive articulator. Most of these places of articulation are familiar to you, but there are some that involve the new active and passive articulators you just learned

about. **Retroflex**, an allophonic place of production for English "r," is a phonemic place of articulation in many languages. The active articulator for retroflex sounds is in the underside of the tongue. During a retroflex consonant production, the tongue tip is up and the underside of the tongue tip approximates or touches the post-alveolar region. **Uvular** consonants are those where the back of the tongue approximates the uvula. In uvular sounds, the back of the tongue is active and the uvula is passive. Consonants produced in the pharyngeal cavity are called **pharyngeal**, noting the movement of the active articulator, the tongue root or the epiglottis, to the passive articulator, the pharyngeal wall. Even though both the tongue root and the epiglottis can move to the pharyngeal wall, the single place category is pharyngeal, similar to the use of the tip or blade of the tongue as an active articulator in alveolar sounds.

Manner of Articulation. English utilizes many of the possible phonemic manner categories. These include plosives, nasals, glides, fricatives, and liquids. The International Phonetic Association does

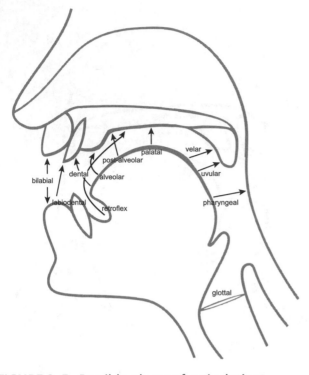

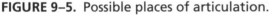

FIGURE 9–5. Possible places of articulation.

approximant or fricative production or escape centrally after the obstruction related to plosive or affricate production is released.

Now that you have learned the possible place and manner categories for consonants, we will look at manner differences across languages by place category, reviewing English categories at the same time.

? 9–3. Did You Get It?

1. Two place categories that are phonemic in other languages but are not used in English are _____ and _____ .

2. Two manner categories that are phonemic in other languages but are not used in English are _____ and _____ .

3. Phonemes produced with central obstruction while air is released on the sides of the tongue are called _____ .

---

not officially recognize affricates as a unique manner category but considers the affricate a composite speech sound. Affricates are considered phonemic in English and are an important phonemic category in speech-language pathology in English.

Consonants can be made by constricting or obstructing air in ways beyond those of English. **Trills** are produced by approximating two articulators and setting one of them in motion. Taps, used allophonically in English, are phonemic in many languages. As you have learned, taps are produced by quickly and lightly bringing one articulator to the other, obstructing air very briefly without the burst characteristic of stops.

Centrality. Central versus lateral release is a final distinction necessary to differentiate consonant obstruction in other languages. In English, /l/ is the only phoneme that has a lateral release of air. During the production of [l], the tongue tip is brought to the alveolar ridge while air escapes laterally. All other consonants in English have a central release, either allowing air to escape centrally during an

Place and Manner Combinations. Bilabial phonemes are sounds produced with both lips. English has bilabial plosives /p, b/, a nasal /m/, and the labial-velar glide /w/. Other languages have voiceless and voiced bilabial fricatives: /ɸ, β/. Bilabial fricatives are produced by bringing the lips close together, but not letting them touch, and allowing air to pass between them. The voiced bilabial fricative, /β/, is phonemic in a few languages, such as Ewe, spoken in Ghana. In Ewe, /β/ phonemically contrasts with /v/ and /w/. Typically, though, [β] is allophonic in languages. [β] is an allophone of /b/ in intervocalic position in Spanish in words like *saber (to know)*, phonemically transcribed as /saber/, but often produced [saβer]. /ɸ/ is a voiceless bilabial fricative, most typically an allophonic production of /f/ or /p/. The bilabial trill, /ʙ/, is produced by allowing air to pass through the lips while the lips are brought together, causing the lips to vibrate. /ʙ/ is a phoneme in the Brazilian language, Wari. Some people will know the bilabial trill as the Bronx cheer or a raspberry, a sound used by some to suggest derision or to mimic a horse sound; it also is a bilabial sound made by infants.

Labiodental sounds are produced by bringing the lower lip to the upper teeth. Labiodental phonemes in English are the fricatives /f, v/. Many languages have at least one of these two fricatives. The IPA does not recognize labiodental stops. Try producing one: obstruct air by bringing your lower lip to your upper teeth. Did you find it hard to completely obstruct air? More likely you produced a fricative instead, not fully obstructing airflow. If you were successful in blocking airflow, it probably sounds a lot like /p/, another reason it is not used contrastively in languages. It is possible to produce a labiodental nasal; the symbol is [ɱ]. This sound, produced by bringing the lower lip to the upper teeth, is not phonemic in any known language, but is an allophone in many. In English, we produce [ɱ] allophonically for /m/ as a result of coarticulation when a nasal is followed by a labiodental fricative. Try saying *comfort* quickly. Do so again but prolong the nasal consonant. Is your lower lip on your upper teeth? If so, you said [ˈkʌɱ.fɚt]. In Chapter 7, you learned to transcribe this allophone in English using the tooth diacritic under the [m̪]; either way of noting this allophone is correct. Finally, there is a labial affricate, involving a bilabial stop and a labiodental fricative. The voiceless affricate is written [p͡f] and is phonemic in German. The voiced affricate, [b͡v], is rarer, occurring in Tsonga. [b͡v] is an allophone of /v/ in Italian in certain nasal contexts.

As for place of articulation, alveolar is the most popular! It is possible to make a lot of articulatory distinctions at the alveolar ridge. The IPA groups interdental, alveolar, and post-alveolar sounds into a single alveolar category for all but fricatives. English makes use of most of these alveolar region sounds phonemically or allophonically, including the plosives /t, d/, nasal /n/, tap [ɾ], alveolar /ɹ/, and liquid /l/. There are three fricative contrasts in the alveolar region, all of which English uses. Interdental sounds are produced with the tip of the tongue contacting the teeth. In English, we have alveolar fricatives /s, z/, post-alveolar fricatives /ʃ, ʒ/, and interdental fricatives /θ, ð/. Interdental fricatives are quite rare across languages. Languages also have alveolar trills, transcribed /r/. The alveolar trill is produced by raising the tip of the tongue to the alveolar ridge, being sure

to keep the tongue relaxed. Air flows through the obstruction and vibrates the tongue. Alveolar trills occur in many languages, including Russian, Spanish, Arabic, and Hindi. Because of the frequency of alveolar trills across languages, it is important that the English "r" sound be transcribed using the designated /ɹ/ symbol in the IPA, as we have taught you.

As with other consonants produced with the tongue, alveolar sounds can contrast laterality. English does so with the lateral alveolar liquid /l/. There are also the voiceless and voiced lateral fricatives /ɬ, ɮ/.

While there are not different phonetic symbols, there are slight differences in production of phonemes made in the alveolar region. It is possible to differentiate dental, alveolar, and post-alveolar sounds with diacritics. As you learned in Chapter 4, apical, laminal, and dorsal are terms that refer to the part of the tongue used. Apical consonants, made with the tip of the tongue, include dental phonemes, in languages such as Arabic and Russian, as well as rare linguolabial stop, nasal, and fricative phonemes in a few South Pacific island nation languages. /s/ in Castilian Spanish is an apical consonant [s̺], but /s/ is pronounced as a laminal consonant—with the blade of the tongue—in English, [s̻]. Dorsal consonants are produced with the back of the tongue, such as /g/.

Retroflex is not a phonemic place of articulation in English, but is phonemic in many other languages. There are the retroflex voiceless and voiced plosives /ʈ, ɖ/, voiced nasal /ɳ/, rhotic /ɻ/, tap /ɽ/, voiced and voiceless fricatives /ʐ, ʂ/, and lateral /ɭ/. Hindi has many retroflex consonants, including retroflex plosives, nasals, fricatives, affricates, and flaps. English sometimes produces allophonic retroflex taps in certain phonetic contexts, especially when a rhotic vowel is followed by a "d" sound. Say the phrase *hard up*. Did you produce the [d] with the underside of your tongue, as in [hɑɚ.ɽʌp]?

Palatal sounds are limited in English. You have learned /j/ is a palatal glide and the English "r" consonant is a palatal liquid. Other languages have voiced and voiceless palatal plosives /c, ɟ/, fricatives /ç, ʝ /, nasal /ɲ/, and lateral /ʎ/. The palatal nasal occurs in Spanish, in words such as *baño* (*bathroom*), transcribed /baɲo/. Allophonically, English speakers can produce a word like *canyon* with a palatal nasal [kæɲən], changing the CVCCVC word shape to a

CVCVC. And you may remember from Chapter 7 that the velar plosives /k, g/ are produced as palatal stops after a front vowel in words like *keep* and *geese*, or before a front vowel in words like *seek* and *league*. Can you remember the diacritic used to denote these palatal allophones of [k] and [g]? Yes, the palatal allophones can be transcribed as [k̟] and [g̟]. However, in languages that have palatal phonemes, we use their phonetic symbols, as in [cip] (*keep*) and [ɟis] (*geese*). Polish is an example of a language that has palatal nasals, glides, fricatives, and affricates.

Most of the world's languages have a velar plosive, and many have both /k, g/. English also has a velar nasal /ŋ/. Voiced and voiceless velar fricatives also are found in many languages. The voiceless velar fricative /x/ is phonemic in Spanish and German, and the voiced velar fricative /ɣ/ is phonemic in Greek. A few languages also have a velar approximant, /ɰ/. The velar lateral /ʟ/ is extremely rare, occurring in a few Papuan languages. Some linguists capture the English velarized lateral using the /ʟ/ symbol, transcribing words with a velarized-l, such as *silk*, as [sɪʟk], instead of with the velarized diacritic.

Uvular sounds are made with the back of the tongue touching or approximating the uvula. Uvular consonants are rarer than those made farther forward on the tongue, although some languages contrast many uvular sounds phonemically. There are voiceless and voiced uvular plosives /q, ɢ/, nasal /ɴ/, fricatives, /χ, ʁ/, and a trill /ʀ/. The uvular trill is produced in some dialects of German and the uvular fricatives occur in some dialects of Arabic. Some dialects of Inuit, spoken in the Arctic, contrast uvular plosive, fricative, and nasal consonants.

It is not possible to produce many manner categories at the pharyngeal place of articulation, because it is too difficult to bring the tongue root to the pharyngeal wall quickly enough for a plosive. We also cannot contrast oral/nasal and central/lateral sounds pharyngeally, because these contrasts require manipulation of the airstream anterior to the pharynx. The most common pharyngeal sounds are the fricatives /ħ, ʕ/. Arabic, Ukrainian, and Hebrew are three languages that contrast voiced and voiceless pharyngeal fricatives. Can you produce a pharyngeal sound? It is easiest to try by producing fricative [h] with a low back vowel, intentionally moving the tongue root posteriorly during the vowel production while bringing the root to the pharyngeal wall. It is a new movement for English speakers, but with practice you should be able to make the sound less effortful and more phoneme-like. Still, it is good to listen to the sound produced as a phoneme in languages to remind you that it can sound as natural as a /d/ does in English. It just takes practice and exposure.

Finally, plosives and fricatives can be made at the glottal place of articulation. English has the allophonic glottal stop [ʔ], used phonemically in many languages, and the voiceless glottal fricative /h/. The voiced glottal fricative /ɦ/ is found in many languages, including Czech, Polish, and Zulu.

? | 9–4. Did You Get It?

1. Laminal sounds are made with the _____ of the tongue.

2. Apical sounds are made with the _____ of the tongue.

3. What part of the tongue is used for the following three sounds, in order?
   /ʃ/, /k/, /n/

Airstream Source and Direction

In English, all consonant and vowel productions are superimposed on air exhaled from the lungs. Speech sounds produced with air leaving the lungs and flowing out of the body are called pulmonic **egressives**, with pulmonic defining the airstream source for the sound as the lungs, and egressive indicating that the airstream direction is outward. Vowels and sonorant and fricative consonants can only be made as pulmonic egressives.

There are other airstream sources and airstream directions that can be manipulated to make sound in the vocal cavity. For example, you can puff up your cheeks and slowly release that air, making a squeaking sound like a balloon. You can make a lot of animal sounds, too, such as chirping, squawking, and reciting the alphabet on a burp even. Languages make use of some but not all the vocal tract's sound possibilities. While languages do not make use of these noise-making possibilities, many languages contrast speech sounds using other airstream sources for sound and using other airstream directions. For example, many languages have sounds made with bilabial obstruction, like English, but use a different airstream to alter the sound phonemically.

To identify the airstream used for a speech sound, we need to determine two things: where is the airstream source for the sound, and in which direction is that air going? The airstream sources used in speech are pulmonic, glottalic, and velaric. The different airstream directions are egressive and ingressive, or inward and outward airflow. Below we explore these different airstream mechanisms and the airstream directions and the speech sounds they produce.

We produce speech sounds in English by obstructing air as it travels outward from the lungs. Why does that air rush out audibly, resulting in the sound we identify with the phoneme? When we close our articulators, that air is still flowing from the lungs and the pressure in our oral cavity increases. When we release our articulators, one of the basic laws of thermodynamics takes effect. That law states that energy will travel from an area of high pressure to an area of low pressure, attempting to achieve equilibrium in air pressure. If air traveling from the lungs through the vocal tract is blocked by articulator obstruction, air pressure in the oral cavity will increase. And when the obstruction is released, the blocked air will audibly rush outward to decrease pressure in the oral cavity. This process describes egressive airflow. However, producing speech on an ingressive airflow is also possible, as we first introduced in Chapter 4. Ingressive airflow will occur when the pressure between the airstream mechanism and the articulators decreases, resulting in airflow into the oral cavity to equalize pressure.

Pulmonic egressive stops, or plosives, are the most common consonant sounds in languages. Other stop consonants are called clicks, ejectives, and implosives. Below we explore these three non-pulmonic sound categories, how they are produced, how they are transcribed, and examples of how they contrast phonemically within languages. Figure 9–6 shows the IPA phonetic symbols for these non-pulmonic sounds.

Glottalic sounds, while still having airflow from the lungs as their primary source, result from closure at the glottis and in manipulating the larynx so that the trapped air is either sucked in (ingressive)

CONSONANTS (NON-PULMONIC)

Clicks		Voiced implosives		Ejectives	
ʘ	Bilabial	ɓ	Bilabial	ʼ	Examples:
ǀ	Dental	ɗ	Dental/alveolar	pʼ	Bilabial
ǃ	(Post)alveolar	ʄ	Palatal	tʼ	Dental/alveolar
ǂ	Palatoalveolar	ɠ	Velar	kʼ	Velar
ǁ	Alveolar lateral	ʛ	Uvular	sʼ	Alveolar fricative

FIGURE 9–6. IPA symbols for non-pulmonic consonants. *Source:* Copyright © 2015 International Phonetic Association. Available under a Creative Commons Attribution-Sharealike 3.0 Unported License.

or the trapped air is forced out (egressive). The glottis serves as an airstream source for two types of speech sounds: ejectives and implosives.

Ejectives. Ejective stops and affricates are produced with a glottalic egressive airstream. How does this work? Air flowing from the lungs travels into the oral cavity. Articulators come together at the same time as the vocal folds adduct, closing the glottis, and the velum is raised to block air flow through the nasal cavity. These three simultaneous movements trap air between the articulators and the glottis. This trapped air pressure is increased by raising the larynx with the glottis closed, like a pump. The articulators are then released and the vocal folds are abducted immediately afterward. By first releasing the articulators, the trapped air rushes out of the oral cavity, resulting in the characteristic louder burst of an ejective.

Figure 9–7 demonstrates the production of a voiceless bilabial ejective. See if you can walk through the sequence needed to produce the sound. First, the airstream must be closed off in the oral cavity. This is done by bringing the lips together, abducting the vocal folds, and raising the velum. The trapped air in the oral cavity is then compressed by raising the larynx. Once the air pressure has been increased, the lips are separated, and the air trapped between the glottis and the articulators rushes out.

Ejectives can be produced at any place of articulation that a pulmonic egressive can be produced.

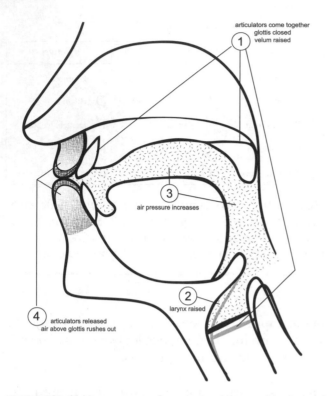

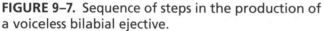

FIGURE 9–7. Sequence of steps in the production of a voiceless bilabial ejective.

Ejectives are voiceless, since the vocal folds cannot vibrate while being closed to increase pressure. Ejectives are written phonetically by adding an apostrophe [ʼ] diacritic to voiceless stop/affricate symbols representing places of articulation. For example, a bilabial ejective is transcribed /pʼ/.

Ejectives occur in about 18% of the world's languages, including many languages indigenous to North and South America. Velar and uvular places of articulation are most common. Peruvian Quechua has four clicks: / pʼ, tʼ, kʼ, t͡ʃʼ/, which contrast with voiceless and voiceless aspirated plosives at the same places of articulation.

While English does not have phonemic ejectives, many English speakers produce ejectives allophonically when they are emphasizing the end of a word. You may produce ejectives yourself for emphasis. Try saying the word *book*, but really holding on to the [k] at the end without releasing it. Instead build up a lot of pressure in your mouth, then release the [k] with a popping sound. Were you able to do this? If so, you produced [kʼ]. Try saying it again, this time with

your fingers placed lightly on your larynx. During the production of an ejective you should feel your larynx raise while your glottis is closed and your back of the tongue is raised to the soft palate. Once you can produce an ejective at the end of a word in [bʊkʼ], try saying a vowel afterward, [bʊ.kʼə], and then an initial ejective in the nonsense word [kʼi]. Now try the same with alveolar [tʼ] and bilabial [pʼ].

Implosives. Implosive stops are produced with a glottalic ingressive airstream. Most ingressive sounds are voiced and are produced by closing the articulators while continuing to let air flow through vibrating vocal folds. Continuing to vibrate the vocal folds results in a downward movement of the larynx as air travels through the vibrating vocal folds into the oral cavity. By lowering the larynx, the air pressure decreases slightly in the oral cavity and there is no buildup in pressure. Thus when the articulator is released, there is an inflow of air to the oral cavity.

Figure 9–8 illustrates how a voiced dental implosive is produced. First, the tip of the tongue touches the alveolar ridge with the vocal folds vibrating. As air continues to flow into the vocal tract, the larynx lowers, maintaining equivalent air pressure above and below the vocal folds while creating a resonant quality unique to implosives. The tongue tip is then released from the alveolar ridge, with a slight decrease in pressure in the oral cavity resulting in an inward airflow.

Because implosives are produced by changes in pressure in the oral tract, they can be produced at any place of articulation that a plosive can be produced. Implosives are almost always voiced, since the air continues to flow through the vocal folds while the vocal folds are vibrating. Implosives are written phonetically by adding a right-curve to the top of a phoneme, such as the bilabial implosive /ɓ/.

About 10% of the world's languages have implosive phonemes. Implosives occur in many sub-Saharan African languages and in some Asian languages. Sindhi, spoken in India and Pakistan, has four voiced implosives at the bilabial, alveolar, palatal, and velar places of articulation: /ɓ, ɗ, ʄ, ɠ/.

Like ejectives, we produce implosives allophonically in English. Try doing so by making a long voiced stop at the beginning of a word. Say a word like *bike*, but do not let the lips go on the [b], making the closure for the [b] really long. Air will continue

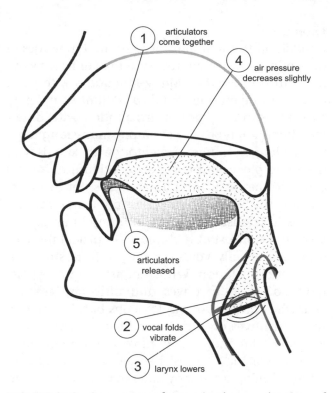

FIGURE 9–8. Sequence of steps in the production of a voiced alveolar implosive.

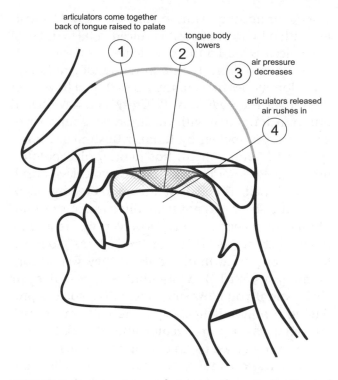

FIGURE 9–9. Sequence of steps in the production of a voiceless post-alveolar click.

traveling through your vocal folds so that when you release the articulators for the [b], it should have a unique resonant quality. Does it? If so, you have produced the allophone [ɓ]. Try producing it again, this time with your hand on your larynx. You should feel the larynx lowering. And now try making a bilabial implosive in the middle of the word, really delaying release of the articulators as you produce it: [a.ɓa].

Clicks. Clicks are produced on an ingressive velaric airstream. To produce clicks, the articulators come together at the same time that the back of the tongue is raised to the velum, trapping air between the articulators and the velum. The tongue body is then lowered between the articulators and the velum, decreasing pressure in this space in the oral cavity. Next the articulators are released, with the velum released immediately after the articulators. The decreased pressure anterior to the velum causes air to rush inward and results in a clicking sound.

Figure 9–9 illustrates the production of a post-alveolar click. In producing this click, the following steps are taken. The blade of the tongue is raised to the post-alveolar place of articulation at the same time that the back of the tongue is raised to the velum. These simultaneous movements trap air above the tongue. The tongue body is lowered, decreasing the pressure of the trapped air. When the articulator is released from the post-alveolar region, air rushes in to equalize pressure and give the click its characteristic clicking sound.

Note that the place of articulation for all clicks is anterior to the closed velum. Clicks can be voiced, voiceless, and nasal, because the airstream source, the velum, is anterior and independent of the vocal folds and the oro-nasal juncture.

Velaric ingressive clicks have unique phonetic symbols representing place of articulation that are combined with velar symbols to indicate voicing and nasality. For example, the symbol for a bilabial click is /ʘ/. The symbols for clicks by place of articulation are bilabial, /ʘ/; dental, /ǀ/; post-alveolar /ǃ/; palato-alveolar /ǂ/; and lateral, /ǁ/. Each click must be accompanied by a velar symbol to indicate voicing or nasality. Thus, a voiced click will be written with a [g] to indicate it is voiced, a [k] to indicate it is voiceless, and a [ŋ] to indicate it is nasal.

Clicks are relatively rare in languages, although some languages have many clicks. If you have seen the movie *The Gods Must Be Crazy,* you have heard !Kung, a language with an impressive number of clicks that is spoken by Kalahir Bushmen. Xhosa, spoken in South Africa, has dental, alveopalatal, and alveolar lateral clicks that are voiceless, nasal, and aspirated, as well as breathy and breathy nasal.

In English, we do not typically use clicks as allophones of speech sounds. However, we frequently make click noises. Think of the "tsk tsk" sound a teacher or parent might make if they were disappointed in your behavior—that is a post-alveolar click. And if you blow someone a kiss, you are producing a bilabial click. Trying to call your horse? We often use a post-alveolar lateral click for that action. When used as an actual phoneme in a language, clicks are much more natural-sounding and are produced in consonant-vowel syllables easily. Try making some of these sounds with a vowel. Can you say [ʘka], starting with a voiceless bilabial click, followed by a vowel? Or [!ŋi], a nasal version of the elder's disapproval sound?

Phonation

In addition to the respiratory system, languages of the world use the phonatory system in different ways to contrast phonemes. Many languages with large consonant inventories build consonant complexity by contrasting a place of articulation with differing phonation types. For example, many languages build a larger phoneme inventory with sounds with the same place and manner by adding a voicing contrast—between two bilabial stops, for instance, creating the two voiced-voiceless phonemes /b/ and /p/, as in English. Common in many languages is a voicing contrast at both places of articulation, or a pattern of only voiced or only voiceless at each place of articulation. While English contrasts voicing for all stops, fricatives, and affricates, Mexican Spanish contrasts voicing for stops but does not do so for fricatives or affricates, which are only voiceless. Many languages only have voiced phonemes, with no voicing contrast between any phonemes, although allophones may differ in voicing. Ecuadorean Quichua is an example, where the word *father* can be produced [daɪ.da] or [taɪ.ta] without changing meaning.

Voicing is produced along a continuum, from completely voiceless (vocal folds apart), to modal

---

? | 9–5. Did You Get It?

1. If the air pressure inside the lungs is increased, does inhalation or exhalation occur?

2. All phonemes in English are produced on which airstream? _____

3. Clicks are made using which airstream mechanism? _____

4. Plosives are made using which airstream mechanism? _____

5. Ejectives are made using which airstream mechanism? _____

6. Implosives are made using which airstream mechanism? _____

7. Which stop categories can be voiced?
   _____

8. Which stop categories can be voiceless?
   _____

9. What sound do you make if you overemphasize the final /t/ in the word **kite** by producing it with both an alveolar obstruction and simultaneous glottal closure, then releasing the alveolar stop before opening the glottis?

10. The phoneme /ɠ/ is a _____
    _____.

11. The phoneme /ʘŋ/ is a _____
    _____.

or regular voicing, to fully closed, for a glottal stop. Phonemic distinctions are most frequently voiced/voiceless contrasts, as in English. In these cases, the vocal folds are adducted and vibrating or abducted and allowing air to flow through the vocal folds unobstructed. This voicing contrast is most typical with obstruents (stops, fricatives, affricates), although a few languages contrast voiced/voiceless nasals.

Phonation can be phonemically contrasted in other ways. Breathy voice (also called murmured voice) is produced by abducting the vocal folds, but not completely. Thus, there is some vibration, but turbulent air also travels through the vocal folds. This results in more turbulence through the vocal folds and a more breathy quality—like whispering and phonating at the same time. There are actually a few ways to create the quality of breathy voice, since there are different ways to vibrate the vocal folds while simultaneously allowing turbulent air to flow through them.

As you learned in Chapter 4, breathy voice is indicated by two dots under the phoneme. Breathy voice is not phonemic in English but is contrastive in languages such as Khmer, spoken in Cambodia, and Gujarati, spoken in India. Hindi contrasts voiced and breathy stops, and Nepali (spoken in Nepal and nearby countries) contrasts voiced, voiceless, and breathy stops in words.

Creaky voice, also called laryngealized voice, is another phonation type. As with breathy voiced phonemes, there are languages, such as Kambaata in Ethiopia, Mazatec in Mexico, and Hausa in West Africa, that contain creaky phonemes. This phonation type results from the vocal folds being brought tightly together but not fully closed, allowing for vibration, but at a much lower frequency than a speakers' typical F0. Creaky voice is also called vocal fry. Creaky voice is indicated by a tilde below the phoneme as in [l̰]. Stops are less likely to be laryngealized, but liquids are contrasted, such as /l/ and /l̰/ in Kambaata (spoken in Ethiopia).

There are no creaky phonemes in English, although as pointed out in Chapter 4, vocal fry appears to be on the rise in the speech of young women in the U.S. Note that this social creaky voice tends to be whole word and not on single phonemes.

? 9–6. Did You Get It?

1. _____ voice is produced by vibrating the vocal folds while simultaneously allowing turbulent air to flow through.

2. _____ voice is produced by bringing the vocal folds tightly together during phonation.

3. The difference between a consonant made with breathy voice and a consonant made with a creaky voice is

_____.

Voice Onset Time

In Chapter 6 you were introduced to the concept of voice onset time (VOT), used to describe plosive production and the amount of time between the release of the articulators and the start of vocal fold vibration for the following vowel. We learned that VOT is typically 25 to 45 milliseconds longer for English voiceless than English voiced stops. We talk about voiced and voiceless stops in a simplistic way in English, since there is only a two-way contrast for voicing in English. That is, we have referred to /b, d, g/ as voiced, and /p, t, k/ as voiceless. We presented this voicing contrast as a simple relationship between states of the glottis, with voiced consonants produced with the vocal folds together and voiceless consonants having vocal folds apart.

In many cases, referring to voiced stops as voiced is misleading. Go back to Figures 7–11 and 7–13, looking closely at the voiced stops in the spectrograms. Notice that the voicing is really not pronounced in these productions. Often the biggest difference between English voiced and voiceless stops is not whether the stop consonant is voiced, because most English [b]s and all English [p]s are not voiced. What do we hear that tells us a sound is a /b/ or a /p/ in initial word position? It is not whether or not the consonant is voiced. What tells the listener the voicing in English is whether or not there is aspiration. Technically, /b, d, g/ in English are voiceless unaspirated stops and /p, t, k/ are voiceless aspirated stops in initial word position. You read that correctly: voiced stops in English are actually voiceless. What we hear in this difference is the amount of time that passes from the closure of the articulators and the start of vocal fold vibration, or voice onset time.

VOT differs in milliseconds and is not an absolute quality. There are three general categories, though: (1) fully voiced (or prevoiced) stops, where the vocal folds start vibrating before the articulators are released; (2) voiceless stops or partially voiced stops, where the vocal folds begin to vibrate right as the articulators are released, and (3) voiceless aspirated stops where there is a delay in VOT after the articulators are released. The difference in voicing contrasts is milliseconds. Prevoiced stops tend to have 0 or fewer milliseconds of VOT; voiced stops are between 0 and 40 milliseconds; aspirated stops tend to have over 50 milliseconds of VOT. In English, the range for voiced stops is from 0 (or a few milliseconds negative) to about 25 milliseconds for bilabials, 35 milliseconds for alveolars, and 45 milliseconds for velars. Any VOT over these amounts is heard as voiceless stops in English.

Many languages have phonemic voicing contrasts, but the exact VOT and the VOT distinction between the voiced cognates will differ from that of English. This is because what matters for a phonemic voicing distinction is that there is enough of a VOT difference for the listener to easily hear two distinct phoneme categories. As an example, both Spanish and English have voiced and voiceless stops, with the voiced/voiceless distinction in each language resulting from a difference of approximately 40 to 50 milliseconds. However, the voiceless stops in English and Spanish have very different VOT values, as do the voiced stops in both languages. Figure 9–10 compares the VOT of voiced and voiceless stops in Spanish and English. The waveform is of four words *baba* (Spanish for *drool*), *Bobby* (English), *papa* (Spanish for *potato*), and *papa* (English). Phonemically these words are transcribed /ba.ba/, /ba.ba/, /pa.pa/, and /pa.pa/ (Spanish has a low central and not a low back vowel). Note that the VOTs for /b/ in Spanish and English differ quite a bit, as do the VOTs for the voiceless /p/ in each language. Do you notice anything unusual about the VOT? The VOT for /b/ in English and /p/ in Spanish are more similar to each other than the voiced/voiceless sounds are to each

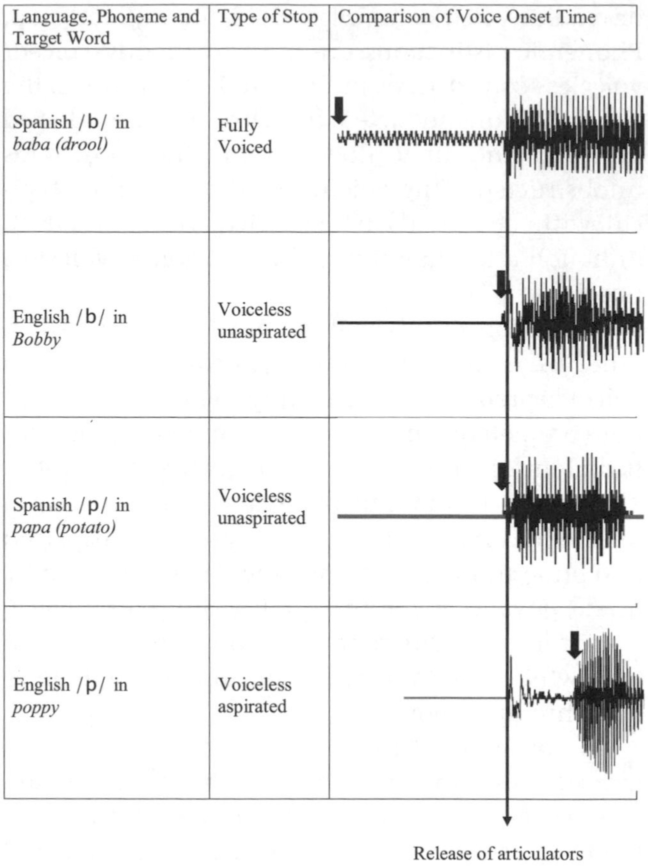

Language, Phoneme and Target Word	Type of Stop	Comparison of Voice Onset Time
Spanish /b/ in *baba (drool)*	Fully Voiced	
English /b/ in *Bobby*	Voiceless unaspirated	
Spanish /p/ in *papa (potato)*	Voiceless unaspirated	
English /p/ in *poppy*	Voiceless aspirated	

Release of articulators

FIGURE 9–10. A waveform comparing VOT between Spanish and English voiced and voiceless bilabial stops. The dark line marks the release of the articulators. The arrows mark the onset of voicing.

other across languages. In Spanish, voiced stops are fully voiced, with vocal fold vibration starting before the articulators are released. Spanish voiceless stops are not aspirated as in English; in fact, the VOT for Spanish /p, t, k/ is around 0 ms, the same VOT as the voiced /b, d, g/ in English.

As a general rule, Germanic languages—English, Dutch, German—have aspirated voiceless stops, whereas few Romance languages, like Spanish, Italian, and French, do. Some languages have even more delayed VOT than the aspirated stops of English. Navajo has a strongly aspirated stop, which has double the aspiration length of English voiceless aspirated stops. Some languages have two or even three phonemic VOT contrasts, contrasting prevoiced, voiceless unaspirated, and voiceless aspirated stops. Hindi contrasts VOT in four ways: voiceless aspirated, /pʰ/, voiceless unaspirated, /p/, voiced /b/, and fully voiced /bʰ/. Sindhi, spoken in Pakistan and India, has a five-way voicing contrast for stops, the same four VOT contrasts, plus the voiced implosive /ɓ/.

? 9–7. Did You Get It?

1. The difference between a slightly aspirated stop and a strongly aspirated stop is _____.

2. Which of the following bilabial stops will have the greatest delay in voice onset time?

   a. an allophonic bilabial implosive stop in *Betty*

   b. the bilabial stop in *buy*

   c. the bilabial stop in *pie*

   d. the bilabial stop in *spy*

Consonant Length

In some languages, consonants that share manner, place, airstream, and voicing are phonemically contrasted by the length or duration of the consonant production. That is, a language may phonemically contrast short and long /b/. When phonemes differ only in length, it is considered a singleton/geminate contrast. A **geminate** is a consonant, or vowel, that is double in length. Geminates are transcribed phonetically with consonant repetition or with the length diacritic [ː]. A language uses geminate contrasts if there are minimal pair words that differ only in length. In Italian, for example, the singleton/geminate /t, tː/ is established by minimal pairs like /fa.to/ *fate*, and /fa.tːo/, *fact*.

Geminate consonants occur with stops, affricates, fricatives, liquids, and nasals. The duration of the articulatory obstruction is longer for geminate than for singleton consonants. The difference in duration between singleton and geminate consonants varies between 30 and 70 milliseconds in length.

There are over 70 languages that have phonemic consonant geminates. These include Italian, Japanese, Estonian, and Arabic. How geminates are used differs markedly across languages. Some languages have a geminate contrast for every consonant in the language's inventory. Dobel, an Austronesian language spoken in the Aru islands of Malaysia, has 14 single consonants, all of which have a geminate contrast, resulting in 28 consonant phonemes: /b t d kw ɸ s m n ŋ l r w j ʔ bː tː dː kwː ɸː sː mː nː ŋː lː rː wː jː ʔː/ Other languages only have geminates of some of their sounds, such as only voiceless stops (Anejom), or only liquids (Palauan), or only voiced stops (Somali) (Blevins, 2008).

Although English does not have phonemic geminates, consonant length differences are produced allophonically as we discussed in Chapter 7. For example, we tend to say the word *misspell* as [mɪ.sːpɛl], even though saying it with a shorter first [s] will not change meaning. We also observed consonant length differences morphologically, [ʌːnæ.ʧɚ.əl] and in compound words, such as roommate,[ɹumːeɪt]. And we do mark meaningful distinctions in length across word boundaries to decrease confusion, as in *white eye* [waɪt.aɪ], and *white tie*, [waɪ.tːaɪ].

Nasal and Lateral Stops

The combination of stop and fricative obstructions results in the affricate manner of articulation. There are a few additional combinations of manner that are used phonemically in other languages.

Some languages combine homorganic nasal and voiced stop obstruction to create phonemes. A **prenasalized stop** is a phoneme comprising a nasal and stop consonant sequence. Languages also have prenasalized affricates. If we did so in English, it would be written *ndo* or *mba*. Like affricates, phonemic combinations of this type have a shorter duration than the nasal and stop produced separately. **Prenasalized stops** are phonemic in many languages. Guarani, spoken in Paraguay, has prenasalized bilabial, alveolar, and velar stops. Some Burmese languages also have prenasalized fricatives and approximants, although these combinations are very rare. Prenasalized stops are transcribed either as the two symbols, with or without a tie bar, or with a superscript nasal in front of the symbol. For example, in the Bantu language Ndebele, spoken in South Africa, the Nd in the language name could be transcribed /nd/, /n͡d/, or /ⁿd/.

Languages also have nasal and lateral release sounds, concepts you learned about in Chapter 4. A nasal release consonant is an allophonic or phonemic combination of a stop consonant released nasally. A lateral release consonant is an allophonic or phonemic combination of a stop consonant released laterally. These consonants are produced when a stop is combined with a homorganic nasal or lateral consonant. You have learned nasal release, or nasal plosion, as allophonic in English, possible in words such as *sudden*, produced [sʌdˀ.n̩], and lateral plosion in words like *subtle*, [sʌdˀ.l̩]. Some languages have initial nasal release (e.g., Russian), and lateral release (e.g., Navajo) stops; however, linguists debate whether these are consonant clusters or individual phonemes. We will not take a stance on these debates. Nevertheless, it is interesting to see that nasal + stop and lateral + stop sequences can occur at the beginning of the syllable in other languages but are not permissible in English phonology.

Summary of Consonant Possibilities

While English has a fair number of consonants, there are languages with many more. Taa dialects, spoken in Botswana and Namibia, are thought to have the most consonants, with over 87 consonants reported by conservative estimates, and other linguists counting well over 100. Of the 600 different consonants used across languages, most are stops. The voiceless stops /p, t, k/ have the greatest frequency, occurring in approximately 98% of the world's languages (Ladefoged, 2005).

As you have seen, there are an impressive number of ways languages vary consonant productions. The greatest variation is in stop production. Stops can be fully voiced, voiceless, aspirated, implosive, ejectives, clicks, breathy voice, creaky voice, affricates, and a multitude of combinations of these differences with different place and manner properties. Table 9–1 summarizes the ways consonants can vary.

? 9–8. Did You Get It?

1. You can now identify multiple properties of any consonant using the IPA chart. You can identify nine properties of consonants regardless of whether you can produce the sound. These properties are airstream source, airstream direction, state of the glottis, part of the tongue involved (or absence of the tongue for sounds made with the lips), place of articulation, manner of articulation, centrality, nasality, and length. Can you identify each of these properties for the phonemes identified below?

   a. /ʝ/

   b. /cː/

   c. /t͡sʼ/

TABLE 9–1. Summary of the Nine Ways Consonants Can Differ

Airstream		Part of Tongue	State of Glottis	Place	Centrality	Nasality	Manner	Length
Source	Direction							
Pulmonic	Egressive	Laminal	Fully Voiced	Bilabial	Central	Oral	Stop	Singleton
Glottalic	Ingressive	Apical	Voiceless Unaspirated	Labiodental	Lateral	Nasal	Fricative	Geminate
Velaric		Dorsal	Voiceless Aspirated	Dental			Affricate	
		NA	Breathy (Murmured)	Alveolar			Approximant	
			Creaky (Laryngealized)	Alveopalatal			(Liquid)	
			Closed	Post-alveolar			(Glide)	
				Retroflex			Trill	
				Palatal			Tap/Flap	
				Velar				
				Uvular				
				Pharyngeal				
				Glottal				

Vowels

To explore vowel contrasts across languages we start with a shape you have become quite familiar with: the vowel quadrilateral. Figure 9–11 is the IPA vowel quadrilateral. We have discussed the vowel space as nine regions, as is typically in clinical phonetics, although the IPA chart is divided a little differently. We can use the vowel quadrilateral to understand vowels in other languages as we have those of English.

Comparing across languages, GAE has a large vowel inventory. Depending on whether words like *caught* and *cot* are pronounced the same or as a minimal pair, GAE has 14 or 15 vowels, including three phonemic diphthongs. And this vowel inventory count does not include rhotic vowels. Most languages in the world have a smaller vowel inventory than English. The majority of languages have five to six vowels, and many have three. Regardless, English does not utilize all the ways vowel phonemes can be contrasted. Let us look at how languages differ in the use of English vowel categories as well as other ways vowels are contrasted.

Tongue Height, Advancement, Tenseness, and Rounding

If we exclude rhotics, English contrasts most vowel phonemes with three properties: tongue height, tongue advancement, and tenseness. The fourth category you learned, rounding, is only needed to contrast /ɝ/ and /ʌ/, because vowels sharing height and advancement are unrounded if they are front or low back and rounded if they are mid or high back places.

As noted, English has front unrounded and back rounded vowels. Other languages combine rounding, height, and advancement differently and have different vowel phonemes. German has four high front vowels, the two unrounded /i/ and /ɪ/, and the front rounded tense and lax vowels /y/ and /ʏ/. And some languages, such as Japanese, have back unrounded vowels such as /ɯ/.

Advanced Versus Retracted Tongue Root

Languages contrast vowels by changing the shape of the vocal tract in different ways. Some languages, like English, contrast vowels by raising the tongue more forward or more back in the mouth. Other languages contrast vowels through advancing or retracting the tongue. This contrasting movement changes the width of the pharynx during vowel production, affecting resonatory properties in a similar way that advancing the tongue does. Tongue root contrasts are used in Kazakh's nine vowel system, for example. Maasai, spoken in Kenya and Tanzania, also has nine vowels, with four sets of vowels that contrast in tongue root.

Nasality

As you have learned, English has allophonic nasal vowels in nasal consonant contexts. Phonemic nasal vowels are actually quite common in languages, contrasting with non-nasal vowels in French, Portuguese, Hindi, Mohawk, Yoruba, and Hmong.

Voicing

No language appears to make a clear voicing distinction in vowels, though it is common, as in Japanese, for phonologically voiced vowels to devoice in certain contexts, such as in final position and when adjacent to voiceless consonants.

Types of voicing are phonemically contrasted for vowels across languages. Some languages contrast modal voice with breathy voice. Gujarati contrasts breathy and voiced vowels in the words [bar] (the number *12*) and [bar̤] (*outside*).

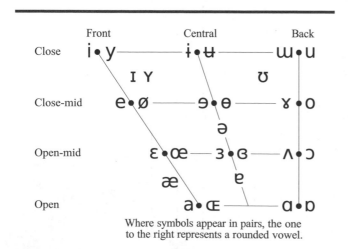

Where symbols appear in pairs, the one to the right represents a rounded vowel.

FIGURE 9–11. The IPA vowel quadrilateral. *Source:* Copyright © 2015 International Phonetic Association. Available under a Creative Commons Attribution-Sharealike 3.0 Unported License.

Creaky vowels are contrasted with voiced vowels in some languages, such as Jalapa Mazatec, which is spoken in Mexico. Interestingly, Jalapa Mazatec contrasts breathy, voiced, and creaky vowels, also nasalizing all three types. This means a Jalapa Mazatec speaker has six ways to contrast a vowel like /a/ phonemically.

Breathy and creaky voice are not phonemic in English but they are allophonic. Try producing some English words in breathy and creaky voice. Produce the word *why* four ways: with regular voicing, whispered, with breathy voice, and with creaky voice. Were you able to contrast these four voicing types?

Vowel Length

Like consonants, vowel length can be contrasted phonemically. We have seen how tense and lax vowels in English are acoustically salient due to length distinctions. In addition, languages can have two vowels with the same tenseness, height, advancement, and rounding, and only contrast them in length of vowel. Geminate vowels are found in diverse languages. Finnish has five front vowels and three back vowels, all of which have phonemic length contrasts. Japanese has five vowels, all of which are also contrasted in length.

? 9–9. Did You Get It?

1. Name three ways languages contrast vowel phonemes that are not used in English.

2. If two vowels are contrasted by increasing the width of the pharynx without tongue movement, we can say that these vowels contrast in _____.

3. In addition to fully voiced vowels, languages can contrast which other vowel voicing types phonemically?

_____

Syllable-Level Differences

In addition to differences in consonant and vowel inventories, languages differ in the ways of conveying meaning at the syllable and word levels. Four ways to do this are stress, tone, phonotactic complexity, and word length.

Stress Patterns

Stress patterns differ across languages, contributing to languages' unique prosodic patterns. As you have learned, English has a variable but rhythmic stress pattern, using stress to indicate new and important information. The English word-level stress pattern is variable, with many words stressed on the first syllable, some on the second syllable, and longer words placing stress on pretty much any syllable. And as you have seen, changing the stress on the same phonemes is used to contrast meaning, such as *the 'content* and *to be con'tent*. In Russian, the stress pattern is even more variable, requiring one to learn the unique stress pattern of each word as it is acquired.

Languages with a fixed stress usually have straightforward rules for stress patterns in words. Many languages always or almost always have stress on the first syllable of a word. Languages with first-syllable stress patterns include Hungarian and Afrikaans. Other languages, like Armenian and Yupik (spoken in Alaska), stress the last syllable of a word, regardless of the word length. In some languages, the stress is on the second to the last syllable, regardless of whether the word has 2 or 15 syllables.

In addition to word-level stress patterns, languages have sentence-level stress patterns. English is considered a stress-timed language. This means that syllables can differ in length but there is a rhythmic occurrence of stressed syllables. In Chapter 8 we learned that in longer sentences, unstressed syllables are shortened and stressed syllables occur at fairly regular intervals. In a longer sentence with a rhythmic pattern of stressed syllables, the syllables in-between will be shortened. In sentences like *Fatemah is my friend* versus *Fatemah is my very best friend,* the word *my* will be shortened in the second sentence so that additional words can be said between the longer stressed words, *Fatemah* and *friend,* without changing the sentence's rhythm.

Syllable Duration Patterns

The particular prosody of a language is also affected by syllable duration. Languages can be syllable-timed, where every syllable is the same length; stress-timed, where stressed syllables are longer and unstressed syllables are shorter; and mora-timed, where certain types of syllables are always longer and others are always shorter. Mora are basically heavy and light syllables and result in some syllables always being shorter and others always being longer. English, with its reduced vowels, is an example of a stress-timed language; German is another stress-timed language. Spanish is syllable-timed. Sanskrit is a mora-timed language, where heavy syllables have long vowels or end in consonants and light syllables have short vowels.

Tone

Pitch can be used different ways to convey information in languages. As you learned in Chapter 5, English pitch is altered at the word or sentence level to convey meaning, but not at the phoneme level. Phrase-level uses of pitch include letting your listener know non-phonemic information, such as whether you are asking a question or making a statement. Changes in pitch are also used in English to convey information the speaker thinks is new and important.

Other languages use pitch to contrast meaning. Syllable-level contrasts in pitch are called tones. Tonal languages use differences in tone to contrast meaning at the syllable level. In a tonal language, the same syllable produced on a high versus a low pitch can mean different things. Tonal languages abound in Asia and Africa; in fact, the majority of the world's languages are tonal.

Tonal languages use tone in different ways. Languages can contrast varying numbers of tones: high/low, or high/mid/low, for example. Xhosa is a two tone language. Tlingit, spoken in Western Canada, has some dialects with two tones and some with three. Tones can also be contoured in the same syllable. Some contoured tones include rising (low to high), falling (high to low), falling-rising, and rising-falling. Mandarin has five tones: a neutral tone, contrasted with a high-level, a rising, a falling, and a falling-rising tone. The same syllable has five different meanings because of tone changes. For example /ma/ means *mother, horse, scold, numb* and indicates a question, depending on whether the tone is high-level, rising-falling, falling, rising, or neutral.

Phonotactic Complexity

Finally, languages have different phonotactic structures and typical word length patterns. English words can have quite complex syllable shapes, as we covered in Chapter 7. Word-initial three-consonant clusters are not uncommon in English; consider *splat, spray,* and *squirt.* And word-final consonant clusters of three or even four consonants are not unusual: *widths, squelched, fixed, strengths.* Other languages have more complex consonant sequences, such as Russian, which has many and frequent four-consonant clusters. In contrast, many languages only permit simple syllable shapes, such as Hmong, which is primarily composed of CV syllable shapes, with only nasal consonants allowed in the coda of a syllable. Hawaiian syllables can only be CV.

? 9–10. Did You Get It?

1. Word level stress patterns are _____ or variable.

2. _____ languages use pitch to convey meaning at the syllable level.

3. Languages that do not vary stress patterns across syllables are called _____.

Language Complexity

It certainly is fascinating that some languages have so few and some have so many sounds. And languages with only three vowels or eight consonants seem to have very simple phonemic systems, whereas languages like Taa, spoken in Botswana, have extremely complicated phonemic systems. Some languages have as many as 140 phonemes! As we conclude our exploration of meaningful sound possibilities, let's consider a few frequent questions out there. Do these different sound inventories mean some languages are harder than others? Do we know why languages end up with such differing sound systems? Let's end your phonetics journey by exploring answers to these questions.

The human species has had a common purpose as languages have evolved. It is the same purpose that infants and toddlers have as their speech capacity grows. Whether it is the evolution of speech across the species or the acquisition of speech in the individual, we are taking advantage of vocal tract capabilities to make sound to communicate. As languages grow and as infants develop into children and then adults, what is communicated becomes more and more complex. To communicate all the things we want to talk about, from—what we want to eat to how quantum physics works—requires us to develop a system that contrasts meaning in a variety of ways. Imagine if we could not contrast many sounds, but if we were only like that newborn infant, producing just a few nasalized vowels and consonants in short little strings. Or even the 6-month-old who can put a few consonants together with vowels in speech-like strings. As infants, and the earlier humans, developed greater cognitive abilities and had more and more things to tell others, they either had to make longer and longer and longer strings of syllables with few consonants and vowels, or needed to come up with new ways to contrast sounds. From what we know about the evolution of language, our early ancestors had to make the same choices, doing so in over 7,000 different ways.

The manner for contrasting meaning differs dramatically across languages and no two languages do so in exactly the same way. Some languages have complex grammars, some complex phonologies, and some unusual ways of creating words. There are an infinite number of ways we can contrast meaning within languages. For the sake of a phonetics course, we will stick with ways sounds can be contrasted.

Despite the existence of over 600 consonants possible, different languages and different language families share many sounds. In explaining how sound systems are developed, Lindblom (1986) noted, "spoken language tends to evolve sound systems . . . that can be explained, at least in part, with reference to the fact [the language] is spoken." Thus sound system similarities reflect the premise we started this book with: languages use a speech system that balances the ease of articulation and perceptual distance of sounds so that the speakers can communicate effectively with listeners.

How are sounds similar across languages? All languages appear to have at their base easier sounds that are very distinct from each other. The easier sounds tend to be consonants that involve simple ballistic movements: making a sound by bringing two articulators together and closing and opening the mouth. Thus all languages have stops and most have nasals, sounds that also predominate in children's babbling and early word productions across languages. Sounds made at the front of the mouth—with the lips and the tip and blade of the tongue—are also shared across languages and observed in developing speech productions. Because it is easier to move the front than the back of the tongue in many directions, it is hypothesized that these sounds are easier to make.

Lindblom spent a lot of his career studying why languages end up with the speech sounds they have. It turns out that the phonological system of languages is functional and systematic, not random. There is typically a predictable system to the sounds in a language, and computers can predict fairly accurately what sounds languages of different sizes will have. At the core is the principle that ease of articulation and sufficient perceptual contrast guide the development of small and large phonological inventories. Below we see how this works.

The most frequent vowel inventory in languages is a five-vowel system, typically comprising /i, e, a, o, u/. From a purely phonological perspective, there is not a rationale for why languages would end up with these same five vowels. You could have any combination! Why not have /u, ae, ɛ̃ ɪ, ɝ/ combining breathy, creaky, rhotic, nasal, front, back, and rounded vowels? They would sure sound different from each other. But there are not languages with five vowel systems like this. If we instead look at the evolution of vowels in a language as one of efficiency, a language would end up with sounds that are maximally distinctive while not hard to produce. And that is in fact what is observed. In three-vowel languages, maximal and sufficient contrast is achieved through the three vowels at the far corners of the vowel quadrilateral, /i, a, u/. While these three vowels could be even more distinct if they differed in phonation type (modal vs. creaky, for instance), or in voicing, nasality, or rhoticity, /i, a, u/ are easy to hear as distinctive. It is only when languages evolve to have large vowel inventories that more variety is needed.

Thus, languages with very few vowels tend to have the same vowels—those that are perceptually salient. Many five-vowel languages comprise /i, e, a, o, u/. Note that languages with smaller vowel inventories most frequently have the low central vowel /a/, not the low back vowel of GAE.

Figure 9–12 illustrates the most common vowel inventories for languages as the number of vowels grows (Vallée, 1994). As you can see, of the languages Vallée compared, 11 languages have three-vowel systems, and the three vowels are the same. Ecuadorian Quichua is a language with three vowels. Most languages have five-vowel systems, and 92% of them have the same five vowels. These include Spanish, Arabic, and Japanese. Only two other patterns were observed for five vowel systems. It is only when a language has a six-vowel system that there is more variety. Still, even in languages with nine vowels, almost all of the languages maximize acoustic distinctiveness through tongue height and tongue advancement properties. It is only in very complex vowel systems that you see vowels with creaky and breathy voice, or other subtle contrasts, such as vowel geminates.

What about consonant inventories? As Lindblom and Maddieson (1988) noted, if you were going to have a seven-consonant inventory that achieved maximal contrast, it might look like [ɗ, kʼ, tŝ, m, r, ɬ, ɻ]. However, languages with only seven consonants look nothing like this. Instead, consonants build in complexity from basic to elaborated to complex consonant articulations. Lindblom and Maddieson define basic sounds as those that are near default modes of articulation—pure up and down movements of the jaw or tongue, fricatives that are voiceless, etc. Elaborated consonant systems involve departure from basic default modes, such as voicing fricatives, adding new airstream mechanisms, moving beyond basic tongue and lip movements (labiodental, uvular, retroflex, pharyngeal), as well as secondary movements, such as affrication. Complex consonants are those that combine two elaborated systems, such as an ejective lateralized affricate, or a retroflexed consonant produced with creaky voice.

Languages with very large consonant inventories build on basic consonants in perceptually distinct ways. What tends to happen in languages is that

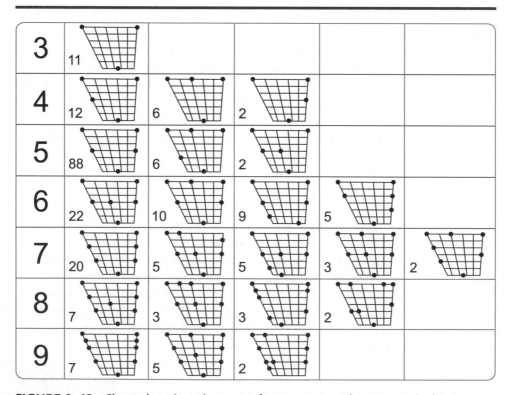

FIGURE 9–12. Chart showing the most frequent vowel contrasts in languages that have three to nine vowel phonemes. The left column indicates the number of vowels in a language. Each square indicates the number of languages that have a particular vowel system (Vallée, 1994).

basic consonants are maximized acoustically before adding elaborated or complex consonants. Thus a language with eight consonants, such as Hawaiian, is correctly predicted to have basic consonants: /p, m, n, t, ?, h, w, l/. Note that while basic consonants, they maximize acoustic distinctions. Languages with complex consonants tend to have a lot of consonants. As noted, Taa dialects are purported to have the largest consonant inventories. Taa consonants contrast four VOT possibilities: voiceless and voiced ejectives and fricatives; two manner categories for nasals, and liquids. In addition, there are clicks overlaid on many of these sound categories, with at least 83 clicks identified in Taa. Most sounds in Taa are bilabial, dental, alveolar, velar, and uvular. Even with this many consonants, Taa does not utilize certain manner and place categories, instead maximizing contrast possibilities at particular places of articulation with different manner, airstreams, and phonations.

In summary, languages with small sound inventories start with vowels that maximize perceptual distinctiveness. Languages with few consonants start with easier to produce consonants that are also perceptually distinct.

Let's return to that complexity question. Languages contrast meaning in ways so that adults in those languages can communicate complex messages in as easy a manner as possible. It is fascinating to see the ways languages achieve this goal. But the question of harder or easier languages is really not answerable. What is true is that languages that are hard in one area tend to be easier in another. For instance, English has a medium consonant inventory and a fairly large vowel inventory. English also utilizes the consonants it has in many ways by combining them into complex consonant strings (clusters) so that English has CCCVCCCC syllable shapes. However, English does not make use of many other speech possibilities that are employed by other languages. Pitch is not used to contrast meaning, nor are different airstreams, voicing types, consonant length, or word length (most words in English are one-syllable). In contrast, some languages have very few phonemes. Pirahã, spoken in Brazil, is considered to have the smallest phonemic inventory, with just 10 phonemes. While phonologically simple, linguists consider Pirahã one of the most difficult languages for non-native speakers to learn. Verb

and grammatical forms are quite complex, and the language is whistled, hummed, or spoken to convey different meaning, without the need for phonemes at all! Pirahã serves as an example of how complexity is achieved in different ways across languages.

Another way to think about complexity is to realize that infants the world over travel from not being able to communicate anything with speech sounds to communicating in fairly complex ways by around 3 or 4 years of age. This rapid sound acquisition occurs regardless of how many sounds a language has.

? 9–11. Did You Get It?

1. The sounds of languages tend to be governed by two principles. These principles are _____ and _____.

2. You have just discovered a new language and are transcribing it. You have determined that this language has five vowel phonemes. Which five vowel phonemes is this language most likely to have? _____

3. Consonants that are produced with simple movements are called _____.

4. Consonants that combine basic and elaborated movements are called _____ consonants.

Putting It All Together

Let's end by applying cross-linguistic information to the field of clinical phonetics. If you are learning English as a second language or are bilingual, the articulatory and phonological aspects of your other language can affect your English. And the older you are when you learn English, the more likely your native language will have an effect. That is, if you are learning English and your first language is Spanish, you might produce English alveolar consonants as dental consonants, given their dental quality in Spanish. Or you may produce words like /bæθ/

as [baθ], /baks/ as [baks], or unaspirated [t] for the allophone [tʰ], demonstrating phonetic properties of Spanish in English. These are examples of language transfer, where properties of one language are transferred to the other language. These examples suggest articulatory transfer, substituting articulations from the first language for new movements in English. Second language learners make speech errors in their new language for phonological reasons as well. These include lack of the phoneme in the first language, allophonic but not phonemic contrast in the first language, phonological substitutions, and different phonotactic structures.

Be careful as a clinical scientist. As we learn differing dialectal information, use the information descriptively rather than assuming a speaker will use certain sounds. Learn how adults around a child talk to determine whether the sounds that child is producing are typical or atypical. You must research other languages and dialects as needed to make sure a difference is not identified as a disorder. Be careful not to pathologize accented speech or different dialect patterns.

You are encouraged to explore the phonemic and allophonic patterns of English dialects, also looking for exceptions to those dialects. Be careful of assuming an individual speaks a certain dialect because of geographic origin or ethnicity. Be aware that dialects change, with older adults often differing from younger members of their community in their sound patterns or preferences. Phonological differences in dialects are not universal, and any individual may use some of the dialect properties but not others.

Your newfound knowledge of how speech is produced, heard, and transcribed is an important skill as a clinical scientist. As you learn more about communication and communication disorders, we hope you put your newly gained tools to good use. Humans and languages have overlaid speech on the physical structures necessary for human survival, supporting breathing, chewing, and swallowing, and maximized their anatomical and physiological capacities for communication with other members of their species. As a clinical scientist, understanding how those speech sounds are produced, other ways sound can be produced, and what the listener is cueing into to understand speech are important tools for assessing and treating speech as well as aural rehabilitation. Sometimes individuals with communication disorders make sounds that are unlike English sounds; however, understanding different airstream and phonatory and articulatory possibilities for speech aids in describing those different sounds. Also understanding how sounds pattern in languages, and how those patterns may differ in other languages or dialects is useful in ascertaining whether a child cannot produce a sound or put a string of sounds together, or whether they are not understanding the rules for the dialect they are learning. This is particularly true for individuals learning English as a second language, who may not have been exposed to specific speech productions or may apply phonological rules for meaningful consonant, vowel, voicing, and tonal contrasts as in their first language, and thus struggle to learn a new pattern in English. And as you work with non-English speakers, you will learn the importance of researching the other language's phonological properties to understand what phonemes the language has, how suprasegmentals are used, and whether some of these properties are applied to English productions. As future audiologists, this information aids in the understanding of important acoustic properties for discriminating and producing English speech sounds and how hearing loss at different frequencies can affect the perception and production of sounds.

It is critical that speech-language pathologists know the phonetic, allophonic, and phonological patterns of a speaker's language and dialect, so that actual speech errors can be determined; otherwise, the speech-language pathologist may incorrectly label a pronunciation as incorrect, when, in fact, it is an acceptable production in the individual's language or dialect. Your newfound skills can take you in different directions: continuing to develop skill in cross-language application of phonetics to further your understanding and practice with the phonetics of English to applying phonetic properties to development and disordered speech in clinical phonetics. Regardless of the ways you apply your phonetic skills, we hope you appreciate the amazing ways that humans have taken their capacity for sound variation to communicate verbally with one other.

? 9–12. Did You Get It?

It is your turn to explore the phonological system of a new language. There are many resources in the *Interest Piqued* section of this chapter that can help you get started. Pick a language or dialect. Research your choice to answer the following questions.

1. What is the vowel inventory of the language? Make note of all ways vowels are contrasted. These could include tongue height, tongue advancement, phonation, length, and many other properties. Find out everything you can.

2. What is the consonant inventory of the language? How does your language or dialect contrast consonants? Use all nine of the consonant categories found in Table 9–1 as you answer this question.

3. How does the language build complexity? Are there complex syllable shapes? Tones? Do words tend to be long or short?

4. Anything else of note about your language?

5. Finally, compare the language you researched with English. Do they share sounds, word shapes, other properties? How do they differ? What might be difficult for speakers of that language as they learn English? Conversely, what would be hard for English speakers about this language?

Applied Science: Revisited

Summary

At the beginning of this chapter, you were introduced to Geovany, a 13-year-old boy who was suspected of having a speech sound disorder. Unusual sounds were noted in his speech, including guttural, clicky, nasal, and breathy sounds. Geovany had only recently come to the United States from Guatemala and speaks three languages, English, Spanish, and K'iche. Because of his multilingual background, you want to make sure his unusual sounds are not a sign of difference rather than disorder. You realized you needed to gather more information on Geovany to make this determination. What did you decide to do?

One Step at a Time

While you do not speak Spanish or K'iche, as his speech-language pathologist and an expert in typical and atypical speech, you need to understand the phonological system of Spanish and K'iche to see if there are cross-language transfer effects of either language to English. You also want to learn more about Geovany's speech and language development from his family.

From your research, you learn that Spanish has 5 vowels and 17 consonants, although the consonant number does differ slightly by dialect. All Spanish phonemes are produced on a pulmonic egressive airstream. Spanish and English consonants use similar places and manners of articulation, although Spanish also has a phonemic trill and tap. There are no differences in phonemic nasal or phonation types. Your research of Spanish does not uncover any reasons for the unusual sounds in Geovany's speech.

You also research K'iche and learn that this language is very different from English. Many dialects of K'iche have 10 vowels, five geminate pairs. There are more consonant places than in English, including retroflex and uvular. Consonant manner categories include velaric ingressive clicks. Phonation and nasality are similar to English.

You also talk to Geovany's parents with the assistance of an interpreter. You learn that Geovany's speech is considered unusual by them, that he has always sounded different from his siblings. They are so happy to have this assessment for him, as they have not worked with a speech-language pathologist before.

After conducting a thorough speech and language assessment with Geovany in all three languages, you feel you have the information you need to determine whether Geovany has a speech and language disorder, and what next steps should be. Can you guess what the conclusion and the next steps are?

Answer

Your original hunch was *partially* correct. That is, the guttural and popping sounds of Geovany's speech reflect two properties of K'iche: uvular sounds and clicks. It is possible that Geovany is carrying these properties over as he gains skill in English. However, two unusual properties in his English cannot be explained by K'iche, or Spanish. Geovany's speech is definitely nasal and breathy. In looking at Geovany's vocal tract anatomy, you notice that the back of his soft palate is split and he actually has two uvulae. Geovany has an unidentified cleft at the back of his palate and you will refer him for a full examination by a physician. This cleft makes it difficult for him to close the oral and nasal cavity for typical stop production and resonatory quality. You realize that the cleft causes the breathiness and hypernasality of his speech, qualities not phonemic to any language he speaks. And with your thorough knowledge of the vocal tract and how sounds are produced, you realize that Geovany may be producing plosives as clicks because he can obstruct air for a click but not for a plosive, given the click is produced in front of his cleft.

Science Applied

You are both embarrassed and proud of yourself, aren't you? While you almost dismissed Geovany's unusual speech as dialectal, you researched his languages and learned that his speech differences could not be explained by K'iche or Spanish. Your careful review of the languages and conversation with Geovany's parents assured that you correctly identified which properties of his speech were expected and which were signs of a speech sound disorder. Great job!

References

Blevins, J. (2008). *Explaining diversity in geminate consonant inventories: An evolutionary approach.* http://www
.eva.mpg.de/lingua/conference/08_springschool/pdf/
course_materials/blevins _evening_lecture.pdf

IPA Chart. http://www.internationalphoneticassociation
.org/content/ipa-chart. Available under a Creative
Commons Attribution-Sharealike 3.0 Unported License.
Copyright © 2015 International Phonetic Association.

Lindblom, B., (1986). Phonetic universals in vowel systems. In J. J. Ohala & J. J. Jaeger (Eds.), *Experimental
phonology* (pp. 13–44).

Lindblom, B., & Maddieson, I. (1988). Phonetic univer-
sals in consonant systems. In L. M. Hyman & C. N. Li
(Eds.), *Language, speech, and mind: Studies in Honor of
V. A. Fromkin.* London, UK and New York, NY: Routledge.

Vallée, N. (1994). *Système vocaliques: de la typologie aux
predictions.* Université Stendhal Grenoble, Grenoble,
France. Ph.D., Language Science.

Interest Piqued?

Recommended materials to further your understanding of topics covered in this chapter.

Print Resources

Erard, M. (2012). *Babel no more: The search for the
world's most extraordinary language learners.* New
York, NY: Free Press.

Everett, D. (2008). *Don't sleep there are snakes: Life
and language in the Amazonian jungle.* New York,
NY: Pantheon Books.

Labov, W. (2014). *Dialect diversity in America: The politics of language change.* Charlottesville: University
of Virginia Press.

Labov, W., Ash, S., & Boberg, C. (2005). *Atlas of North
American English.* Berlin, Germany: De Gruyter.

Ladefoged, P., & Disner, S. F. (2012). *Vowels and consonants: An introduction to the sounds of languages*
(3rd ed.). Malden, MA: Blackwell.

Ladefoged, P., & Johnson, K. (2014). *A course in phonetics* (7th ed.). Belmont, CA: Wadsworth.

Ladefoged, P., & Maddieson, I. (1996). *The sounds of
the world's languages.* Oxford, UK: Blackwell.

Munson, B. (2013). Phonetic variation. In L. D. Shri-
berg & R. D. Kent, *Clinical phonetics* (pp. 165–179).
Boston, MA: Pearson Educational.

Online Resources

http://accent.gmu.edu/

Website with many samples of non-native English
speakers reading English passages.

http://aschmann.net/AmEng/

Lots of information on various dialects of English.

https://www.britannica.com/topic/
Khoisan-languages

Information and audio examples of clicks and
audio examples.

http://www.dialectsarchive.com/

Primary-source archive of recordings of English
dialects and accents, with 1,300 samples from 120
countries.

http://www.internationalphoneticassociation.org/
content/ipa-chart

The official International Phonetic Association IPA
chart.

http://www.ipachart.com/

An interactive IPA chart. If you click on the
symbols you can hear most sounds produced in CV
and VCV contexts.

https://www.pdx.edu/multicultural-topics-
communication-sciences-disorders/

Multicultural topics in communication sciences
and disorders. A website summarizing information
for clinical use.

http://soundsofspeech.uiowa.edu/#

Sounds of Speech App that shows the production
of sounds of English, Spanish, Chinese, and
Korean.

http://web.uvic.ca/ling/resources/ipa/charts/
IPAlab/IPAlab.htm

Phonetic symbols in the IPA chart connected to
production information.

https://www.youtube.com/watch?v=f62dqc-L36o

Examples of different types of phonation.

https://www.youtube.com/watch?v=JKP10ARLnzM
Video of an English speaker explaining the production of non-pulmonic sounds.

http://wals.info/
The world atlas of language structures (WALS). A database of structural properties of languages.

? Did You Get It?

ANSWER KEY

9–1.

1. Variants of a language that are mutually intelligible are called <u>dialects</u>.

2. Which type of dialect is Chicano English? <u>social</u>

3. Which type of dialect is Appalachian English? <u>regional</u>

4. Languages that share a proto-language are called a <u>language family</u>.

5. If people who speak two different languages share a third language to speak to each other, that shared language is called a <u>lingua franca</u>.

9–2.

1. As an articulator for speech sounds, the hard palate is:
   d. <u>a passive upper surface structure</u>

2. The following is a passive articulator:
   a. <u>the uvula</u>

9–3.

1. Two place categories that are phonemic in other languages but are not used in English are <u>uvular</u> and <u>pharyngeal</u>.

2. Two manner categories that are phonemic in other languages but are not used in English are <u>taps</u>, and <u>trills</u>.

3. Phonemes produced with central obstruction while air is released on the sides of the tongue are called <u>laterals</u>.

9–4.

1. Laminal sounds are made with the <u>blade</u> of the tongue.

2. Apical sounds are made with the <u>tip</u> of the tongue.

3. What part of the tongue is used for the following three sounds, in order? /ʃ/, /k/, /n/ <u>laminal, dorsal, apical (or blade, back, tip of tongue)</u>

9–5.

1. If the air pressure inside the lungs is increased, does inhalation or exhalation occur? <u>exhalation</u>

2. All phonemes in English are produced on which airstream? <u>pulmonic egressive</u>

3. Clicks are made using which airstream mechanism? <u>velaric ingressive</u>

4. Plosives are made using which airstream mechanism? <u>pulmonic egressive</u>

5. Ejectives are made using which airstream mechanism? <u>glottalic egressive</u>

6. Implosives are made using which airstream mechanism? <u>glottalic ingressive</u>

7. Which stop categories can be voiced? <u>plosives, implosives, clicks</u>

8. Which stop categories can be voiceless? <u>plosives, ejectives, clicks</u>

9. What sound do you make if you over-emphasize the final /t/ in the word **kite** by producing it with both an alveolar obstruction and simultaneous glottal closure, then releasing the alveolar stop before opening the glottis? <u>glottalic egressive ejective</u>

10. The phoneme /ʄ/ is a <u>voiced glottalic ingressive velar implosive</u>

11. The phoneme /ʘŋ/ is a <u>velaric ingressive bilabial nasal click.</u>

9–6.

1. <u>Breathy (or murmured)</u> voice is produced by vibrating the vocal folds while simultaneously allowing turbulent air to flow through.

2. <u>Creaky (or laryngealized)</u> voice is produced by bringing the vocal folds tightly together during phonation.

3. The difference between a consonant made with breathy voice and a consonant made with a creaky voice is <u>vocal fold tension</u>

9–7.

1. The difference between a slightly aspirated stop and a strongly aspirated stop is <u>voice onset time</u>.

2. Which bilabial stop has the greatest delay in voice onset time?
c. <u>the bilabial stop in **"pie"**</u>

9–8.

Can you identify the nine properties for the consonant phonemes identified below?

1. /ɮ/
<u>pulmonic, egressive, fully voiced, laminal, alveolar, oral, lateral, singleton, fricative</u>

2. /cː/
<u>pulmonic, egressive, voiceless, dorsal, palatal, oral, central, geminate, stop</u>

3. /tŝʼ/
<u>glottalic, egressive, voiceless, apical, alveolar, oral, central, singleton, affricate</u>

9–9.

1. Name three ways languages contrast vowel phonemes that are not used in English.
<u>Three of the following: length, tongue root advancement, nasality, breathy voice, creaky voice.</u>

2. If two vowels are contrasted by increasing the width of the pharynx without tongue movement, we can say that these vowels contrast in <u>advanced tongue root</u>.

3. In addition to fully voiced vowels, languages can contrast which other vowel voicing types phonemically? <u>breathy, creaky.</u>

9–10.

1. Word-level stress patterns are <u>fixed</u> and variable.

2. <u>Tonal</u> languages use pitch to convey meaning at the syllable level.

3. Languages that do not vary stress patterns across syllables are called <u>fixed stress</u>.

9–11.

1. The sounds of languages tend to be governed by two principles. These principles are <u>ease of articulation</u> and <u>perceptual distance</u>.

2. You have just discovered a new language and are transcribing it. You have determined that this language has five vowel phonemes. Which five vowel phonemes is this language most likely to have? <u>/i, e, a, o, u/</u>

3. Consonants that are produced with simple movements are called <u>basic</u>.

4. Consonants that combine basic and elaborated movements are called <u>complex</u> consonants.

9–12.

Answers will vary depending on the language investigated by the student.

abduction: to move apart, as in pulling the vocal folds apart to open them

acoustic phonetics: the branch of phonetics that is focused on the physical properties of speech sounds

acoustics: the branch of physics that is focused on the physical properties of sound

active articulator: the articulator that moves to touch or approximate the other articulator

adduction: to bring together, as in bringing the vocal folds together to close them

affricate: a consonant sound produced by rapidly sequencing a stop and a fricative produced in the same place

allophone: variations of a phone

alveolar: a consonant produced with the tongue tip or blade on or near the upper gum (i.e., alveolar) ridge

alveolar ridge: the bony ridges behind the upper and lower incisors; also called the gums

alveolar tap: a voiced allophone of /t/ and /d/ in English; made by striking the tongue tip against the alveolar ridge one time

alveoli: tiny air sacs found in the lung tissue

ambisyllabic: a consonant sound that crosses two syllables

amplitude: the intensity (i.e., loudness) of a sound wave; represented on the *y*-axis on a waveform

anticipatory coarticulation: when a sound's production is modified because of a sound yet to be articulated

antiresonance: a decrease in resonance at certain frequencies

aperiodic wave: a wave with no repeating pattern of vibration; perceived as noisy and hiss-like (i.e., white noise)

apical: a consonant produced using the tip of the tongue

approximant: a superordinate manner category consisting of glides and liquids

articulate: to produce speech

articulatory phonetics: the branch of phonetics that is focused on speech production

articulatory system: the process of pronouncing sounds using structures in the vocal tract

aspiration: the turbulent noise after the release of a stop consonant

auditory phonetics: the branch of phonetics that is focused on speech perception

back vowel: a vowel produced with the highest place of the tongue raised posteriorly (i.e., toward the velum/soft palate)

Bernoulli principle: an aerodynamic effect of pressure decreasing when the speed of a fluid, such as air, increases; used to describe vocal fold motion

bilabial: a consonant produced using both lips

bilingual: a person who communicates using two languages

bunched-r: an articulatory variation of the rhotic consonant; produced with the tongue tip lowered and the tongue body raised

brackets: symbols (i.e., [ ]) used to enclose the phonetic transcription of spoken words and sounds

breathy voice: see "murmured voice"

carryover coarticulation: when a sound's production is modified because of a sound that was just articulated; also called retentive or perseverative coarticulation

central: a consonant produced with air flowing over the middle of the tongue; describes all the consonants in English except for /l/

central vowel: a vowel produced with the body of the tongue raised in a neutral position (i.e., in the center of the mouth)

citation form: overarticulated speech that is produced with precise movements

click: stop or affricate consonant produced on a velaric ingressive airstream

coarticulation: the overlapping of speech movements in connected speech

coda: consonants and consonant clusters in syllable-arresting position

cognate consonants: a pair of consonants that share place and manner of articulation but differ in voicing

cognate vowels: a pair of vowels that share tongue height, tongue advancement, and lip rounding but differ in tenseness

complementary distribution: allophones that occur in one specific phonetic context and only in that specific context

complex wave: multiple simple waves traveling simultaneously at many different frequencies

compression: period of high pressure created when molecules are pushed away from the disturbance and closer to a neighboring molecule

contrastive distribution: when two phonemes occur in minimal pairs that establish them as phonemes

contrastive stress: emphasizing a sound, syllable, or word, indicating its relative importance to the speaker

creaky voice: voicing produced by the vocal folds when the anterior portion of the folds are closed tightly, permitting only the posterior edges to vibrate

cycle: period of time it takes for a pressure wave to go from resting position to maximal compression and rarefaction dispersion

decibels: measurement unit for intensity (i.e., loudness) of a sound wave; abbreviated dB

declination: a sentence with a falling pitch pattern

dental: a consonant produced using the tip or blade of the tongue against the upper teeth

diacritics: small marks placed on, under, or next to a phonetic symbol to detail articulatory characteristics of that sound's production

dialect: a mutually intelligible variant of a language

diaphragm: the dome-shaped muscle used in respiration; relaxing the diaphragm pushes air out of the lungs and through the vocal folds

digraph: a pair of symbols used to represent a single sound

diphthong: a single vowel produced with two rapidly articulated vowel gestures

displacement: distance from original position

disyllabic: a word containing two syllables

duration: the length of a sound as measured in time units (e.g., milliseconds, seconds)

dynamic vowel: a vowel that is the product of multiple articulatory movements

economy of articulation: the principle of producing speech using only as much articulatory precision as is needed to be understood; also called ease of articulation

ejective: stop or affricate consonant produced on a glottalic egressive airstream

elasticity: ability of a physical substance to return to its original shape or position after being stretched or displaced

epiglottis: cartilage that protects our airway by covering the larynx during swallowing

exhalation: the process of moving air out of the lungs; also called expiration

formant: a group of harmonics that form a band of acoustic energy that corresponds to a resonating frequency of the air in the vocal tract; sound characteristics of a particular vowel or voiced consonant

Fourier analysis: method of separating a complex non-sinusoidal wave into its constituent sine waves of different frequencies, amplitudes, and phases

free variation: when a sound can be produced in various ways without changing the meaning of a word

frequency: the number of times a compression-rarefaction cycle occurs in one second; objective measurement of pitch; measured in hertz

fricative: a consonant sound produced by the partial obstruction of airflow by two articulators closely approximating one another to create turbulence

front vowel: a vowel produced with the tongue anterior in the mouth

fundamental frequency: the number of vocal fold vibratory cycles over time in seconds; the objective measurement of pitch; measured in hertz

geminate: the doubling in length of a consonant or vowel

glide: a consonant sound produced with minimal friction by the smooth and rapid movement of the articulators

glottal: a consonant produced by the vocal folds

glottal stop: a voiceless consonant produced by closing and quickly opening the vocal folds

glottis: space between the vocal folds

grammatical stress: the stress pattern in a word that indicates its linguistic function (e.g., noun versus verb)

harmonics: whole number multiples of the fundamental frequency that decrease in amplitude as they increase in frequency; also called overtones

hertz: measurement unit for frequency of a sound wave; measured in cycles per second; abbreviated Hz

high vowel: a vowel produced with the tongue raised close to the palate

homographs: words that are spelled the same way but that have different meanings

homophones: words that are spelled differently but that are pronounced the same way

hypernasality: speech produced with excessive nasal resonance

hyponasality: speech produced with too little nasal resonance

implosive: stop consonant produced on a glottalic ingressive airstream

impressionistic transcription: to use phonetic symbols to transcribe spoken forms of words

inhalation: the process of breathing air into the lungs; also called inspiration

intensity: how high or low the pressure changes in a sound wave are; also referred to as amplitude of air pressure variations; objective measurement of loudness; measured in decibels, abbreviated dB

interdental: a consonant produced with the tongue tip or blade lightly touching the upper teeth and protruding slightly through the upper and lower incisors

interdental lisp: an interdental placement of the tongue tip or blade for a non-interdental consonant

intervocalic: a consonant occurring between two vowels

intrusive-r: a rhotic vowel produced in some nonrhotic dialects of English when a word ending in a vowel is followed by a word that starts with a vowel

labial spreading: producing a sound with the lips spread widely

labiodental: a consonant produced with the upper incisors resting on the lower lip

laminal: a consonant produced using the blade of the tongue

language: a community's shared communication system of words and the rules for combining and producing those words

language family: group of related languages that share linguistic properties

language isolate: a language that does not share a proto-language with any other languages

lateral: a consonant produced with air flowing over the sides of the tongue; consists of only [l] in English

lateral release: a consonant produced with air flowing over the sides of the tongue at the release of the sound; an allophonic or phonemic combination of a stop consonant released laterally

larynx: the anatomical structure that houses the vocal folds; also called the voice box

lax vowel: contrasts with tense vowel; production is more centralized

lexical stress: the inherent stress pattern of a word

ligature: the raised symbol placed over two phonetic symbols to indicate that they are part of the articulation of a single phone; also called a tie bar

lingua franca: language used to communicate between individuals who do not share their first language

linguistic phonetics: the branch of phonetics that is focused on the production, perception, and use of speech sounds in different languages

linking-r: a rhotic vowel produced in some nonrhotic dialects of English when the following word begins with a vowel; used to differentiate two consecutive vowel phonemes

linguolabial: a consonant produced with the tongue tip touching the upper lip

lip rounding: results in vocal tract lengthening and significantly changes the acoustic quality (resonance) of vowels

liquid: a consonant sound produced with minimal friction by the smooth movement of the articulators, with variable types and places of articulation

loanword: a word adopted into one language from another language

longitudinal wave: a wave produced by molecules colliding in the same direction as the direction of the wave

loudness: the subjective perceptual measurement of intensity

low vowel: a vowel produced with the tongue low in the mouth

mandible: the lower jaw

manner of articulation: how a sound is produced

medium: the matter through which air molecules travel (i.e., solids, liquids, and gases)

mid vowel: a vowel produced with the tongue body and jaw in neutral positions

minimal pair: two words that differ by only a single consonant or vowel sound

misarticulate: to mispronounce a sound

monophthong: a steady-state vowel produced with a single articulatory gesture that can be produced indefinitely

monosyllabic: a word containing one syllable

morphology: the linguistic study of word structure and how words are formed

multilingual: a person who communicates using more than two languages

multisyllabic: a word with more than one syllable

murmured voice: voicing produced with the vocal folds loosely vibrating, creating a breathy voice

narrowband spectrogram: a type of spectrogram that provides fine-grained frequency details (i.e., fundamental frequency and harmonics), but less fine-grained temporal details

nasal: a consonant sound produced by two articulators touching while the velum is lowered, so air travels into the nasal cavity

nasal bar: the nasal resonant characteristic that results in a relatively low F1, usually below 250 hertz

nasal cavity: the nose region

nasal release: an allophonic or phonemic combination of a stop consonant released nasally

nasal sound: a speech sound that resonates primarily in the nasal cavity

nonphonemic: a variation of a phone that does not change meaning; also called allophonic changes

nonsibilant fricative: fricatives produced without a hissing quality ([f, v, θ, ð])

nonsinusoidal wave: a complex wave comprising multiple sine waves

nucleus: central part of a syllable; can be a vowel or a syllabic consonant

obstruent: a speech sound produced with a relatively obstructed airway, includes stops, fricatives, and affricates

occlusion: to temporarily block airflow

offglide: the ending articulatory position when producing a diphthong

onglide: the starting articulatory position when producing a diphthong

onset: consonants and consonant clusters in syllable-initiating position

oral cavity: the mouth region

oral sound: a speech sound that resonates primarily in the oral cavity

oro-nasal system: how air flows through the oral and nasal cavity, controlled by raising and lowering the velum

orthography: alphabetic writing

palatals: consonants produced with the front of the tongue near the hard palate

passive articulator: an articulator that does not move

period: the time it takes a wave to complete one full cycle; measured in time (e.g., milliseconds, seconds)

periodic wave: a wave with a rhythmic, repeating pattern, in which each cycle is a repetition of the preceding and following cycle

periodicity: having periodic cycles

perturbation: movement from resting position resulting from an external influence

pharyngeal: a consonant made by bringing the tongue root or the epiglottis to the pharyngeal wall

pharynx: the throat region

phasing: timing of cycles of complex sound waves

phonatory system: the anatomy and physiology of producing sound by the vocal folds; provides the source of sound for all voiced speech sounds

phone: the spoken form of a speech sound; transcribed using brackets: [ ]

phoneme: the mental representation of a speech sound that can be used to establish meaning in words; transcribed using virgules: / /

phonemic diphthong: a vowel phoneme in which the entire diphthong must be produced to understand the phoneme or vowel meaning

phonetic context: the consonant and vowel makeup of a word, including the individual sounds and their order of sequence

phonetician: a scholar who studies phonetics

phonetics: the field of linguistics focused on the study of speech sounds

phonology: the field of linguistics focused on the study of phonemes and the set of rules governing their use in a language

phonotactics: the sound structure of syllables and words; also called syllable and word shape

post-alveolar: a consonant produced with the tongue blade just behind the alveolar ridge, ending with the tongue front near the hard palate

pitch: the subjective and psychological measurement of frequency

pitch accent: the stressed word in an utterance that carries the accent

place of articulation: where in the vocal tract a sound is produced

plosive: stop consonant produced on a pulmonic egressive airstream; also called stop when referring to English plosives

primary stress: the syllable in a word that has the most prominent stress

prenasalized stop: a phoneme comprising a nasal and stop consonant sequence

prevocalic: a consonant occurring before a vowel

postvocalic: a consonant occurring after a vowel

propagation of sound: displacement of molecules by movement of the sound source

proto-language: a hypothesized language that is the predecessor of all languages in a language family

pulmonic air: air from the lungs

quadrant: provides a visual representation of vowels that is highly accurate in describing vowel acoustic qualities

rarefaction: the period of low pressure in a pressure wave that results from the molecules behind the wave of compression being farther apart

register: a style of speaking; varies on a continuum from formal to casual styles

retroflex: a consonant made by bringing the underside of the tongue tip to the post-alveolar region

retroflex-r: an articulatory variation of the rhotic consonant; produced with the tongue tip curled up and back

resonation: the amplification of sound as it travels through sympathetically vibrating structures of the vocal tract

respiratory system: the anatomy and physiology of breathing; provides the power for sound production

rhotic: a consonant or vowel produced with rhoticity

rhoticity: having an r-like auditory quality

rhythm: the stress pattern of an utterance

rime: the part of a syllable that contains the nucleus and the coda

rounded: an articulatory position based on lip posture; rounding results in vocal tract lengthening, which affects the resonant quality of rounded vowels

schwa: the unstressed allophone of the central monophthong; transcribed [ə]

schwar: a central vowel with stressed and unstressed allophonic variations; stressed schwar is a mid central rounded tense vowel and unstressed schwar is a mid central unrounded lax vowel

segmental system: comprises consonants and vowels and their sequencing into syllables and words

sentential stress: the pattern of stress extending over an utterance

sibilant: a fricative sound with a hissing quality; includes [s, z, ʃ, ʒ]

sine wave: smooth, repeating sound wave, does not occur in speech; also called sinusoid

sliding: two rapid articulations that result in a consonant diphthong

sonorant: a high-amplitude sound, such as a vowel, nasal, glide, or liquid, produced with a relatively unobstructed airway

sound source: repeated vibration of an entity, e.g., a string, an engine, a tuning fork, the vocal folds

source-filter theory: the concept that a sound originates at a source, which provides its spectral shape; the sound is then filtered by the vocal tract, resulting in the sound's characteristic resonant qualities

spectrogram: a visual representation of the frequency of sound over time, with frequency on the *y*-axis and time on the *x*-axis

spectrum: a visual representation of sound that graphs a single moment in time, with amplitude on the *y*-axis and frequency on the *x*-axis

speech system: the combination of processes used to produce speech; includes respiratory, phonatory, resonatory, articulatory, auditory, and neurophysiological processes

spherical: the multidirectional travel of sound as it leaves a source

spoonerisms: a specific type of speech error when one sound switches syllable place with another sound in the same syllable position

states of the glottis: variations in vocal fold activity based on how far apart or close they are in relation to one another; the aperture size determines the vocal quality of the sound be produced

steady-state vowel: a vowel that requires a single articulatory movement to produce

stop: an oral consonant sound produced by two articulators touching and temporarily stopping airflow while the velum is raised, resulting in a sudden release of air that travels through the mouth; also called a plosive

stress: the amount of emphasis we place on a syllable; achieved by increasing loudness, pitch, and/or articulatory precision

striations: vertical lines on the spectrogram representing vocal fold vibration

suprasegmental system: aspects of speech production in addition to the consonants and vowels; includes intonation, stress, loudness, etc.

surface wave: a wave created by molecules moving back and forth around the same spot, generating waves that travel in all directions

syllabic consonant: when the weak vowel in a syllable is omitted, and a sonorant consonant serves as the nucleus of the syllable

syllabification: the process of dividing words into syllables

syllable shape: see "phonotactics"

systematic transcription: to use phonemic symbols to transcribe mental representations of words

tap: a consonant produced by quickly and lightly bringing one articulator to the other, obstructing air very briefly

tense: a vowel that is produced with more extreme articulation (i.e., farther forward for front vowels and farther back for back vowels)

thorax: the chest region that houses the rib cage and lungs

tie bar: see "ligature"

tone: a pitch pattern on a syllable that contrasts meaning

tongue advancement: where in the oral tract the tongue is raised on an anterior/posterior (i.e., front/back) scale; also called tongue frontness

tongue height: how near to the roof of the mouth the tongue is during the articulation of vowels

trachea: the anatomical tube-like structure that extends from the top of the lungs to the larynx; also called the windpipe

transverse wave: a wave created by molecules moving in a perpendicular direction compared with the direction of another wave

trigraph: a sequence of three symbols used to represent a single sound

trill: a consonant made by approximating two articulators and vibrating them

triphthong: a single vowel produced with three rapidly articulated vowel gestures

trisyllabic: a word containing three syllables

unrounded: a lip posture ranging from lips in a neutral position to a spread position

uvular: a consonant made by bringing the back of the tongue to the uvula

velar pinch: the joining of the second and third formants in an articulatory transition from a vowel to a velar consonant that can be seen on a spectrogram

velars: consonants produced with the back of the tongue near the soft palate

velum: soft tissue that makes up the posterior portion of the roof of the mouth; used to allow or seal off airflow into the nasal cavity

virgules: symbols (i.e., / /) used to enclose the phonemic transcription of words; also called slashes

vocal folds: a pair of muscular tissues housed in the larynx that produce sound when they vibrate

vocal tract: the anatomical region from the larynx to the oral and nasal cavities where sound is produced

voice bar: a dark band of periodic energy at or below about 200 hertz

voice onset time: the length of time after the release of a stop consonant and before the start of vocal fold vibration for the following vowel; also called VOT

voicing: a sound that is produced while the vocal folds are vibrating

vowel quadrilateral: a visual representation of the place of articulation of vowels

waveform: a graph showing air pressure changes over time, with the x-axis representing time and the y-axis representing pressure/amplitude

wideband spectrograms: a type of spectrogram that provides fine-grained temporal details but less fine-grained frequency details

word shape: see "phonotactics"

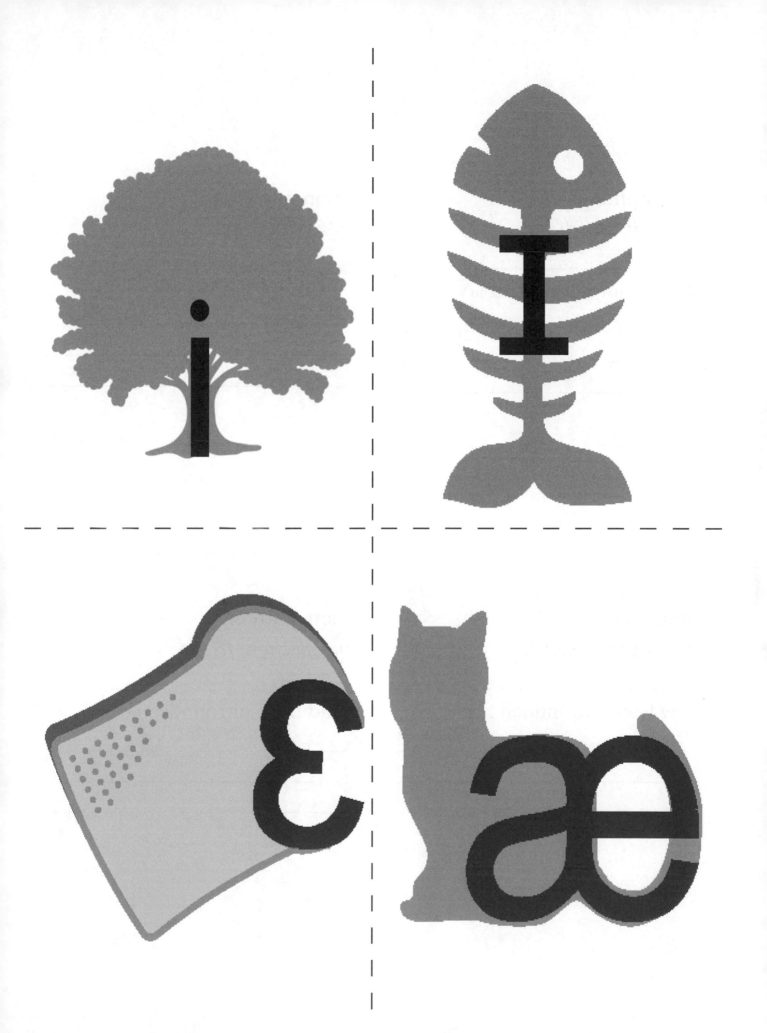

monophthong
*fish, h*i*t, sw*i*tch*

---

high front unrounded lax

---

monophthong
*tree, ch*ie*f, k*e*y*

---

high front unrounded tense

---

monophthong
*c*a*t, wr*a*pped, h*a*tch*

---

low front unrounded lax

---

monophthong
*br*ea*d, ch*e*st, fr*ie*nd*

---

mid front unrounded lax

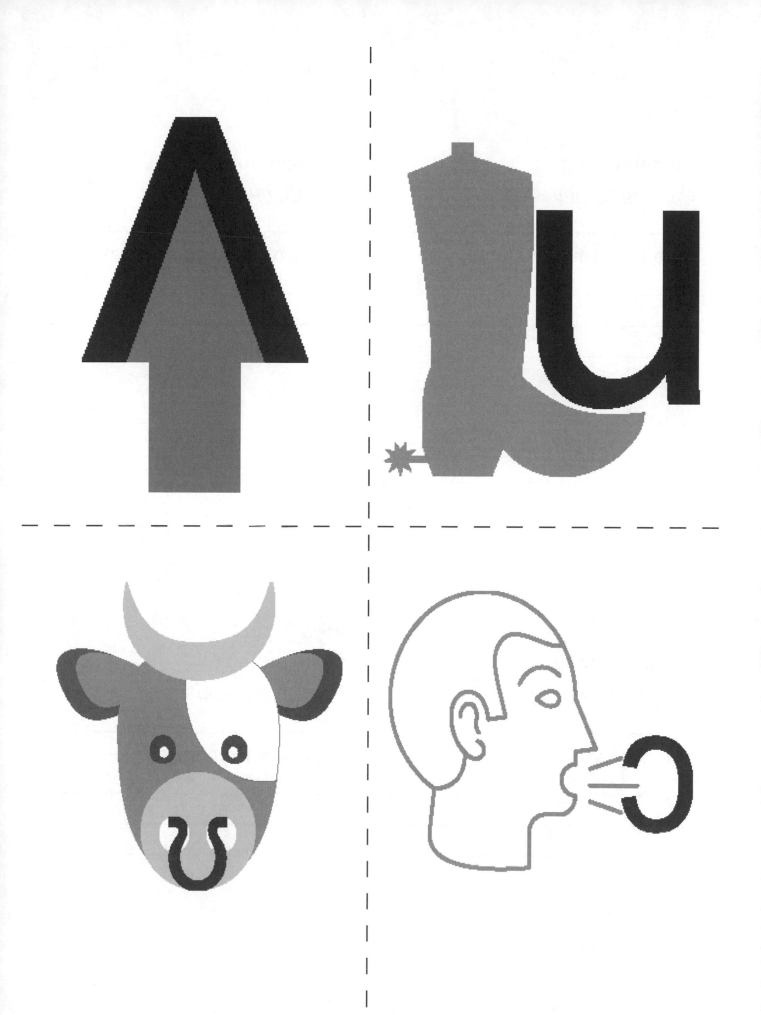

monophthong
sh<u>oe</u>, j<u>ui</u>ce, l<u>oo</u>p

---

high back rounded tense

---

monophthong
<u>u</u>p, n<u>u</u>t, h<u>u</u>sh

---

mid central unrounded lax

---

monophthong
c<u>ough</u>, c<u>au</u>ght, l<u>o</u>g

---

mid back rounded lax

---

monophthong
h<u>oo</u>k, p<u>u</u>sh, g<u>oo</u>d

---

high back rounded lax

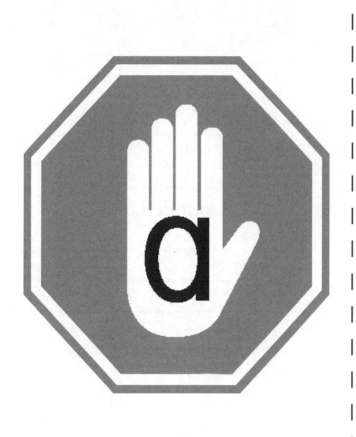

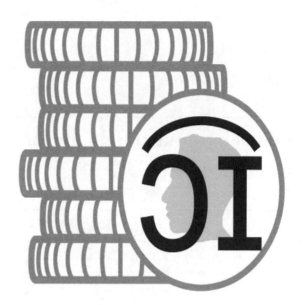

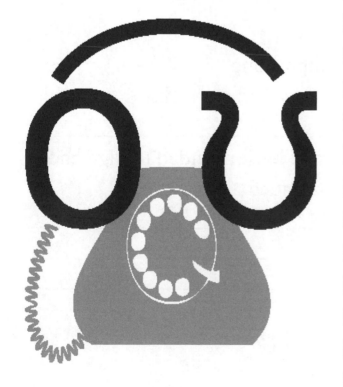

diphthong
coins, foil, choice

_____

mid back rounded to high front
unrounded

_____

_____

_____

monophthong
stop, bought, hot

_____

low back unrounded tense

_____

_____

_____

diphthong
owl, how, shout

_____

low central unrounded to high
back rounded

_____

_____

_____

diphthong
telephone, nope, rose

_____

mid back rounded to high back
rounded

_____

_____

_____

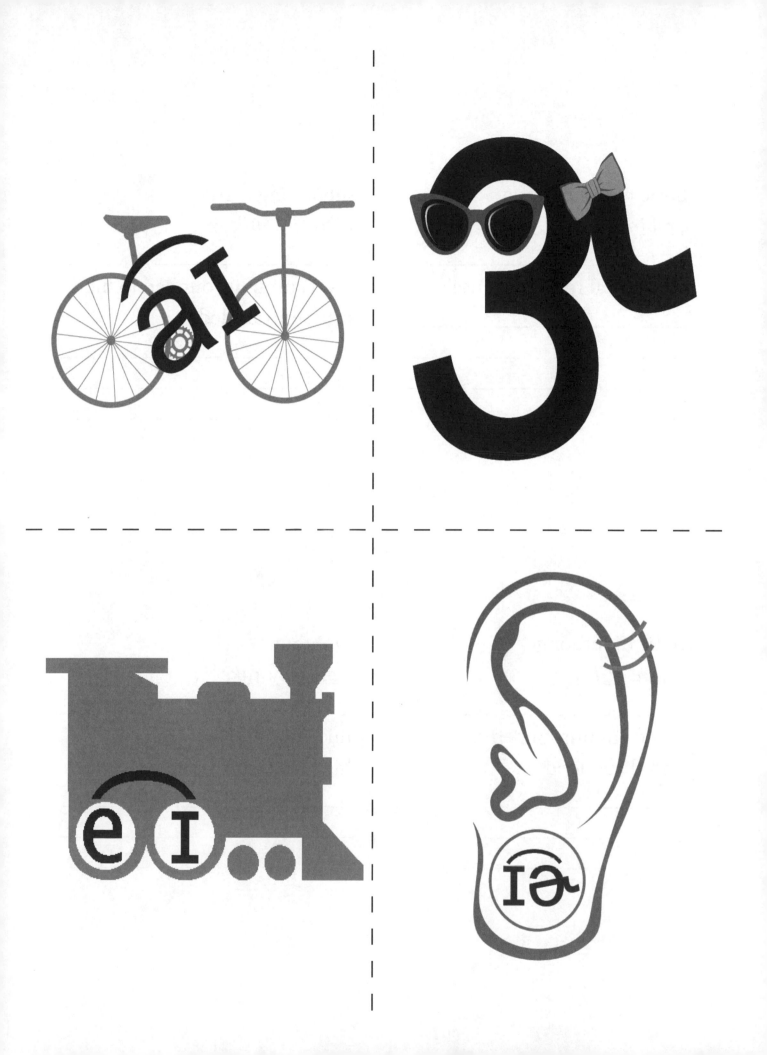

rhotic monophthong
h<u>er</u>, b<u>ir</u>d, w<u>or</u>d

---

mid central rounded tense

---

diphthong
b<u>i</u>ke, sh<u>y</u>, m<u>i</u>le

---

low central unrounded to high
front unrounded

---

rhotic diphthong
<u>ear</u>, sn<u>eer</u>, f<u>ear</u>

---

high front unrounded to mid
central rounded

---

diphthong
tr<u>ai</u>n, s<u>ay</u>, r<u>a</u>ke

---

mid front unrounded to
high front unrounded

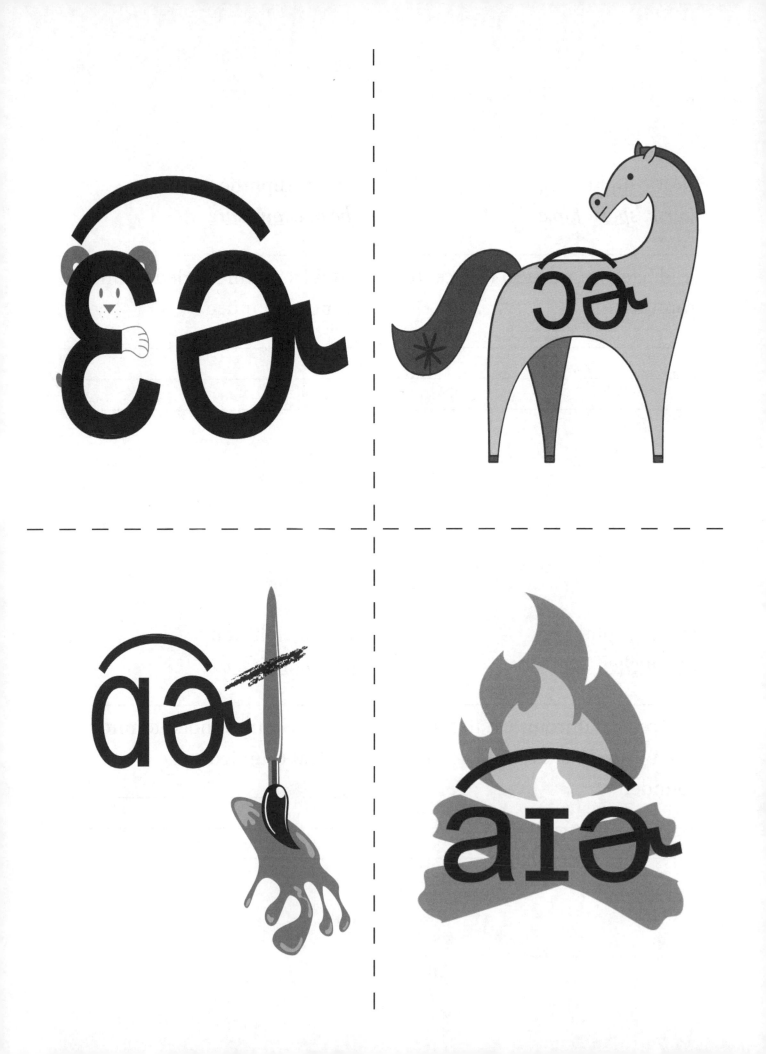

rhotic diphthong
*h**or**se, sp**or**t, f**or**ce*

_____

mid back rounded to mid central
rounded

_____

_____

_____

rhotic diphthong
*b**ear**, ch**air**, h**are***

_____

mid front unrounded to mid
central rounded

_____

_____

_____

rhotic triphthong
*f**ire**, h**igher**, l**iar***

_____

low central unrounded to high
front unrounded to mid central
rounded

_____

_____

rhotic diphthong
*art, sh**ar**k, f**ar**m*

_____

low back unrounded to mid
central rounded

_____

_____

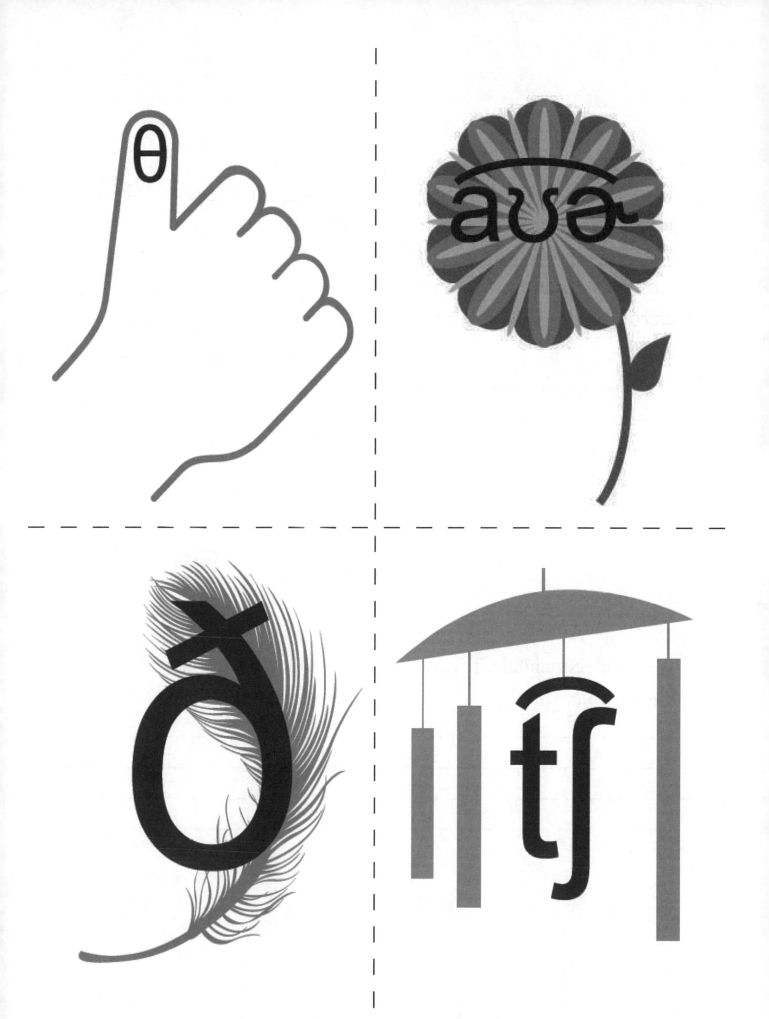

rhotic triphthong
flower, showers, hour

_____

low central unrounded to high
back rounded to mid central
rounded

_____

_____

_____

voiceless interdental fricative
thumb, something, bath

_____

_____

_____

_____

voiceless alveopalatal affricate
chimes, achoo, which

_____

_____

_____

_____

voiced interdental fricative
this, feather, bathe

_____

_____

_____

_____

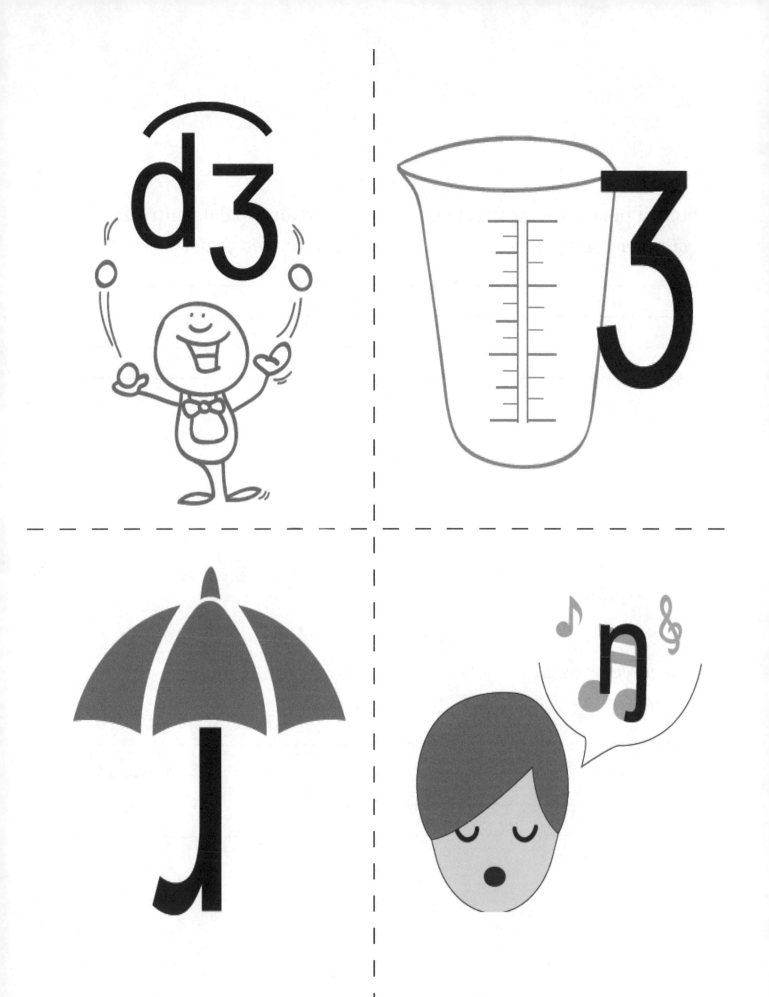

voiced post-alveolar fricative
genre, mea<u>*s*</u>*ure, bei*<u>*ge*</u>

_____

_____

_____

_____

voiced alveopalatal affricate
<u>*j*</u>*uggle, ma*<u>*g*</u>*ic, fri*<u>*dg*</u>*e*

_____

_____

_____

_____

voiced velar nasal
gi<u>*ng*</u>*ham, si*<u>*ng*</u>

_____

_____

_____

_____

voiced palatal liquid
<u>*r*</u>*isk, umb*<u>*r*</u>*ella*

_____

_____

_____

_____

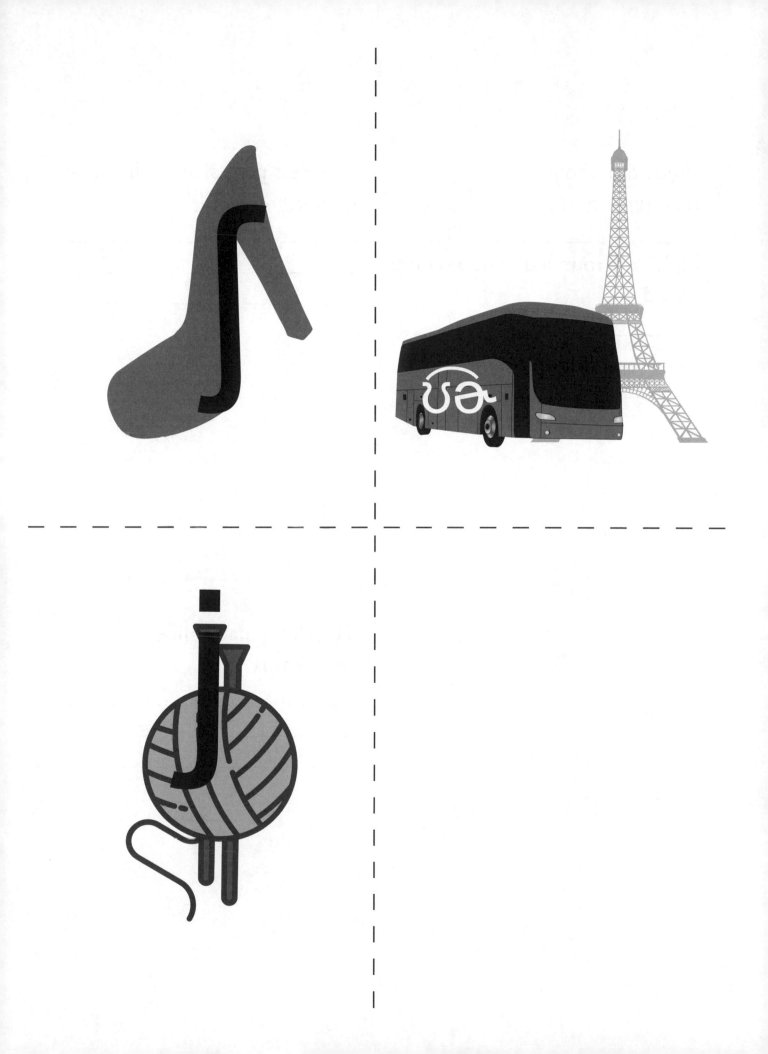

rhotic diphthong
tour, lure, sure

_____

high back rounded to mid central rounded

_____

_____

Voiceless post-alveolar fricative
shoe, fishing, hush

_____

_____

_____

Voiceless palatal glide
yarn, kayak

_____

_____

_____

Note: Page numbers in **bold** reference non-text material.

A

AAVE. *See* African American Vernacular English

Abdominal area, 23

Abdominal muscles, 22

Abduction of vocal folds, 24, **24**

Abutting vowels, 105

Accented speech, pathologizing, 288

Acoustic phonetics, 143–186
  about, 145–146
  consonants, 172–179
  vowels, 163–165

Acoustics
  basic principles of, 146–151, **147–151**
  speech signal, 150
  wave motion, 147
  See also Sound waves

Active articulators, 268, **269**

Acute accent mark, 109

Adduction of vocal folds, 24–25, **24**

Adjectives, stress in two-syllable adjectives, 14

Advanced pattern consonants, **203**, 207, 208

Adverbs, stress in two-syllable adverbs, 14

Affricate consonants, 43, **43**, 48, **48**, **51**
  allophonic patterns of, 219, **219**
  identifying on a waveform, 158
  manner of articulation, 175, 177, 270
  spectrogram, 175, 177, **177**

Affricated patterns, **203**, 209–210, **210**

African American Vernacular English (AAVE), 254, 265

Afrikaans (language), 283

Airflow and speech production, 22–24, 25
  articulation of consonants, 43–51, **202**
  articulation of vowels, 63–90
  consonant diacritics for normal speech, 111, **111**, **115**
  diacritics for disordered speech, 120, **121**
  exhalation, 23, 24, 63, 120
  ingressive air, 120, **121**

Airstream mechanisms, for consonants, 111, **111**, **115**, **121**, 272–276, **281**

Allophones, 192, 195

consonant allophones, 107–108, **108**, 201–225
  affricates, 219, **219**
  approximants, 224–225, **224**
  disordered speech, 226
  fricative consonants, 215, **216–218**, 217–218
  nasals, 219–222, **220–223**
  stops, 202, 204, 206–214

context-dependent allophones, 196

defined, 3

manner of articulation, **203**, 209–211, **210**, **211**

phonetic transcription of, **108**

vowel allophones, 238–244
  in multisyllabic words, 238–241, **238–240**, **242**, 243, **255**
  tense vs. lax vowels, 244, **245**

Alveolar consonants
  interdental lisp, 121, **121**
  manner of articulation, 172
    fricatives, 47, **47**
    nasals, 45, **45**
    stops, 44, **44**, 173
  place of articulation, 29, **29**, 33–34, **33**, **34**, 41, **42**

Alveolar region sounds, 271

Alveolar ridge
  consonant articulation
    alveolars, 29, **29**, 33–34, **33**, **34**
    alveopalatal, 29, **29**, 36–37, **37**
    post-alveolars, 29, **29**, 35–36, **36**
  speech production and, 26, 27, **27**

Alveolar tap, 107

Alveolar trill, 271

Alveoli, 23

Alveopalatal consonants
  manner of articulation, 48, **48**
  place of articulation, 29, **29**, 36–37, **37**, **42**

Ambisyllabic consonants, 10

American English
  consonants in, 22
    manner of articulation, 22, 41, 43–51, **43**, **51**
    place of articulation, 29–41, **42**
  glottal stops in, 107